the principles of PSYCHIATRIC REHABILITATION

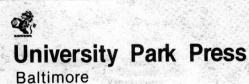

University Park Press

Baltimore

William A. Anthony, Ph.D.

UNIVERSITY PARK PRESS
International Publishers in Science, Medicine, and Education
233 East Redwood Street
Baltimore, Maryland 21202

International Standard Book Number: 0-914234-86-2
Library of Congress Number: 78-59285
First Printing — November, 1978

Parts of this work were sup-
ported by a Public Health Service
Research Training Grant No. T21
MH 14502-02 from the National
Institute of Mental Health.

Designed and Illustrated by Tom Capolongo

1.5

ABOUT THE AUTHOR

Dr. William A. Anthony is an Associate Professor and Director of Clinical Training in the Department of Rehabilitation Counseling, Sargent College of Allied Health Professions, Boston University, Massachusetts. Dr. Anthony is also currently Project Director of a National Institute of Mental Health grant designed to develop and evaluate training materials for persons studying and practicing in the field of Psychiatric Rehabilitation. Dr. Anthony has been involved in the field of Psychiatric Rehabilitation in several different capacities. He has been a practitioner in several mental health settings, both in-patient and out-patient; he has trained students from a variety of disciplines in the skills and knowledge of psychiatric rehabilitation; he has served as a consultant to numerous rehabilitation settings and has researched various aspects of psychiatric rehabilitation practice. Furthermore, Dr. Anthony has authored a number of highly acclaimed articles about psychiatric rehabilitation which have appeared in such professional journals as: "The American Psychologist", "Schizophrenia Bulletin", and "The Community Mental Health Journal". During 1977, Dr. Anthony was selected by the President's Commission on Mental Health to serve on its Task Force on Deinstitutionalization, Rehabilitation and Aftercare. This present text reflects Dr. Anthony's commitment to the practice of Psychiatric Rehabilitation as a developing, viable component of a comprehensive mental health delivery system.

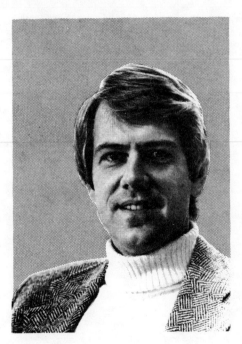

the principles of PSYCHIATRIC REHABILITATION

TABLE OF CONTENTS

CHAPTER VI

CHAPTER VII

CHAPTER VIII

CHAPTER IX

CHAPTER X

FOREWORD[1]

The field of mental health is experiencing a multitude of growing pains as it passes through the current decade. It is an exciting time which offers new opportunities to respond to the changing needs of the psychiatrically disabled. But, as with any alteration of the status quo, it is potentially a disorienting and therefore frightening period.

Many of our beliefs about the treatment of mental patients stem from experience in long-stay, institutional settings which emphasize the medical model. Work with patients in such settings has not usually stressed the development of functional skills. Rather, treatment has been viewed as a circumscribed event focused on the removal of psychopathology — the assumption being that the control of symptomatology will lead to the restoration of normal community functioning. The few inpatient programs aimed at developing functional skills have had discouraging results: behaviors learned in a hospital setting are often not transferable when the patient is discharged to the community.

But the once chronically hospitalized psychiatric population is now largely living in the community. A policy of deinstitutionalization has been adopted nationwide, with consequences that seem not to have been anticipated by its advocates. In a period of rapid change, deinstitutionalized patients, mental health works, and members of the community have proved ill-equipped to deal with their altered circumstances. Ex-patients, whose compliance and dependency had long been fostered in authoritarian institutional settings, found themselves handicapped by these behavior patterns in their new community environment. Mental health workers, who tended to be either vehemently opposed or complacently approving of the migration of patients to the community, made little effort to adapt the existing community service delivery system to the special needs of the large numbers of discharged patients that suddenly confronted them. Similarly, the response of the community members to the ex-patients suddenly in their midst was, at best, indifference and, at worst, outright hostility and rejection. Inevitably, this generalized failure of preparation and response had damaging results, which have been well documented in the press.

Although the early crises of the deinstitutionalization movement found the mental health community in disarray, workers in the field were eventually able to regroup, marshal their forces, and move forward with innovative efforts to address the needs of discharged patients. One of the most compelling of these responses is described in this book. Dr. Anthony and his colleagues have developed a thoughtful, comprehensive, and practical approach to the rehabilitation of the psychiatrically disabled. Focusing on the skilled behaviors patients need to function effectively in the community, they emphasize those islands of competency that we all need in order to live rewarding and satisfactory lives. They have shifted their clinical emphasis from symptoms of psychopathology (which are only weakly correlated with community tenure) to indicators of the patient's functional capacity — the key to his or her survival in the community. Anthony and his colleagues, in their functional approach to assessment, not only provide us with a valid concept but with the knowledge, principles, and skills necessary to implement their program. By ignoring the siren song of causality, they do not find themselves trapped into a program of merely

i

removing their clients' psychopathologic symptoms but rather take incremental steps toward building positive and adaptive skills.

It is always refreshing to read that someone does not claim to have all the answers to a given problem. The authors of this book take a modest, sensible, and practical approach to their goals. In doing so, they do not have to rely on charismatic zeal to carry their plan forward. They have developed a technology that is relevant to the needs of their target population. Their approach takes into account the need to document successes and failures, and allows the flexibility to refine their methods over time. We recognize the care, effort, and thought that went into the writing of this book, and hope that it will be read with those same qualities.

Samuel J. Keith, M.D.
Assistant Chief, Center for Studies of Schizophrenia
Clinical Research Branch
National Institute of Mental Health/ADAMHA/PHS/HEW

Judith C. Turner
Chief, Community Support Program
Division of Mental Health Service Programs
National Institute of Mental Health/ADAMHA/PHS/HEW

May, 1978

---

[1]The opinions expressed in the Foreword are those of the authors and do not necessarily represent any official position of the National Institute of Mental Health or the U.S. Department of Health, Education, and Welfare.

PREFACE

This is indeed the era of rehabilitation. Helping professionals in many different fields speak of "rehabilitating" drug addicts, alcoholics, the criminal offender, the physically disabled, and the psychiatrically disabled. Historically, however, the term *rehabilitation* has been used primarily to describe those professional activities whose main goal has been the employment restoration of the physically disabled. It is only within the last several decades that the "rehabilitation of the psychiatrically disabled" has become a viable concept.

Yet, the popularity of the **concept** of psychiatric rehabilitation does not mean that the competent **practice** of psychiatric rehabilitation is in fact occurring. The gap between concept and practice is great, and it can only be successfully bridged by knowledgeable and skilled practitioners. The purpose of the present text is to assist professionals in bridging this gap, and thus improve the practice of psychiatric rehabilitation.

To accomplish this purpose, the text first explores the present state of psychiatric rehabilitation, then identifies what the unique goals of psychiatric rehabilitation can be, and lastly delineates the unique practitioner skills and programs which can help achieve these rehabilitation goals.

The preparation of this text involved the assistance of a number of persons. Main contributions were provided by the following persons: Mikal Cohen, Linda Boucher, Roger Davies, Marianne Farkas, Bernard Greenberg, Keith Hume, Christopher Ross, and Raphael Vitalo. The author especially wishes to acknowledge the contribution and stimulation of Dr. Robert Carkhuff, whose path-finding efforts in the areas of therapy and education form the foundation for this text.

Boston University   W.A.A.

September, 1978

CHAPTER I

An Introduction
to the Field of
Psychiatric Rehabilitation

This book represents a beginning step toward defining the unique knowledge and principles of psychiatric rehabilitation. Outlined in this book are the necessary skills required of its practitioners; skills which are distinct from the skills required to practice psychiatric therapy. Although the total treatment process of the psychiatrically disabled helpee combines both therapy and rehabilitation, it is important that they be separated conceptually so that the rehabilitation process receives the emphasis necessary to develop its own unique contribution to patient care. From this conceptual difference will develop the knowledge, principles, and skills unique to the practice of psychiatric rehabilitation.

Throughout the book the term *psychiatrically disabled* helpee, patient, or client is used in place of more common terms such as "mentally ill," "schizophrenic," or "psychotic." No one term can adequately describe those individuals who have been labeled as "mentally ill," however, some term must be used to identify those persons who are the recipients of psychiatric rehabilitation services. For lack of a better descriptive phrase, the term *psychiatrically disabled helpee* has been used to describe a person who wants or needs help due to his or her inability to function effectively in the emotional-interpersonal area. Unlike some of the more common psychiatric labels, the term *psychiatric disability* connotes less stigma and is obviously less esoteric than many psychiatric terms. In addition, the term *disability* is a common rehabilitation word and implies the definite possibility of constructive helpee change. In rehabilitation, a disabling condition can be overcome by developing new abilities and skills or by making the necessary environmental modifications for rehabilitation. There is no need for labels such as "schizophrenia in remission"; once helpees overcome their disability they essentially become "psychiatrically able."

PSYCHIATRIC REHABILITATION AND PSYCHIATRIC TREATMENT

The practice of psychiatric rehabilitation and the practice of psychiatric treatment (e.g., psychotherapy, chemotherapy) do possess some similarities. In terms of timing, psychiatric therapy and psychiatric rehabilitation procedures ideally occur simultaneously or in close sequence. In terms of the setting, therapeutic techniques and rehabilitation techniques are often carried out in the same facility or separate facilities run by the same agency. In terms of the helping person, psychiatric therapy and psychiatric rehabilitation are often conducted by the same helper.

However, distinctions can and must be made between therapy and rehabilitation if the field of psychiatric rehabilitation hopes to contribute fully and effectively to the needs of the psychiatrically disabled helpee. Maximal contributions by psychiatric rehabilitation practitioners cannot occur if the field of psychiatric rehabilitation continues to be perceived as the poor sister of psychiatric therapy. All too frequently, psychiatric rehabilitation is considered only after the therapy process has concluded or as an alternative when therapy has failed. At present, many of the principles and programs of psychiatric rehabilitation are not unique to psychiatric rehabilitation but have been borrowed from psychiatric therapy. This lack of uniqueness is clearly illustrated by the fact that in many rehabilitation settings (e.g., half-way houses) the main treatment modality is apt to be chemotherapy combined with individual or group therapy (sometimes euphemistically called "group discussion"). In addition, psychiatric rehabilitation professionals are often overly concerned with the helpee's psychiatric diagnosis, even though rehabilitation research indicates that the diagnostic label provides the staff with no information relevant to rehabilitation outcome. Furthermore, the staff members of rehabilitation facilities and rehabilitation programs are often selected for their training in the use of therapeutic techniques and not for their expertise in psychiatric rehabilitation.

At present, psychiatric rehabilitation can be most facetiously described as *the development of nontraditional settings for the purpose of using traditional tech-*

niques by traditionally trained profession-als (Anthony, 1977). While the place and time of rehabilitation treatment and perhaps the name of the treatment are different, closer examination often reveals that *the difference between therapy and rehabilitation does not extend to what is actually being done.* Only the location of the game and the positions of the players have changed; the rules remain the same. In fact, rehabilitation workers and agencies still often evaluate themselves in terms of the therapeutic model. Evaluations are positively influenced if the rehabilitation program includes therapy or has highly paid therapeutic consultants. "Therapy" seems to connote more status than "rehabilitation." It is not uncommon for a professional in a psychiatric rehabilitation setting to feel compelled to mention that in addition to his more mundane chores he also "does therapy."

The rehabilitation professional, whether he or she is a psychiatrist, psychologist, social worker, nurse, or counselor, must be able to answer the question: "What can I effectively do for the psychiatrically disabled if I don't do some variation of psychotherapy?" This is a critical concern because the specialty of psychiatric rehabilitation has been typically defined by the absence of a strong therapeutic emphasis. The psychiatric rehabilitation field must now be defined on the basis of what it *is* rather than on the basis of what it is

not. The unique principles and programs of psychiatric rehabilitation must be developed so that prospective rehabilitation professionals can be trained in a specific set of skills built upon the newly developing knowledge of the psychiatric rehabilitation process.

The basic difference between psychiatric therapy and psychiatric rehabilitation has been typically described in terms of philosophical goals. Rehabilitation is considered to be directed primarily at developing the patient's strengths, focusing on the helpee's assets in order to restore his or her capacity to function in the community. In contrast, psychiatric therapy is typically directed at reducing the patient's discomfort; focusing on his liabilities in order to alleviate the patient's symptoms. However, this philosophical distinction has not often been translated into behavioral differences. The skills needed to practice psychiatric rehabilitation remain for the most part the traditional therapeutic skills. The training programs designed to teach psychiatric rehabilitation professionals unique rehabilitation skills still primarily teach the theory and techniques of therapy. The philosophical distinction between therapy and rehabilitation has primarily affected the practice of rehabilitation only to the extent that the setting in which rehabilitation occurs may be different from the therapeutic setting.

PSYCHIATRIC REHABILITATION AND PSYCHIATRIC PREVENTION

In contrast to the rather piecemeal and superficial approach to psychiatric rehabilitation, the last fifteen years have witnessed the rise, and perhaps the beginning of the demise, of psychiatric prevention. In retrospect, it appears that while many people were talking about prevention, few were doing it (NIMH, 1971). Some have argued that preventive psychiatry may have promised too much and delivered too little, perhaps because its goals and techniques were rather vague and confusing, or perhaps because in reality mental health professionals do not have the power to implement large-scale preventive programs (Simon, 1975). Indeed,

large-scale prevention activities seem to be more in the province of educators, social planners, and politicians than in the realm of the mental health professional.

However, a preventive strategy may be accomplished by the mental health professional through comprehensive rehabilitation programming. The ultimate outcome of rehabilitation is the **prevention** of further deterioration or the **prevention** of a reoccurrence of a psychiatric disability. The successful implementation of a rehabilitation program can prevent future treatment episodes. In addition, because successful rehabilitation programming must include elements of intervention in the client's home, school, or work environment, the mental health professional is provided with a credible reason for intervening beyond the office environment and into the community. A rehabilitation intervention may also achieve preventive outcome by minimizing the unhealthy impact of the client on significant others; for example, early intervention may prevent interpersonal difficulty in the family. This contact with the environment could possibly open the door to early intervention in the lives of significant others in the client's life who without this early contact would have been left untreated. Thus, prevention need not be perceived as distinct and separate from rehabilitation; in reality, if psychiatric rehabilitation is able to develop a useful model and set of techniques, it may be the best use of our preventive energies.

In essence, the field of psychiatric prevention, for a variety of reasons, has generated much talk, little energy, and even less outcome. In contrast, the field of psychiatric rehabilitation has generated little talk, a great many rehabilitation environments, and very little energy directed at how to most effectively utilize these rehabilitation environments. The time has come for mental health professionals to focus more of their energies on psychiatric rehabilitation, an area where mental health professionals have a great deal of influence and could have a great deal of impact on outcome figures. But first, mental health professionals must learn to practice a rehabilitation approach to psychiatric rehabilitation.

The stage has been set for a truly rehabilitative approach to emerge within the mental health system. The unmet needs of those persons with psychiatric disability are many. Yet, if the field of psychiatric rehabilitation is going to make a meaningful contribution to the mental health system and its consumers, it must be based on more than propitious timing and individual suffering. For these factors, motivating as they are, offer no guarantee of improved and effective services. The ultimate efficacy of the psychiatric rehabilitation field will be drawn from the knowledge and skills of those who practice it. It is toward this end that the present text is written. The following section overviews the particular rehabilitation content areas to which this text is addressed and which presently comprise the fundamental subject matter of psychiatric rehabilitation practice.

THE UNIQUE CONTENT OF PSYCHIATRIC REHABILITATION

This book essentially consists of three parts: Chapter II, which examines the present state of psychiatric rehabilitation; Chapter III, which describes the potentially unique outcomes of psychiatric rehabilitation; and Chapters IV-XII, which present many of the principles, programs, and skills necessary to move the field from its present level of expertise to its potential level of competence (outlined in Chapter III). In contrast to existing books on psychiatric rehabilitation, this text does not provide detailed descriptions of various rehabilitation environments. Rather, the focus of this book is on those practitioner skills necessary to achieve rehabilitation outcome, the knowledge base underlying these skills, and the principles guiding the future development of the field of psychiatric rehabilitation. This text does not pretend to provide solutions. Instead, it provides a direction and the rationale underlying that direction as comprehensively as the present state of our knowledge will permit.

More specifically, Chapter II analyzes the comparative effectiveness of various psychiatric rehabilitation procedures on post-hospital adjustment using the criteria of hospital recidivism and post-hospital employment. The base line against which the unique effects of rehabilitation procedures can be evaluated is the percentage of psychiatric patients who receive the traditional hospital regimen of drug treatment and perhaps some form of individual or group therapy and who are able to avoid rehospitalization and become employed. Conclusions are then drawn concerning the present efficacy of psychiatric rehabilitation procedures.

In Chapter III the specific outcomes of rehabilitation are outlined. In contrast to the therapist's primary goal of symptom reduction, the rehabilitation practitioner's overall goal is health induction. Specifically, a psychiatric disability may be characterized most comprehensively as a deficit in skilled performance. Rehabilitation procedures are thus directed at increasing and extending the helpee's repertoire of skilled behavior in the physical, emotional, and intellectual areas of functioning for the purpose of providing the helpee with the living, learning, and working skills necessary to function effectively in the community.

Chapter IV describes the rehabilitation diagnostic process as a procedure entirely different from the present psychiatric diagnostic process. A rehabilitation diagnosis describes what the client can and cannot do in terms of skills, focusing specifically on assessing the helpee's present and needed skilled behavior. It requires the diagnostician to use his or her interpersonal skills and goal-setting skills to enter the frame of reference of the helpee rather than forcing the helpee to enter into the frame of reference of the diagnostician's theory. Unlike the psychiatric diagnosis, the rehabilitation diagnosis is relevant to the overall rehabilitation objective in that the information gathered possesses empirical and face validity with various rehabilitation outcome criteria.

Chapter V discusses the procedures necessary to develop psychiatric rehabilitation programs designed to take the psychiatrically disabled helpee from his or her present level of skilled behavior to a more advanced level of skilled performance. The principles of program development and program implementation are outlined, and applications are made to the field of psychiatric rehabilitation. Typical inadequacies in present rehabilitation programs are analyzed and solutions are advanced based on the principles of program development.

Chapter VI addresses an issue which has been almost totally ignored by the practitioners of psychiatric rehabilitation, that is, the level of physical functioning of the psychiatrically disabled helpee. Evidence exists that suggests that physical training programs do affect an individual's emotional and intellectual functioning. Yet psychiatric therapy and rehabilitation settings and programs often not only ignore the helpee's physical functioning, but also inadvertently create an environment which may be physically debilitating. A physical fitness program for patients that is capable of being instituted in most rehabilitation programs is outlined in this chapter.

In contrast to the relative infrequency of physical fitness training for the psychiatrically disabled, Chapter VII deals with an area which has rather consistently been the focus of psychiatric rehabilitation, that is, the psychiatrically disabled person's vocational functioning. Historically, however, the psychiatrically disabled helpee has not been taught any of the specific career-planning and placement skills which the helpee needs to function more independently in a working community. Typically the psychiatrically disabled helpee is counseled and placed in a specific work setting. If problems occur, the helpee must either return for more "rehabilitation" or drop out of the world of work. As opposed to this present state of affairs, this chapter identifies the specific vocational skills which many psychiatrically disabled helpees can be taught. In this way the helpees learn to truly rehabilitate themselves, rather than remain totally dependent upon psychiatric rehabilitation practitioners or agencies.

Chapter VIII focuses on the importance of developing community rehabilitation programs designed to facilitate the helpee's community functioning. As rehabilitation programs attempt to return or keep more psychiatrically disabled helpees in the community, the knowledge and skills of how to use existing community resources and develop new community resources is extremely important in overcoming the anticipated indifference, fear, or antagonism of the community in which the helpee may need to function.

Chapter IX is concerned with the need

of each individual practitioner to develop evaluation skills with which to evaluate psychiatric rehabilitation programs. The field of psychiatric treatment, in general, has been notorious for its inability to document the value of its services in terms of patient benefits. There is no need for the newly developing profession of psychiatric rehabilitation to follow suit. Practitioners equipped with evaluation skills facilitate the development of an agency-wide evaluation system. Such a system helps to insure program accountability; but more importantly an evaluation system provides the data base, the means by which rehabilitation programs can be improved.

Chapter X discusses in greater detail some of the recent applications of a skills-based rehabilitation approach. As a result, Chapter X provides an overview of some of the early successes of a true rehabilitation approach, as well as the difficulties involved in using a rehabilitation model. These applications have occurred in both in-patient and community-based settings.

In Chapter XI, the unique skills of the psychiatric rehabilitation professional are outlined. Unfortunately, professionals in psychiatric rehabilitation have traditionally been trained in the theory and practice of therapy. Knowledge and training in psychiatric rehabilitation has occurred primarily on-the-job. A common core of training experiences is proposed for professionals who wish to specialize in psychiatric rehabilitation; such training would be in addition to the training specific to their unique profession. Lastly, the contributions of the paraprofessional to psychiatric rehabilitation are reviewed and suggestions advanced for the complete utilization of the paraprofessional in rehabilitation.

In Chapter XII, the book concludes with a discussion of the promise of rehabilitation by briefly examining once again the present position of the field of psychiatric rehabilitation, what the unique goals of rehabilitation can be, and the necessary principles and programs to achieve these goals. The Appendices which follow the final chapter provide examples of selected programs useful in psychiatric rehabilitation.

In sum, the promise of psychiatric rehabilitation can be realized in only one way — by hard work — work which is directed at developing new knowledge, new skills, and new programs relevant to the goals of psychiatric rehabilitation.

REFERENCES

Anthony, W. A. Psychological rehabilitation: A concept in need of a method. **American Psychologist**, 1977, *32*: 658-662.

National Institute of Mental Health Biometry Branch. Consultation and education services — community mental health centers, January, 1970. Statistical Note No. 43, USPHS, 1971.

Simon, G. C. Is there progress in community mental health? In **Progress in community mental health**. L. Bellak and H. H. Basten, eds. New York: Bruner/Mazel, 1975, *3*: 3-22.

CHAPTER II
The Efficacy
of
Psychiatric Rehabilitation

In order for psychiatric rehabilitation to develop a unique base upon which unique rehabilitation principles and programs can be built, we must begin by examining the effectiveness of current psychiatric rehabilitation procedures. We must first analyze how well we are doing what we purport to be doing, and identify what works and what doesn't work. Psychiatric rehabilitation cannot charter its course toward meaningful goals without first determining its present capabilities. Direction is meaningless unless one knows where one is, as well as where one wants to go.

Understanding the present capabilities of psychiatric rehabilitation is not an easy process. Very few studies can be found which have systematically evaluated various psychiatric rehabilitation techniques. Hardly any studies exist which have directly compared one rehabilitation technique against another. Because no helping profession may lay unique claim to the field of psychiatric rehabilitation, those research studies which have been done are reported in a wide variety of journals and books.

Other problems exist which further complicate an analysis of the present effectiveness of psychiatric rehabilitation. Evaluation studies use different outcome criteria and different follow-up periods, while others may lack control groups. Thus, comparisons between studies become very difficult. In addition, the characteristics of the subjects vary from study to study; even more difficult to integrate are the reports which do not adequately describe the parameters of the subject population.

However, these difficulties are not insurmountable and it is possible to review comprehensively the field of psychiatric rehabilitation. In 1972, the first comprehensive review of psychiatric rehabilitation was attempted (Anthony, Buell, Sharatt, and Althoff, 1972). Since that time periodic reviews have been published (e.g., Bachrach, 1976; Erikson, 1974) relevant to the issue of psychiatric rehabilitation outcome. In general, these later reviews supported and extended the suggestions formulated by the initial review of Anthony et al. (1972). The original review is reprinted here to provide the reader with an historical research perspective of the first attempt to evaluate the efficacy of psychiatric rehabilitation. In addition, this review serves as an empirical foundation from which some tentative principles may be advanced concerning the current techniques of psychiatric rehabilitation.

THE PRESENT EFFECTIVENESS OF PSYCHIATRIC REHABILITATION[1]

In order to evaluate the psychiatric rehabilitation field, meaningful outcome criteria must be selected. Typically, procedures designed to rehabilitate the psychiatric patient have been evaluated by using a variety of criteria; recidivism, post-hospital employment, hospital discharge rate, and hospital adjustment. Because of the multiplicity of criteria presently used, it is extremely difficult to compare the effectiveness of different programs.

To help overcome this difficulty, both for this present survey and to serve as a basis for future comparisons, two criteria were selected (recidivism and post-hospital employment) and used consistently throughout the survey. Recidivism was defined as the percentage of discharged psychiatric patients who are subsequently rehospitalized. Post-hospital employment, as defined in this survey, refers to the percentage of discharged psychiatric patients who are competitively employed at follow-up, or employed full-time during the entire follow-up period.[2]

In selecting these two criteria, other criteria such as hospital discharge rate and various measures of hospital adjustment were ruled out. The research seems to indicate that the evaluations of rehabilitation efforts made from a hospital base do not appear to be consistently related to functioning in the community and thus are not valid outcome criteria if the goals of rehabilitation are to improve community functioning (Bloom & Lang, 1970; Ellsworth, Foster, Childers, Arthur & Kroeker, 1968; Forsythe & Fairweather, 1961; Paul,

1969; Schaeffer, 1969; Walker & McCourt, 1965; Williams & Walker, 1961).

On the other hand, recidivism and post-hospital employment seem to be criteria which are more commonly used and more easily defined. This does not imply that there are no problems involved in using these criteria as indicators of community functioning (see Ellsworth et al. 1968). However, the selection of recidivism and post-hospital employment as the basic criteria to be used does seem to make sense both economically and psychologically. Concerning recidivism, most would agree that one is psychologically "better off" if he can avoid returning to a psychiatric institution; economically, it is less expensive for the taxpayer if the patient remains out of the hospital. Concerning employment, many would agree that working has psychological benefits; economically, work produces tax dollars and avoids government aid payments.

BASE RATE

In order to evaluate the unique effects of rehabilitation procedures, the effects of traditional hospital treatment on recidivism and post-hospital employment must be established as a base line. That is, what is the percentage of psychiatric patients who receive the traditional hospital regimen of drug treatment and perhaps some form of individual or group psychotherapy that are able to remain out of the hospital or find employment. Knowing this base rate, the efficacy of specific rehabilitation procedures can be evaluated by comparing the results obtained by specific rehabilitation procedures with the results obtained by traditional hospital treatment.

Recidivism Base Rate

Several studies provide estimates of the recidivism base rate for hospitalized psychiatric patients. Though the studies differ in years sampled, geographic location and type of institution, their results are remarkably similar and suggest a recidivism rate for a one year period of approximately 40-50%.

For example, Miller (1966, 1967) and

Savino and Schlamp (1968) reported recidivism rates in California for 1956, 1963, 1965, and 1966 to be 40%, 40%, 48%, and 53% respectively. A study of Chicago residents (Orlinsky & D'Elia, 1964) found a recidivism rate of 46% for a group of patients who received traditional care. A study based at a Cleveland hospital reported 50% readmissions in the first year (Friedman, vonMering, & Hinko, 1966), while an extensive study of Massachusetts' hospitals (Freeman & Simmons, 1963) found a one year recidivism rate of 38%.

Other studies not specifically concerned with rate of recidivism report data from which a base rate may be computed. Results of Bloom and Land (1970) suggest a base rate of 42%, Lorei (1967) a base rate of 39%, while Wilder, Levin, and Zwerling (1966) reported a 45% readmission rate between one and two years after discharge.

Some researchers have also examined recidivism rates of less than or more than one year and typically have reported data which suggests a continual increase in recidivism as time from discharge increases. Within three months, reported rates of return were 15% (Orlinsky & D'Elia, 1964), within six months, 40%, 33%, and 30% (Fairweather, et al. 1960; Friedman et al. 1966; Orlinsky & D'Elia, 1964), within three years, 65% (Olshansky, 1968) and within five years, 67%, 70%, and 75% (Friedman et al. 1966; Miller, 1966, 1967).

Employment Base Rate

The employment data suggest that during the year following discharge approximately 20-30% of the ex-patients work either full-time throughout the year or were employed at the one year follow-up date. For example, Hall, Smith and Shimkunas (1966) classified 28% of their sample as "steady workers," i.e., "employed at time of follow-up and had been working continuously on a single job without serious absenteeism." Similarly, Lorei (1967) reported that 24% of their sample had worked full time for at least one year. At one year follow-up, Freeman and Simmons (1963) found that 60% of the nonrecidivist patients were still working, or roughly 20% of the total sample of discharged patients.

Base-rate figures for time periods of less or more than one year are at best tentative. The only long-term study from which base-rate data can be gleaned was a three-year employment follow-up which found 25% of the initial sample of hospitalized patients living in the community and competitively employed (Walker, Williams & Kelley, 1960).

Unfortunately, employment data for a time period of six months do not seem to be reported in full-time employment figures. For example, Olshansky (1966) stated that of a sample of 3,248 patients released from twelve V. A. hospitals, 33% worked more than one month during the six months following discharge. Fairweather (1964) reported 38% of his traditionally treated hospital patients were employed "some of the time," while Walker and McCourt (1965) found that 47% of their sample of V. A. patients had experienced "some employment." However, when Walker and McCourt (1965) used full-time employment as their criterion, the percentage originally classified as employed was decreased by about one-half to 23%.

Thus, the combined base-rate percentages for employment would suggest that during the first six months after discharge 30-50% of the patients become gainfully employed. When employment percentages are based on either employment status at follow-up or full-time employment during the entire follow-up period the base-rate appears to fall between 20-30% regardless of the time period sampled.

Table 2-I presents a summary of the base rate percentages for both the employment and recidivism criteria.[3] Using the base-rate percentage for comparative purposes when necessary, the effectiveness of various rehabilitation procedures can now be surveyed. For purposes of discussion, rehabilitation techniques were divided into two main categories depending on when and where the rehabilitation efforts took place — in the hospital prior to discharge, or after discharge on an outpatient basis.

TABLE 2-I
Suggested Base-Rate Data for Recidivism and Employment

Time Since Discharge	Recidivism	Full-time Employment
6 months	30-40%	30-50%[a]
12 months	40-50%	20-30%
3-5 years	65-75%	25%[b]

[a] Percentage of those who become gainfully employed. Rate similar to 12 months figures when criterion is entire six months of employment.

[b] Based on only one study.

IN-PATIENT REHABILITATION

The hospital rehabilitation programs were further divided into four categories: 1) traditional hospital treatment, 2) work therapy, 3) "total push" therapy, and 4) non-traditional groups.

Traditional Hospital Treatment

It does not seem to matter whether hospitalized psychiatric patients receive eclectically-oriented group therapy (Haven & Wood, 1970) psychoanalytically-oriented individual or group therapy (Walker & Kelley, 1963), individual or group therapy (Fairweather et al., 1960; Fairweather & Simon, 1963), or drugs, shock, individual, or group therapy (Freeman & Simmons, 1963). Regardless of the type of traditional therapy patients receive, their recidivism and employment rates are not differentially affected. In the preceding studies of outcome in specific treatment modalities, the recidivism rates were similar to the base-rate figures for hospitalized patients, ranging from a low of 38% for one year (Freeman & Simmons, 1963) to a high of 73% for three years (Walker & Kelley, 1963). Full-time employment percentages ranged from a high of 42%[4] at six months (Fairweather et al. 1960) to a low of 23% at three years (Walker & Kelley, 1963).

Work Therapy

Kunce (1970) surveyed the literature on work therapy and concluded that the research does not support the idea that work therapy can be therapeutic. He estimated that regardless of whether patients receive work therapy or not, 33% will become employed; a finding consistent with the base-rate data presented here. A recent study (Walker, Winick, Frost, & Lieberman, 1969) which contrasted two types of work therapy reported that at six months follow-up, 36% of both groups "held regular competitive work at some time during the six months."

Some researchers (Barbee, Berry and Micek, 1969) have suggested that work therapy may foster institutional dependency. Their results indicated that patients participating in work therapy remained hospitalized longer than nonparticipants. During the two-year follow-up, 46% of the work therapy group and 23% of the nonparticipants were readmitted to the same hospital. However, when readmission to all psychiatric facilities was examined, there were no significant differences between groups.

Another study (Johnson & Lee, 1965) investigated the effects of a hospital program in which work therapy, rehabilitation counseling, and work placement were emphasized. While those investigators did not present figures for recidivism and employment *per se*, they did report no difference from a control group in mean number of weeks out of the hospital or community adjustment as rated by heads of the household.

Several studies of work therapy (Cheney & Kish, 1970; Hoffman, 1965) have presented follow-up employment figures considerably better than the base rate. However, these investigators included in their figures only those patients who successfully completed their therapy program or were placed after therapy ended. For example, Hoffman (1965) reported that 76% of the patients completing the vocational program at a state hospital were gainfully employed, but when the total population entering the program is included in the analysis, the success figure drops to approximately 36%. Perhaps these programs are counting as successful the 30-50% who would have found some type of employment even without a hospital based work therapy program.

The evidence to date indicates that work therapy alone does not increase the patients' probability of remaining in the community or obtaining employment. These conclusions are consistent with the data of Walker & McCourt (1965) who found no relationship between work-like activity in the hospital and later community employment.

Total Push Therapy

As defined in this paper, total push therapy procedures attempt to structure the total hospital environment so that most of the patients' waking hours are directed at therapeutic ends. Although these procedures (variously described as milieu therapy, attitude therapy, social learning therapy and token economies) differ in terms of their theoretical base, the techniques used to facilitate change and the systematization of their application, they are in agreement about the necessity of therapeutically structuring the patient's total hospital environment.

In terms of the topic of this paper, these programs are similar in an even more basic way. While all these approaches have been able to demonstrate positive effects on within hospital behavior, they have as yet not demonstrated their effects on measures of community adjustment, such as rehospitalization rates (Paul, 1969). The outcome studies that have been done typically confined their analysis to changes in the patients' ward behavior (e.g., Foreyt & Felton, 1970).

The only total push treatment program which seems to present favorable community outcome data describes itself as a "behavior-milieu" therapy program (Heap, Boblitt, Moore, & Hord, 1970). This treatment approach consists of a combination of behavior therapy, a token economy, patient government, attitude therapy and other adjunctive programs such as vocational training or psychotherapy. After thirty-five consecutive months of operation, the behavior-milieu therapy ward's recidivism rate was only 14% as compared to 50% for the rest of the hospital.

The authors were careful to point out that it was difficult to differentiate the unique effects of each treatment. In addition, they suggested that the ultimate clinical effects may not be primarily due to the specific techniques but to the fact that these techniques . . . "set in motion more diffuse interpersonal and social processes that may have powerful and pervasive therapeutic effects" (Heap et al. 1970).

Nontraditional Groups

Included in this category are all group approaches, exclusive of group therapy, which seek to improve the patients' interpersonal skills. Fairweather (1964) reported slight support for the use of autonomous problem-solving patient groups in combination with a system in which passes and other responsibilities were contingent upon appropriate behavior. Compared to group therapy patients six months after discharge, more of the nontraditional group patients had become "employed some of the time" (54% vs. 38%) and less tended to be rehospitalized (36% vs. 46%).

Proponents of human relations training groups have reported an effect on both in-hospital behavior and post-hospital employment and recidivism rates (Hanson, Rothaus, Johnson, & Lyle, 1966; Johnson, Hanson, Rothaus, Morton, Lyle & Moyer, 1965). Compared to a control group of traditional group therapy patients, the training group had more employed (65% vs. 50%) and less rehospitalized (16% vs.

26%) at ten month follow-up. Particularly striking is the unusual finding that even the control group patients' community adjustment seems to be better than the base-rate figures. This inconsistency appears to be due to the fact that the data was obtained by a questionnaire to which only 68% of the total sample responded. Because the control group percentages are incongruent with previously reported base-rate figures, the appropriateness of the experimental group percentages certainly becomes questionable.

Several recent studies (Carkhuff, 1969; Pierce & Drasgow, 1969; Vitalo, 1971) have investigated the effectiveness of systematically training psychiatric patients to function in a more interpersonally facilitative manner and have found that the more structured training group approaches were able to positively affect the within hospital interpersonal behavior of psychiatric patients. In an extension of this work with adult psychiatric patients to an institutionalized juvenile population, the staff rather than the treatment population was initially trained in interpersonal and program development skills (Carkhuff, 1974). The staff then trained the juveniles in more than eighty skills training programs. In addition to significant improvement on indices of the juveniles' physical, emotional, and intellectual functioning, the one year recidivism rate was reduced from 40% to 27%.

OUTPATIENT REHABILITATION

Rather than trying to prepare the hospitalized patient for community life, a number of programs have been developed which treat the patient after discharge. These programs may be loosely categorized in terms of the amount of community support which they provide the patient.

Drug Maintenance

Perhaps the minimum expression of support a hospital may provide a discharged patient is to give a prescription for continuation on medication. However, Williams and Walker (1961) found that the " . . . presence or absence of a prescription for tranquilizing drugs, and a report by the patient and relatives that the drugs were taken regularly as prescribed did not differentiate the recidivists from the non-recidivists." The one year recidivism rates for a psychiatrically similar group of drug taking and non-drug taking patients were 43% and 39% respectively. Another study (Walker, Williams & Kelley, 1960) examined the effects of maintenance medication on the community adjustment of primarily acute schizophrenics three months after discharge. Recidivism and employment data did not differentiate the group discharged on drugs from a group discharged without medication.

Two additional investigations compared the rehospitalization rates of a group of patients treated before the use of drugs with a group of patients treated with drugs (Ellsworth & Clayton, 1960; Michtom, Goldberg, Offenkrantz, & Whittier, 1959). Once again, recidivism rates did not differentiate between the two groups.

Aftercare Clinics

Outpatient or aftercare clinics typically provide the patient with a brief interview plus a review or manipulation of the present level of medication. Although the amount of contact varies somewhat, generally attendance is at least once a month.

Research on these clinics has indicated a significant decrease in recidivism rates for those who attend. Within six months to one year after discharge, reported recidivism rates have been no higher than 26% and typically less than 20% (Hornstra & McPartland, 1963; Kris & Carmichael, 1956; Orlinsky & D'Elia, 1964; Mendel & Rapport, 1963; Pollack, 1958; Vitale & Steinback, 1965). For three and five years, reported rates of recidivism were respectively 20% (Mendel & Rapport, 1963), and 37% (Kris, 1963), well under the three to five year base-rate of 65-75%.

Although patients who attend aftercare clinics are less apt to become rehospitalized, it is not clear why this is so. Clinics differ in terms of their emphasis, such as a brief interview (Hornstra & McPartland, 1963), existential therapy (Men-

del & Rapport, 1963), or home visits by a social worker (Pollack, 1958), yet they all report lower recidivism rates. The one consistent type of treatment is medication, but to explain the reduction in recidivism on the basis of drug treatment alone is to overlook the confounding of this interpretation by patient motivation. That is, the patient's motivation to attend the aftercare clinic may be an expression of his or her desire to become or stay healthy, and this patient characteristic could be more important than the treatment which he or she receives.

Planned Follow-up Counseling

This category differs from aftercare clinics in several ways. First, the treatment philosophy centers less around drug manipulation and more around counseling activities. Secondly, the analysis of results includes all patients discharged from the hospital into the program, and not just patients motivated enough to participate.

Caffey, Galbrecht, and Klett (1971) randomly assigned patients to two types of aftercare — one group was merely referred to an agency after discharge, while the other group received follow-up counseling, including contact with a social worker who counseled the patient and the individual with whom he or she was living, monthly contact with the patient's physician, and continued drug treatment. The recidivism rates reported are slightly lower than the base rate, probably because the patients were screened before they were included in the study. No significant difference in one year recidivism rates was found, although the rates did favor the follow-up counseling group (23% to 34%).

The only other investigation of professional follow-up counseling did not report the time period studied so base-rate comparisons cannot be made (Purvis & Miskimins, 1970). Of interest, however, is the authors' examination of the relationship between amount of patient participation in the follow-up program and recidivism. They concluded that the optimum situation for community adjustment "involves a person who is independent enough to accept some risk (i.e., the separation from the hospital) combined with moderate support. A group in the community or minimum counselor contact represents this type of moderate support . . . "

Summarily, these two studies provide only modest support for the effectiveness of follow-up counseling. The relationship between patient participation in follow-up counseling and recidivism, combined with the positive results of aftercare clinics, seem to suggest that programs with moderate types of community intervention are more apt to exhibit lower rates of recidivism. But once again, this may be due to the characteristics of the patient who seeks mild community support rather than the particular support which he or she receives.

Dramatic evidence for the effectiveness of follow-up counseling is provided by an investigation of follow-up counseling conducted by non-professional volunteers (Katkin, Ginsburg, Rifkin, & Scott, 1971). The treatment approach differed from the previous studies in that unlike the professionals, the volunteer counselors often became extremely involved in many aspects of the patient's life.

The one year recidivism rate for female schizophrenics receiving follow-up counseling from the volunteers was 11%, as compared to 34% for a non-counseled control group. This significant difference contrasts sharply with the previous follow-up counseling studies which found a relatively minor effect for less intensive types of community support. Taken together, these three studies seem to suggest that in order to have a dramatic effect on recidivism, follow-up counseling must be flexible enough to provide all levels of community intervention. Discharged psychiatric patients vary in terms of their needs and follow-up counseling must be capable of adapting to a wide variety of patient needs.

Transitional Facilities

Falling under this rubric are programs such as family care, half-way houses, sheltered workshops and day care centers. For some transitional programs the goal is to enable the patient to become independent of the transitional facility itself, while for others an equally important goal is to enable the patient to become an adjusted member of the transitional facility. Based on this difference in goals, transitional facilities judge their effectiveness at two different times, either after the patient has left the transitional facility or while he or she still remains dependent upon the transitional facility.

Several studies (Lamp & Goertzel, 1971; Wilder, Kessel, & Caulfield, 1968) have followed up patients who have "graduated" from half-way houses to independent living. Recidivism rates were 40% six months after departure from the half-way houses (Wilder et al. 1968), and 50% at eighteen months (Lamb & Goertzel, 1971), a relapse rate similar to base-rate data. In a more positive vein, Wilder et al. (1968) also reported a full-time employment rate of 53% at six month follow-up, a figure considerably better than the base rate.

Rehabilitation programs defined as family care traditionally consist of placing a discharged patient in a private home, a transitional facility which seems to be transitional in a dual sense. That is, one to two years after discharge only a minority (20-30%) of discharged patients still remain in the home; approximately 30-35% leave to return to the hospital and about 40% leave to live independently in the community (Cunningham, Botwinik, Polson & Weickert, 1969; Molholm & Barton, 1941; Ullmann & Berkman, 1959). By combining those who are living independently with those who are still living in the home, Ullmann & Berkman (1959) interpret the effect of family care placement positively, i.e., they note that about 65% are able to stay in the community. Other researchers, however, question whether patients placed in homes are truly participating in community affairs (Lamb & Goertzel, 1971).

Those studies which evaluate the patient's functioning while he or she is still a member of the transitional facility report favorable data for recidivism but not for community employment. One study (Beard, Pitt, Fisher, & Goertzel, 1963) of a facility which offered day and evening services reported a slight effect over control group figures for one year recidivism rates (35% vs. 51%), but no impact on the employment criterion (26% vs. 34%). Similarly, Vitale and Steinback (1965) reported a six month recidivism rate of only 17% for their day care patients, but also found that only 17% of their day care patients had become employed some of the time.

Meltzoff and Blumenthal (1966) reported on the effectiveness of a day treatment center for patients either referred by an outpatient mental hygiene department or on a trial visit from a hospital. At eighteen month follow-up the recidivism rate for the same type of patients who had received only conventional outpatient treatment was 64% as compared to 30% for the day treatment center patients. No conclusions could be drawn about the center's effort on the patient's long term vocational adjustment.

The most extensive study of a transitional facility compared traditional outpatient aftercare with a "community lodge," where patients lived together as a family, engaged in a group occupational endeavor, and were gradually weaned from most all staff contact (Fairweather, Sanders, Maynard & Cressler, 1969). The employment criterion was the "median percentage of time spent in employment" and the results significantly favored the community lodge group. They point out that this result is to be expected because the "... experimental plans deliberately created a situation permitting fulltime employment." However, the patients' employability did not transfer to competitive employment — of the patients who left the lodge "... their employment record outside the lodge strongly resembled that of the control group."

Fairweather et al. (1969) did not report recidivism rates; instead they reported a significant difference in favor of the lodge group for the cumulative number of days an ex-patient remained in the community. However, by combining various numbers from different tables it is possible to compute recidivism rates for both the control and lodge groups; they are practically iden-

tical — 38% for the control group and 40% for the lodge group.

In trying to summarize the effect of transitional facilities, several consistent findings emerge. Transitional facilities reduce recidivism as long as the patients remain members of the facility. Except for one study (Wilder et al., 1968) no research has demonstrated an effect on competitive community employment once the patient tried to function independently of the transitional facility.

Most transitional facilities, whether they are family care homes, half-way houses, day centers or lodges, appear to be "transitional" in the sense that the patient "transfers" his dependency from one facility (the hospital) to another (the transitional facility). The main benefits to the discharged patient seems to include more freedom and less stigma; for society, the benefits are somewhat more tangible — it's cheaper (Fairweather et al. 1969).

CONCLUSIONS AND IMPLICATIONS

1. Although the current emphasis, as exemplified by the Community Mental Health Center, is toward avoiding psychiatric hospitalization, it appears that unless mental hospitals close their doors individuals will continue to be hospitalized and thus need to be reintegrated back into the community. While concerted efforts to treat all psychiatric problems on an outpatient basis have been able to significantly reduce the number of people hospitalized (Flomenhaft, Kaplan, & Langsley, 1969; Pasamanick, Scarpitti & Kinitz, 1967), a significant number of individuals are eventually hospitalized.

2. Traditional methods of treating hospitalized psychiatric patients, including individual therapy, group therapy, work therapy, and drug therapy, do not differentially affect the discharged patients' community functioning as measured by recidivism and post-hospital employment.

3. Most all types of inpatient treatment innovations improve the patients' in-hospital behavior. Yet only two programs, extremely comprehensive in nature have demonstrated an effect on community functioning (Carkhuff, 1974, Heap et al. 1970). The research does not support the

belief that any one of the unique approaches to treatment can singularly affect post-hospital adjustment.

4. Aftercare clinics and other forms of moderate community support reduce recidivism. Whether this positive effect is due to the medication administered, the other kinds of services offered, or the type of patient who attends, is not yet clear.

5. Various types of transitional facilities are successful in reducing recidivism but have demonstrated little effect in enabling the patient to function independently in the community as measured by post-hospital employment.

6. One of the advantages of the establishment of specific base-rate figures is that it can help identify outcome studies which have used a more rehabilitative sample or committed a methodological error. This possibility should be examined when the control group has a recidivism or post-hospital employment rate which is higher than the base-rate figures presented in this survey.

7. The primary usefulness of specific base-rate criteria is that they provide a basis by which to evaluate and compare existing and future studies in hopes that consistent findings might emerge. The present authors suspect that some of the unique criteria developed by different investigators may be employed *post hoc* to maximize the treatment effect. For example, in Fairweather's latest studies (1964-1969) his experimental group in the first study appears to become his control group in the second. Yet he chose to report his employment and recidivism data differently in each study. Thus 54% of the experimental group in the first study were "employed some of the time", but when essentially the same treatment group became the control group for his second study on transitional facilities, the "median percentage of time spent in full time employment" for the controls was zero.

The point is not that different methods of follow-up should not be tried, but that as unique methods of follow-up are used they should be used in conjunction with the two criteria outlined in this survey. Although the efficacy of rehabilitation pro-

cedures has been evaluated by extensive and well designed studies, until some uniformity in reporting results is achieved, the field remains in many ways an interpretive nightmare. Hopefully, when various rehabilitation programs examine their effects in some consistent manner, more meaningful comparisons of effectiveness can be made between various rehabilitation procedures.[1]

For the first time, the present state of psychiatric rehabilitation has been systematically examined. This initial attempt at analyzing existing competencies has revealed both bright spots and sore spots. However, a review of the present state of the field must do more than provide us with the opportunity to congratulate or flagellate. History is irrelevant unless we learn from it.

It appears that the preceding survey of the studies concerned with psychiatric rehabilitation procedures contains sufficient consistencies from which to develop tentative principles. These principles are meant to serve as fundamental guidelines upon which psychiatric rehabilitation research and practice can be based. The principles which follow are divided into those principles relevant to the rehabilitation of helpees presently hospitalized and those principles pertinent to the rehabilitation of outpatients.

Principles of Inpatient Rehabilitation

1. **Traditional Methods of Psychiatric Therapy Do Not Effect Rehabilitation Outcome**

   While these methods may successfully reduce the helpee's symptoms, they do not increase the .helpee's chances of becoming employed or remaining out of the hospital. The goals of traditional therapy are limited and no evidence exists which suggests that they can do more than these methods were originally designed to achieve, i.e., symptom reduction.

2. **Unique Inpatient Treatment Innovations Can Not Singularly Effect Rehabilitation Outcome.**

   Although new treatment techniques have been able to dramatically improve the patients' in-hospital behavior, they have as yet not demonstrated a similar effect on community functioning. The enthusiasm engendered by the well-documented in-hospital impact should not be allowed to implicitly indicate a positive effect on rehabilitation outcome without being equally well-documented. However, at a minimum, these innovative approaches do allow for some optimism in that they typically research their efforts, and will no doubt eventually direct their research attention toward evaluating the efficacy of their approach in terms of rehabilitation goals.

3. **In-Hospital Behavior Does Not Correlate With Community Behavior**

For example, patients who engage in work-like activities in the hospital are not more likely to work after discharge. While at first glance this principle may seem surprising, it is in fact common sense. The behaviors demanded in the hospital do not resemble the behaviors necessary to function adequately in the community. Just as school excellence does not predict work excellence, neither does hospital adjustment predict community adjustment. The behavior of psychiatrically disabled helpees is to a large extent situationally determined and inpatient rehabilitation programs must be aware of that fact.

4. **Inpatient Rehabilitation Programs Must Be Extremely Comprehensive in Order to Have an Effect on Community Functioning**

Inpatient facilities must be structured so as to involve the patient in a wide array of services and programs. Rehabilitation programs need to be directed at the helpee's physical, emotional, and intellectual functioning. It is apparent from the preceding review that rehabilitation outcome can not be easily or simply effected on an inpatient basis without an eclectic approach to the problem.

A more recent study of institutionally based rehabilitation problems has re-affirmed the importance of this principle. Becker and Bayer (1975) have reported on a comprehensive inpatient rehabilitation approach which has resulted in a recidivism rate of 12% averaged over a three month to five year follow-up period. Elements of this program include such components as a token economy, milieu treatment, and skills training classes.

5. **The Need For Psychiatric Hospitalization or a Facsimile of It Will Not Disappear Within the Near Future**

Even though community based treatment, as illustrated by the Community Mental Health Center, is the current thrust in psychiatric therapy and rehabilitation, it appears that psychiatric hospitalization has remained the treatment of choice for many helpees, their helpers, and their families. Even though the number of outpatient treatment episodes has skyrocketed, the number of inpatient treatment episodes has also increased within the last several decades. More people were hospitalized in 1971, than in 1955 (NIMH, 1973). The reasons for the continued use of hospitalization as a treatment alternative are no doubt varied, but perhaps may be most simply explained by the fact that our society has traditionally preferred institutional placement as the most expedient way to deal with many of our problems. The public has favored the idea of the need for psychiatric hospitalization just as they have accepted the need for other institutions such as jails, reform schools, and more recently, nursing homes.

Psychiatric hospitalization, by itself, does not need to have an adverse effect on the helpee. Conversely, neither will community based treatment, by itself, have a positive effect on the helpee. Institutions have been evaluated, and Community Mental Health Centers need to be evaluated on the basis of outcome, on the basis of *what* they do rather than *where* they do it. By adopting new programs based on the principles outlined in this book, institutions as well as outpatient facilities could more often become the treatment of choice for reasons of efficacy rather than for reasons of tradition and expediency.

Principles of Outpatient Rehabilitation

1. **Psychiatric Recidivism Can Be Effected by Various Types of Community Support.**

The existence of a person or facility in the community which provides services for the psychiatric disabled helpee increases the helpee's chances of remaining out of the hospital. However, the essential ingredients of community support are not readily apparent. Recidivism can be reduced by a variety of contacts, including aftercare clinics, transitional facilities, and non-professional counseling. One of the difficulties in providing community support is that patients either reject or ignore the possible help available from community personnel and facilities.

One recent study found that the initiation of aftercare programs in a three-county area did not reduce the county--wide recidivism rates. However, a more detailed analysis of one of the counties indicated that recidivism was substantially lower for individuals who contacted the aftercare program versus those who did not. The authors hypothesized that the aftercare programs were not contacting a large enough proportion of released patients to result in a county-wide reduction in recidivism rates (McNees, Hannah, Schnelle, and Bratton, 1977). In a study with similar implications, Wolkon (1970) found that over two-thirds of the psychiatric patients referred to aftercare clinics did not choose to attend. The need for an effective program to insure the use of community facilities is apparent and will be discussed further in Chapter VII.

2. **Psychiatric Recidivism Can Be Reduced by Contacts with Non-Professionals.**

There is evidence to suggest that the psychiatric rehabilitation goal of adequate community functioning can be effectively influenced by non-professionals, just as previous research has shown that the psychotherapeutic goal of symptom reduction can also be positively effected by non-professionals (Carkhuff & Truax, 1965, Poser, 1966).

The effective training and utilization of the non-professional will be outlined extensively in Chapter XI. It appears that rehabilitation programs can increase their efficacy by creatively capitalizing on the potential contributions of the non-professional.

3. **The Outcome Of Psychiatric Rehabilitation Must Be Evaluated by Both**

Traditional and Unique Measures of Community Functioning.

Even for inpatient programs as well, the *ultimate* test must be what the helpee can and cannot do after he or she has left the hospital. Thus, one fact is certain, the historical outcome criteria of hospital discharge rate is not a viable criteria of rehabilitation success (Erickson, 1974). When discharge rates become a matter of public policy rather than a reflection of patient functioning, discharge rates become useless outcome criteria. Cumming & Markson (1975) have presented considerable data which seem to indicate that the most important factors in determining hospital discharge rates are the norms and values of the hospital rather than the patient's level of functioning.

In contrast to hospital discharge rate the traditional measures of recidivism and employment do have some validity as outcome criteria. However, as Anthony et al. (1972) originally suggested and others have reiterated (Bachrach, 1976; Erickson, 1974) other outcome measures must be developed. The value of recidivism and employment as outcome criteria has been their consistent use over several decades. Thus, they allow the future studies of psychiatric rehabilitation to compare their results, at least in a gross way, with studies done previously. At the same time, however, future studies must develop criteria more capable of measuring unique aspects of a helpee's psychosocial functioning. The issue of evaluating psychiatric rehabilitation outcome using such non-traditional and unique criteria will be explored more comprehensively in Chapter IX.

The characteristic that makes recidivism and employment useful criteria, in spite of the grossness of their measurement is their remarkable consistency. The base-rate figures initially suggested by Anthony et al. (1972) have continued to be supported by more recent surveys. That is, later attempts at reviewing the literature have essentially led to the same conclusions (Anthony, Cohen & Vitalo, 1978; Bachrach, 1976; Erickson, 1974). While pointing to the need for additional follow-up data, Bachrach stated that:

"The conclusions drawn by Anthony and associates are roughly but essentially supported by much of the literature searched in preparation for the present report." (p. 74) Erickson's (1974) review provided some additional long-term follow-up data, indicating a recidivism rate of 77% over a ten-year follow-up period.

Thus the outcomes of recidivism and employment remain legitimate but general rehabilitation goals. The next chapter will move from these general outcome measures to a more detailed analysis of more patient-specific rehabilitation goals.

ENDNOTES

1. Reprinted in part from **Psychological Bulletin,** 1972, *78:* 447-456, where it first appeared as "The Efficacy of Psychiatric Rehabilitation". by W. A. Anthony, G. J. Buell, S. Sharratt, and M. E. Althoff.

2. It should be pointed out that recidivism and post-hospital employment are essentially two different criteria. Rehabilitation programs which attempt to have an effect on post-hospital employment cannot assume that they will also have an effect on recidivism (Fairweather, 1964; Freeman & Simmons, 1963; Paul, 1969).

3. The base-rate data was derived from studies on hospitalized psychiatric patients in general (typically schizophrenics). One researcher (Fairweather, 1964; Fairweather et al. 1960; Fairweather & Simon, 1963) has consistently found that acute psychotics fare better in the community than either hospitalized nonpsychotics or chronic psychotics. If treatment programs deliberately select less severe patients their recidivism and employment rates should be better than the baseline data presented here.

4. The validity of this somewhat higher than base-rate percentage is suspect. It was the only one of nine variables which differentiated between treatment groups. Furthermore, by eighteen months follow-up the difference in employment had disappeared (Fairweather & Simon, 1963).

REFERENCES

Anthony, W. A., Buell, G. J., Sharratt, S. and Althoff, M.E. The Efficacy of psychiatric rehabilitation. **Psychological Bulletin,** 1972, *78:* 447-456.

Anthony, W. A., Cohen, M. R. and Vitalo, R. The measurement of rehabilitations outcome. **Schizophrenia Bulletin,** in press, 1978.

Bachrach, L. L. A note on some recent studies of released mental hospital patients in the community. **American Journal of Psychiatry,** 1976, *133:* 73-75.

Barbee, M. S., Berry, K. L. and Micek, L.A. Relationship of work therapy to psychiatric length of stay and readmission. **Journal of Consulting and Clinical Psychology,** 1969, *33:* 735-738.

Beard, J. H., Pitt, R. B., Fisher, S. H., and Goertzel, V. Evaluating the effectiveness of a psychiatric rehabilitation program. **American Journal of Orthopsychiatry,** 1963, *33:* 701-712.

Becker, P. and Bayer, C. Preparing chronic patients for community placement: A four stage treatment program. **Hospital and Community Psychiatry,** 1975, *26:* 448-450.

Bloom, L. B. and Lang, M. E. Factors associated with accuracy of prediction of posthospitalization adjustment. **Journal of Abnormal Psychology,** 1970, *76:* 243-249.

Boudewyns, P. A. and Wilson, A. E. Implosive therapy and desensitization therapy using free association in the treatment of inpatients. **Journal of Abnormal Psychology,** 1972, *79:* 259-268.

Caffey, E. M., Galbrecht, C. R. and Klett, C. H. Brief hospitalization and aftercare in the treatment of schizophrenia. **Archives of General Psychiatry,** 1971, *24:* 81-86.

Carkhuff, R. R. **Helping and human relations. Vols. I and II.** New York: Holt, Rinehart & Winston, 1969.

Carkhuff, R. R. **Cry twice! From custody to treatment — The story of institutional change.** Amherst, Ma: Human Resource Development Press, 1974.

Cheney, M. T. and Kish, B. G. Job development in a VA hospital. **The Vocational Guidance Quarterly,** 1970, *19:* 61-65.

Cumming, J. and Markson, E. The impact of mass transfer on patient release. **Archives of General Psychiatry,** 1975, *32:* 804-809.

Cunningham, M. R., Botwinick, W. I., Polson, J. A. and Weickert, A. A. Community placement of released mental patients: A five-year study. **Social Work,** 1969, *14:* 54-62.

Ellsworth, R. B. and Clayton, W. H. The effects of chemotherapy on length of stay and rate of return for psychiatrically hospitalized patients. **Journal of Consulting Psychology,** 1960, *24:* 50-53.

Ellsworth, R. B., Foster, L., Childers, B., Arthur, G. and Kroeker, D. Hospital and community adjustment as perceived by psychiatric patients, their families, and staff. **Journal of Consulting and Clinical Psychology Monograph Supplement,** 1968, *32:* Part 2.

Erickson, R. Outcome studies in mental hospitals: A review. **Psychological Bulletin,** 1975, *82:* 514-540.

Fairweather, G. W. ed. **Social psychology in treating mental illness.** New York: Wiley, 1964.

Fairweather, G. W., Sanders, D. H., Maynard, H. and Cressler, D. L. **Community life for the mentally ill: An alternative to institutional care.** Chicago: Aldine, 1969.

Fairweather, G. W. and Simon, R. A. further follow-up comparison of psychotherapeutic programs. **Journal of Consulting Psychology,** 1963. *27:* 186.

Fairweather, G. W., Simon, R., Gebhard, M.E., Weingarten, E., Holland, J. L., Sanders, R., Stone, G. B. and Reahl, J. E. Relative effectiveness of psychotherapeutic programs: A multicriteria comparison of four programs for three different patient groups. **Psychological Monographs,** 1960, *74,* (5, Whole No. 492).

Flomenhaft, D., Kaplan, M. D. and Langley, G. D. Avoiding psychiatric hospitalization. **Social Work,** 1969, *14:* 38-44.

Foreyt, J. P. and Felton, G. S. Change in behavior of hospitalized psychiatric patients in a milieu therapy setting, **Psychotherapy: Theory Research and Practice**, 1970, *7:* 139-141.

Freeman, H. E. and Simmons, O.G. **The mental patient comes home.** New York: Wiley, 1963.

Friedman, I., Von Mering, O. and Hinko, E. N. Intermittent patienthood: The hospital career of today's mental patient. **Archives of General Psychiatry**, 1966, *14:* 386-392.

Hall, J. C., Smith, K. and Shimkunkas, A. Employment problems of schizophrenic patients. **American Journal of Psychiatry**, 1966, *123:* 536-540.

Hanson, P. G., Rothhaus, P. M., Johnson, D. L. and Lyle, F. A. Autonomous groups in human relations training for psychiatric patients. **Journal of Applied Behavioral Science**, 1966, *2:* 305-324.

Haven, G. A. and Wood, B. S. The effectiveness of eclectic group psychotherapy in reducing recidivism in hospitalized patients. **Psychotherapy: Theory, Research and Practice**, 1970, *7:* 153-154.

Heap, F. R., Boblitt, E. W., Moore, H. and Hord, E. J. Behavior milieu therapy with chronic neuropsychiatric patients. **Journal of Abnormal Psychology**, 1970, *76:* 349-354.

Hoffman, J. J. Paid employment as a rehabilitative technique in a state hospital. A demonstration. **Mental Hygiene**, 1965, *49:* 193-207.

Hornstra, R. K. and McPartland, T. S. Aspects of psychiatric aftercare, **International Journal of Social Psychiatry**, 1963, *9:* 135-142.

Johnson, D. L., Hanson, P. G., Rothaus, P., Morton, R. B., Lyle, F. A. and Moyer, R. Follow-up evaluation of human relations training for psychiatric patients. E. H. Schein & W. G. Bennis, eds. **Personal and organizational change through group methods.** New York: Wiley, 1965.

Johnson, R. G. and Lee, H. Rehabilitation of chronic schizophrenics: Major results of a three-year program. **Archives of General Psychiatry**, 1965, *12:* 237-240.

Katkin, S., Ginsburg, M., Rifkin, M. J. and Scott, J. T. Effectiveness of female volunteers in the treatment of outpatients. **Journal of Counseling Psychology**, 1971, *18:* 97-100.

Kris, E. B. Five-year community follow-up of patients discharged from a mental hospital. **Current Therapeutic Research**, 1963, *5:* 451-462.

Kris, E. B. and Carmichael, D. D. Follow-up study on patients treated with thorazine. **American Journal of Psychiatry**, 1965, *112:* 1022.

Kunce, J. T. Is work therapy really therapeutic? **Rehabilitation Literature**, 1970, *31:* 297-299.

Lamb, H. R. and Goertzel, V. Discharged mental patients — are they really in the community? **Archives of General Psychiatry**, 1971, *24:* 29-34.

Lorei, T. W. Prediction of community stay and employment for released psychiatric patients. **Journal of Consulting Psychology,** 1967, *31:* 349-357.

McNees, M. P., Hannah, J. T., Schnelle, J. F. and Bratton, K. M. The effects of aftercare programs on institutional recidivism. **Journal of Community Psychology,** 1977, *5:* 128-133.

Meltzoff, J. and Blumental, R. L. **The day treatment center: Principles, application, and evaluation.** Springfield, Ill.: Charles C. Thomas 1966.

Mendel, W. M. and Rapport, S. Outpatient treatment for chronic schizophrenic patients. **Archives of General Psychiatry,** 1963, *8:* 190-196.

Michtom, J., Goldberg, N., Offenkrantz, W. and Whittier, J. Readmission rates for state mental hospital patients discharged on maintenance ataractics. **Journal of Nervous and Mental Disease,** 1957, *125:* 478-480.

Miller, D. Alternatives to mental patient rehospitalization. **Community Mental Health Journal,** 1966, *2:* 124-128.

Miller, D. Retrospective analysis of post-hospital mental patients' worlds. **Journal of Health & Social Behavior,** 1967, *8:* 136-140.

Molholm, H. B. and Barton, W. E. Family care, a community resource in the rehabilitation of mental patients. **American Journal of Psychiatry,** 1941, *98:* 33-41.

Mosher, L. R., Feinsilver, D., Katz, M. M. and Weinckowski, L. A. **Special report on schizophrenia.** Bethesda, Md.: National Institute of Mental Health, 1970.

National Institute of Mental Health Biometry Branch, Patient care episodes in psychiatric sources. United States, 1971. Statistical Note No. 92, USPHS, 1973.

Olshansky, S. The vocational rehabilitation of ex-psychiatric patients. **Mental Hygiene,** 1968, *52:* 536:561.

Orlinsky, N. and D'Elia, E. Rehospitalization of the schizophrenic patient. **Archives of General Psychiatry,** 1964, *10:* 47-54.

Pasamanick, B., Scarpitti, F. R. and Dinitz, S. **Schizophrenics in the community.** New York: Appleton-Century-Crofts, 1967.

Paul, L. Chronic mental patient: Current status-future directions. **Psychological Bulletin,** 1969, *71:* 81-94.

Pierce, R. M. and Drasgow, J. Teaching facilitative interpersonal functioning to psychiatric inpatients. **Journal of Counseling Psychology,** 1969, *16:* 295-298.

Pollack, B. The effect of chlorpromazine in reducing the relapse rate in 716 released patients: Study 3. **American Journal of Psychiatry,** 1958, *114:* 749-751.

Purvis, S. A. and Miskimins, R. W. Effects of community follow-up on post-hospital adjustment of psychiatric patients. **Community Mental Health Journal,** 1970, *6:* 374-382.

Savino, M. T. and Schlamp, F. T. The use of non-professional rehabilitation aides in decreasing rehospitalization. **Journal of Rehabilitation**, 1968, *34:* 28-31.

Ulmann, L. P. and Berkman, V. C. Efficacy of placement of neuropsychiatric patients in family care. **Archives of General Psychiatry**, 1959, *1:* 273-274.

Vitale, J. H. and Steinback, M. The prevention of relapse of chronic mental patients. **International Journal of Social Psychiatry**, 1965, *11:* 85-95.

Vitalo, R. L. Teaching improved interpersonal functioning as a preferred mode of treatment. **Journal of Clinical Psychology**, 1971, *27:* 166-171.

Walker, R. G. and Kelley, F. E. Short-term psychotherapy with schizophrenic patients evaluated over a three-year follow-up period. **Journal of Nervous and Mental Disease**, 1963, *137:* 348-352.

Walker, R. & McCourt, J. Employment experience among 200 schizophrenic patients in hospital and after discharge. **American Journal of Psychiatry**, 1965, *121:* 316-319.

Walker, R. G., Williams R. G. and Kelley, F. E. An evaluation of maintenance medication in the post-hospital adjustment of 66 schizophrenic patients. **Journal of Clinical and Experimental Psychopathology**, 1960, *21:* 304-308.

Walker, R., Winick, W., Frost, E. S. and Lieberman, J. M. Social restoration of hospitalized psychiatric patients through a program of special employment in industry. **Rehabilitation Literature**, 1969, *30:* 297-303.

Wilder, J., Kessel, M. and Caulfield, S. Follow-up of a "high-expectations" half-way house. **American Journal of Psychiatry**, 1968, *124:* 1035-1091.

Wilder, J. F., Levin, G. and Zwerling, L. A two year follow-up evaluation of acute psychotic patients treated in a day hospital. **American Journal of Psychiatry**, 1966, *122:* 1095-1101.

Williams, R. A. and Walker, R. G. Schizophrenics at time of discharge. **Archives of General Psychiatry**, 1961, *4:* 87-90.

Wolkon, G. Characteristics of clients and continuity of care in the community. **Community Mental Health Journal**, 1970, *6:* 215-221.

CHAPTER III

The Unique Outcomes
of
Psychiatric Rehabilitation

Psychiatric rehabilitation has its roots in two distinct specialty areas: psychiatric (psychological) treatment and physical rehabilitation. Each of these specialties has approached the issue of outcome quite differently.

The field of psychiatric treatment, of which psychiatric rehabilitation is currently a part, has traditionally not defined its goals in very specific or observable terms. As a matter of fact, many mental health professionals and their respective agencies do not really understand the concept of a goal or a behavioral objective. For example, this author was involved in a project in which a group of professionals representing a variety of mental health agencies were asked what their agencies' outcomes or goals were for their particular helpees. The overwhelming majority of these professionals responded with a description of their agency's activities, what the agency does, rather than what it hopes to achieve. For example, an answer such as "our goal is to provide a wide range of therapeutic services to our clients" is simply a description of process rather than outcome. Other psychiatric treatment facilities avoid the issue of goals entirely by asserting that their goals are never explicitly stated but implicitly defined by their treatment approach.

In contrast to the field of psychiatric treatment and its incomplete understanding of goal setting, the field of physical rehabilitation has consistently attempted to define its goals in observable terms. Individuals with physical disabilities who are involved in a rehabilitation program are almost always working toward an observable, functional goal. The goals for each physically disabled helpee vary widely, for example, crutch walking using the two-point alternate crutch gait, maintaining full range of motion in joints, able to transfer from bed to wheelchair, able to button a shirt, etc.

Originally, the term *rehabilitation* referred almost exclusively to the treatment provided to individuals with physical disabilities. Now however, rehabilitation alludes to work with drug addicts, alcoholics, the "culturally disadvantaged," psychiatrically disabled, and others. As the concept of rehabilitation encompasses an ever widening spectrum of helpees, the practitioners of rehabilitation have become increasingly less able to define their outcomes in the same manner as their predecessors in physical rehabilitation. While the vagueness in goal definition may have been inevitable, as professionals in the mental health professions rushed to join the rehabilitation bandwagon, it need not be irreversible.

The rehabilitation concept has developed on a wave of popularity, with the popularity developing faster than its programs. Eventually, rehabilitation must survive in a wave of accountability. To do so it must be able to specifically define what it can and cannot achieve.

This chapter examines the potential unique contributions of psychiatric rehabilitation to the psychiatric treatment process. Initially, several reasons are advanced for the necessity of spelling out the unique outcome of psychiatric rehabilitation in observable terms. Next, the rather abstract overall goal of psychiatric rehabilitation as it has been traditionally discussed is contrasted with the overall goal of psychiatric therapy. The next section examines the major innovations in psychiatric treatment and their relevance to the overall goal of psychiatric rehabilitation. The following section specifically defines what the overall goal of rehabilitation needs to be, in hopes that new developments in the mental health system recognize the critical nature of a psychiatric rehabilitation component. The final section gives examples of some specific rehabilitation outcomes.

THE NEED FOR OBSERVABLE OUTCOMES

In order to develop specific rehabilitation principles and programs, we must first determine what the practitioners of psychiatric rehabilitation hope to achieve for their helpees. In other words, rehabilitation goals must precede the planning of the rehabilitation programs, i.e., we must first know where we are going before we can map out a course to get us there. Systematic program development (discussed extensively in Chapter V) cannot occur unless we define the program goals in observable terms, for without an observable goal it becomes difficult to determine whether a particular program step is moving the helpee toward or away from the goal. For example, if the rehabilitation goal is vaguely defined as aiding the helpee to become an "adequately adjusted outpatient," it would be difficult to determine which of the following three behaviors is closer to the goal: watching TV, going to a movie, or going bowling. However, if the rehabilitation goal had been specifically defined as "the ex-psychiatric patient will participate at least ten hours a week in non-passive activities away from the home," it is fairly easy to rank the behaviors in terms of proximity to the goal, with going bowling most closely approximating the goal followed by going to the movies and watching TV.

THE NECESSITY OF IDENTIFYING OBSERVABLE CLIENT OUTCOMES

(Case Illustration 3-1)

During their last several sessions, Ellen had helped Barbara to explore and organize a whole list of specific strengths and deficits relevant to her living environment. Barbara would have to deal with each of these skill behaviors as soon as she was ready to leave the hospital and resume her regular life.

"I guess my biggest problem is with my family," Barbara said. "I just couldn't seem to get along with them when I was at home. Jim always had to have everything just right — dinner ready when he came home, everything just where it was supposed to be. The kids were always racing around. They never listened to a word I said. And Jim's mother — listen, either she and I wouldn't talk at all or we'd end up arguing about the dumbest things. Like how long soft-boiled eggs are supposed to cook, for God's sake!" Barbara sighed. "If I could just keep things on an even keel with my family, I know I could work out all the other things we've talked about."

"You're right," Ellen told her. "I think developing a really good relationship with all the people in your family has got to be a major goal."

They spent the remainder of that session talking about different aspects of Barbara's present relationship with her family. Her two boys were ten and twelve, ages where they had far more energy and enthusiasm than self-control. Jim, Barbara's husband, was a hard-working guy but one who had trouble recognizing other people's needs. Barbara described how he had often yelled at her until she broke down and wept over some simple affair like weak coffee, or a newspaper that had been left out in the rain instead of brought inside. Then there was old Mrs. Savage, Jim's mother. Apparently she saw Barbara's most recent hospitalization as proof positive that her son had made a bad mistake when he married. Even now, Barbara's voice trembled when she talked about her relationship with the older woman.

The next session followed much the same pattern. And the one after that. Ellen worked with Barbara to try to pin down the problem that existed in the latter's relationship with her family. She told Barbara that she must exercise firmer control over her children — "Tell them just what you expect of them and then make them stick to it." She encouraged Barbara to talk out her problems with Jim — "Just sit down with him and tell him how you get upset sometimes when he gets angry with you. He probably doesn't even realize how you feel. . . ." She outlined vague strategies of dealing with Jim's mother — "Try to get her involved in activities outside the house that she might enjoy — anything to get her out of your hair!"

Everything that Ellen said was well-intentioned. Some of it was even mildly constructive. Yet despite this, Barbara found it harder and harder to grab hold of any particular strategy or course of action.

She knew she had to work to develop better relationships within her family. But she still couldn't see how she was supposed to do this. Most important of all, she didn't have any clear idea of just what a "good relationship" was. How then, was she supposed to know exactly what to do or whether or not she was getting closer to her goal?

The longer her sessions with Ellen dragged on, the worse Barbara seemed to feel. Each day brought her closer to the time when she would be home again — and yet she didn't feel any closer to a solution to her major concern. What was she supposed to do? How would she know when she had done it?

For her part, Ellen suspected that things weren't going as well as they might. The big shock, however, came the morning that Barbara failed to show up for her regular session. Ellen called the ward and learned that Barbara was asleep.

"We had to give her extra medication," Ellen was told. "She got pretty up-tight last night — running around and upsetting everyone including herself. I'm afraid it may be a few days before she's ready to start working with you again."

Now it was Ellen's turn to worry. Where had she gone wrong? Everything had gone so well right up to the last minute. Barbara had agreed that working for a better family relationship had to be a major goal. What had gone wrong?

What had gone wrong, of course, was that the "goal" which Ellen had developed was actually not a goal at all, but merely a vague direction. If a client is to work toward and achieve a goal, he or she must have a clear understanding of the specific, concrete things that the goal involves. When the goal is achieved, what will the client be *doing* or able to do? What will others be *doing*?

A goal is a target. The less clear, tangible, and concrete it is, the greater the chance that the client will never achieve or "hit" it. Given the vague, general quality of the "goal" that Ellen developed, Barbara had no chance at all!

Another reason why psychiatric rehabilitation goals must be specifically defined is related to the need to know if the rehabilitation program has successfully achieved the rehabilitation objectives. For example, it is very difficult to determine when the psychiatrically disabled helpee has finally become "more motivated." However, it is certainly easy to ascertain when a helpee "earns a minimum monthly income of $500," or "works a minimum of 35 hours a week." Only to the extent that psychiatric rehabilitation goals are spelled out in observable, measurable terms, will there be a way of determining whether a particular rehabilitation program has achieved its goal.

Furthermore, the value of psychiatric rehabilitation to the welfare of the psychiatrically disabled helpee and to society in general can be ascertained only if the unique goals of rehabilitation are first defined. To define rehabilitation goals vaguely is to repeat the error of the proponents of psychiatric treatment. One of the reasons why the continual challenges to the efficacy of psychotherapy (Eysenck, 1952, 1960, 1972, Levitt, 1957) cannot be completely answered is due to the fact that the practitioners of psychiatric treatment typically do not define their therapeutic goals in observable terms. Thus, even if psychotherapy was having a positive impact on its helpees, the adherents of psychotherapy would still be unable to demonstrate the capabilities of their methods without first defining their goals in observable terms. The critics of psychotherapy have not claimed that psychotherapy *is ineffective*; rather they have pointed out that the evidence which does exist has failed to indicate that psychotherapy *is effective* (Eysenck, 1972). In other words the burden of proof is on the provider of the service; very little evidence pertaining to the efficacy of psychotherapy can ever be provided by the advocates of psychotherapy unless therapeutic goals are first defined in observable terms.

Although an examination of the controversy concerned with the efficacy of psychotherapy remains neither the interest nor the intent of this book, the field of psychiatric rehabilitation can learn from the historical shortcomings of psychotherapy. The failure to define rehabilitation goals in observable terms will inevitably lead to an inability to make clear to ourselves, other professionals, laymen, and our helpees the value of rehabilitation. Goal definition is necessary for both ethical and economic reasons. Ethically, the psychiatrically disabled helpee and his or her family have a right to know what the goals of the rehabilitation program are. Economically, the buyer of the service, whether it be the helpee, his or her family, or the taxpayer, has a right to know how effective these services are. Knowledge of effectiveness can not be provided without observable goals and comprehensive follow-up. Comprehensive follow-up cannot be undertaken unless the psychiatric rehabilitation goals are observable and measurable.

IDENTIFYING THE OVERALL GOAL OF PSYCHIATRIC REHABILITATION

General agreement seems to exist as to the overall goal of psychiatric rehabilitation and how the rehabilitation goal compares with the overall goal of psychiatric therapy. Typically, practitioners of rehabilitation conceive of their goal as restoring the helpee's former capacity to function in the community, or, as reintegrating the helpee back into the community.

To achieve this reintegration, rehabilitation practitioners focus their efforts on increasing or maximizing the psychiatrically disabled helpee's strengths and assets. In contrast, the goal of psychiatric treatment is often considered to be aimed at alleviating the patient's discomfort, reducing the patient's symptoms, and minimizing the patient's "sickness." Martin (1959) uses the term rehabilitation to refer to those "...activities which attempt to discover and develop patient's assets in contrast to treatment which is a direct attack on the patient's disability" (p 56). Leitner and Drasgow (1972) succinctly characterize the rehabilitation goal as "health induction," in contrast to the psychiatric treatment goal of "sickness reduction."

However, in spite of this philosophical agreement about the difference in goals between practitioners in rehabilitation and psychiatric therapy, rehabilitation programs are still often directed at symptom reduction rather than health induction. As Leitner and Drasgow (1972) point out "... our attempts to help are directed more at *minimizing* sickness than towards *maximizing* health." Furthermore, these authors argue that rehabilitation must give up the assumption "... that removing or suppressing sickness automatically leads directly to healthy living. It is just not so! By removing or suppressing illness, we have an end product that is less sick, and that is all. ..." If that is all, it is certainly not enough. The recidivism and unemployment figures of psychiatrically disabled helpees (reviewed in Chapter II) are an indication of the fact that more is needed.

This philosophical distinction in overall goals has not often been translated into a difference in programs because the field of psychiatric rehabilitation has not broken down the overall rehabilitation goal of health induction into terms that are specific and observable. By neglecting to emphasize the observable behavioral goals of rehabilitation, the difference in general goals between psychiatric rehabilitation and psychiatric therapy has remained primarily a philosophical distinction rather than a functional distinction. Many rehabilitation programs attempt to induce health in their helpees by minimizing the sickness of the *environment* in which the helpee works and lives (half-way houses, sheltered employment, day hospitals, etc.). Although this may be an important step in a rehabilitation program designed to increase the health of the psychiatrically disabled helpee, it can not usually be considered the whole program. Maximizing the health of the environment does not automatically lead to maximizing the health of the psychiatrically disabled helpee, just as symptom reduction does not automatically lead to health induction. The overall goal of increasing health must be broken down into specific observable goals before rehabilitation programs can be developed to achieve these goals. The phenomenally high rehospitalization and jobless rates among psychiatrically disabled helpees illustrate the fact that the abstract goal of health induction must be spelled out more specifically if effective rehabilitation programs are to be developed.

MAJOR INNOVATIONS IN PSYCHIATRIC TREATMENT

The treatment of the psychiatrically disabled has been marked by at least four major innovations within the last one hundred years. While these innovations may have achieved some therapeutic goals, it is questionable whether these new methods of treatment had any positive effect on the health of psychiatrically disabled helpees. It is not the purpose of this section to provide a comprehensive overview of the history of psychiatric treatment; such a review has been provided many times elsewhere (Joint Commission, 1961; Angrist, 1963; Deutsch, 1949). Instead, the major innovations in the care of the psychiatrically disabled are analyzed so as to determine the relevance of these innovations to the overall goal of rehabilitation. The present analysis examines the effect of these innovations on increasing the health of psychiatrically disabled helpees. In other words, did the advances in psychiatric treatment also advance the field of psychiatric rehabilitation?

Within the last one hundred years, four major innovations in the area of the psychiatrically disabled helpee are generally recognized: 1) the development of the mental hospital, 2) the development of psychoanalytically oriented psychotherapy, 3) the development of drug therapy, and 4) the development of community-based treatment.

1. **The Development of Mental Hospitals**

The construction of large, government-financed hospitals for the psychiatrically disabled is in large part credited to the industriousness of Dorthea Dix (Felix, 1967). During the mid-nineteenth century her tremendous efforts toward obtaining better conditions for the "mentally ill" heralded an optimistic future for the treatment of the psychiatrically disabled helpee. No longer would the psychiatrically disabled have to be confined to prisons and poorhouses; instead, brand new institutions, often set in peaceful, country surroundings were built for the benefit of the psychiatrically disabled.

Unfortunately, the change in setting without a major accompanying change in goals turned the promises of institutional treatment into a bitter reality. Psychiatric institutions became overcrowded, isolated facilities, in which the psychiatrically disabled helpees received custodial treatment. The nineteenth-century dream of institutional living evolved into the twentieth-century nightmare of institutionalization. Psychiatric rehabilitation has reaped the bitter fruits sown by the humanitarians of the nineteenth century because in part there were no rehabilitation goals incorporated into the development of large institutions for the psychiatrically disabled.

What in fact were the main observable goals, either implicitly or explicitly stated, of the institutionalization of the psychiatrically disabled? As Dix intended, the number of psychiatrically disabled helpees residing in prisons and poorhouses was reduced, and thus the number of interactions between the psychiatrically disabled and "deviants" such as prisoners and paupers was decreased. However, no equally diligent attempts were made to increase the number of interactions between the psychiatrically disabled and non-deviant members of society; rather the implicit goal of psychiatric institutions seemed to be to keep the opportunity for contact between disabled and non-disabled individuals at a minimum. Another implicit goal seemed to be a reduction in the number of injuries caused by psychiatrically disabled helpees, either to themselves, hospital staff, or society. An isolated setting, fences, locked doors, and other physical restraints reflect the pursuit of this goal.

26

From our present historical perspective, it is apparent that none of the goals of the movement to construct large mental hospitals explicitly achieved the rehabilitation goal of health induction. In fact, the construction of mental hospitals was not really addressed to the therapeutic goal of sickness reduction; it primarily addressed the sickness of the patients' environment.

2. The Development of a Psychoanalytic Approach to Psychotherapy

By the mid 1940s the theories and concepts of Freud were the dominant force in the training of American psychiatrists. Because psychiatrists dominated the top-level positions in the mental hospital system, Freudian theory and techniques became the *sine qua non* of psychiatric treatment. Even though the psychoanalytic technique was of debatable effectiveness within most mental hospital settings, its influence on the thinking of mental health professionals has been pronounced. Its long-term nature and excessive cost meant that only a small percentage of mental hospital patients ever received a thorough psychoanalytic intervention. However, Freud's comprehensive theory of personality and psychopathology has played and continues to play a pervasive role in the development of insight-oriented psychotherapeutic approaches.

The research relevant to the inability of the insight-oriented therapies to effect rehabilitation outcome was summarized in Chapter II. Also mentioned earlier in this chapter was the debate over whether the pure insight-oriented approaches have been able to document their effectiveness in terms of symptom or sickness reduction (Eysenck, 1972). It is probably reasonable to conclude that the impact of psychoanalytic theory has had a more dramatic observable effect on the **training outcome** of mental health professionals than the **rehabilitation outcome** of their patients. Based on Freud's creative thinking and working, mental health professionals have changed their vocabularies, their training experiences, and the techniques they use to interact with a minority of psychiatrically disabled helpees. Unfortunately, Freud's contributions have not been able to significantly change the rehabilitation outcome for the overwhelming majority of psychiatrically disabled helpees.

3. The Development of Drug Therapy

Few would quarrel with the statement that the drug revolution has had a dramatic effect on the manner in which the psychiatrically disabled helpee is treated. For approximately the last two decades, the majority of psychiatric patients and virtually all of the most seriously disabled patients have been treated with some form of drug therapy. Felix (1967) characterizes the effects of drugs on the functioning of the mental hospital in this way:

"The drugs have been a significant factor in bringing about profound changes in the structure and administration of the mental hospital itself. No longer is it necessary to keep patients behind locked doors. More and more the open hospital is coming into use, and in some states . . . entire hospitals are now open. Because the patients are calm and can be cared for as any other ill individual, it has been possible to do many things to make the hospital more cheerful and livable." (p. 88)

Furthermore, Felix (1967) notes that one of the results of drug therapy was to make patients more amenable to other forms of psychiatric therapy, which ". . . could be effective at attacking the roots of their problems" (p. 87). The actual goals achieved by drug therapy are essentially fourfold: 1) reduced the psychiatrically disabled helpee's symptoms, 2) reduced the number of physical restraints used on a psychiatric ward, 3) increased the time psychiatrically disabled helpees spend in various forms of psychiatric therapy, and 4) increased the number of patients discharged from the psychiatric hospital.

However, the psychiatric rehabilitation goal of health induction was neither a goal nor a by-product of the drug revolution of psychiatric treatment. Perhaps this was due to the unbridled enthusiasm surrounding the advent of drug therapy.

"(these new drugs) were hailed as the solution to the problems of nearly all mental illness — they were the panacea, and to the more enthusiastic, they

were the means by which most if not all previous forms of treatment could be eliminated and mental illnesses could be eradicated. The popular press was filled with dramatic examples of work done with the drugs." (Felix, 1967, p. 86)

Two decades later it is apparent that although drug therapy effectively reduces the helpee's symptoms (Cole and Davis, 1969) and perhaps indirectly reduces the discomfort of the significant others in the helpee's life, there is little available evidence to indicate that drug therapy increases the psychiatrically disabled helpee's strengths and assets. (See Chapter V for additional references on drug therapy and rehabilitation outcome.) While drug therapy does allow more in-patients to receive more types of therapy, the research presented in Chapter II indicates that the typical in-hospital therapeutic techniques do not affect community behavior. In general, effective comprehensive rehabilitation treatment programs which could capitalize on the symptom reducing capability of drug therapy have not been immediately forthcoming. Instead, a simultaneous increase in discharges and admissions to psychiatric hospitals has accompanied the popularity of drug therapy. However, the "revolving door" helpee which has resulted (reflected by the recidivism rates presented in Chapter II) has provided some of the impetus for the most recent innovation in the care of the psychiatrically disabled.

4. The Development of Community-Based Treatment

The basic philosophy which best characterizes the early development of community-based treatment is that most anything helpful that can be done in a psychiatric institution can be done in the community, and with better results. At the present state of our knowledge (ignorance?), this belief still remains more a statement of hope than a statement of fact.

Community-based treatment became an overwhelmingly popular idea in 1963 when President Kennedy issued his *Message on Mental Illness and Mental Retardation* (Kennedy, 1963), which subsequently resulted in the U. S. Congress passing a bill to provide financial assistance for the construction and initial operation of community mental health centers (U. S. House of Representatives, 1963). In pressing for a community-based approach, President Kennedy (1963) stated that "Merely pouring federal funds into a continuation of the outmoded type of institutional care which now prevails would make little difference." Instead, he recommended, and Congress funded, community-based facilities whose goals would include provisions ". . . for early diagnosis and continuous and comprehensive care, in the community, of those suffering from these disorders" (Kennedy, 1963).

The stated goals of these community-based treatment facilities (which have been named Community Mental Health Centers), are essentially to provide certain essential services to the psychiatrically disabled helpees and to the community in which they live. The initial legislation required five essential services: inpatient services, outpatient services, partial hospitalization, emergency services, and consultation and educational services to community agencies and personnel. Thus, these stated goals are not really explicit goals but merely descriptions of activities. The stated goal of "comprehensive community care" can be broken down into the following four specific observable goals: 1) spend money, 2) build facilities, 3) train professionals, and 4) increase the number of contact hours between the psychiatrically disabled community members and new staff in the new facilities. As these seem to be the implicit observable goals they must also be the primary basis on which community-based treatment has been initially evaluated. Thus, the most important evaluative statistics were those that indicated the amount of money spent, buildings built, professionals trained, and amount of contact with community members. Strikingly absent are statistics which indicate the rehabilitation effectiveness of the increased money, new buildings, more professionals, and more contact hours.

(Case Illustration 3-2)

Jane and her family have a history of interaction with every type of mental health service available. Her parents are alcoholics and have been "treated" in three in-patient alcohol units. They left dry and sober each time. The third time they "slipped," they did not go back. Jane's father was jailed on the charges of beating up his wife and extinguishing cigarette butts on his children's arms. Jane's mother deserted the five children. She was 21. Jane's father was 22.

The social service community stepped in, placing the children first in foster homes (five different ones in an eighteen-month period); then in various halfway houses, group homes, etc. All four of Jane's brothers and sisters graduated from group homes, to psychiatrists, to juvenile court, and then to adult court. At age twelve, Jane took her place with the rest of her family, in court, charged with theft; and again at thirteen and fourteen. Each time, an assessment was done, and "therapeutic" interventions were tried. When she was fifteen Jane ran from the community home to which she had been sent for the last time.

Today, at sixteen, Jane works in a downtown massage parlor and is kept by her pimp. Obviously for Jane and her family the number of services received provides no true index of the *outcome* of the services received.

Unlike the other three major innovations, the community-based treatment innovation at least acknowledges the importance of rehabilitation. However, rehabilitation was initially described only as a service and not in terms of specific observable goals. Unfortunately there seems to be a disturbing similarity between the building of large institutions in the nineteenth century and the building of Community Mental Health Centers in the twentieth century. Once again money is being spent on a new type of facility without an equal emphasis on new types of rehabilitation programs and goals. The most drastic change is an architectural change in the type of building or location where the services are provided rather than in the goals of the services, which to this day remain rather vague and ill-defined.

As a matter of fact, it is extremely distressing to review the major innovations in the treatment of psychiatrically disabled helpees from a rehabilitation perspective. Psychiatrically disabled helpees were removed from prisons and poorhouses to elegant settings which, because of lack of adequate treatment, soon became too overcrowded. Apologists for the hospitals then stated that the crowded conditions thwarted their attempts at providing effective treatment and psychotherapy. Drug therapy, hailed incorrectly by some as the ultimate cure, was able to reduce both the overcrowding the the helpee's symptoms. However, the hoped-for treatment which could now take place because the overcrowding had been alleviated was not forthcoming. Instead, the mental hospital was declared "outmoded" and major efforts were turned toward building and staffing a new facility.

Where will the cycle end? Chances are that it won't unless psychiatric rehabilitation assumes the initiative and defines specific observable rehabilitation goals designed to measure the psychiatrically disabled helpee's strengths. History is telling us that new buildings and new techniques and services designed to reduce symptoms are not enough.

Where must a new direction begin? By first specifying exactly what is meant by rehabilitation outcome, so that the goals of rehabilitation are specific and observable. Without this beginning there can be no systematic rehabilitation programs nor program evaluation. Without these programmatic and evaluative components, the sense of direction becomes more tenuous, and past mistakes are repeated by practitioners incapable of realizing that the historical direction of psychiatric treatment as it relates to psychiatric rehabilitation is becoming increasingly circuitous.

Up until this point the overall goal of psychiatric rehabilitation has been discussed in rather general terms, indicating that the overall goal of rehabilitation is to increase the psychiatrically disabled helpee's strengths or assets, or more simply, health induction.

Identifying the rehabilitation goal as health induction implies that the helpee's present level of assets, i.e., skills, are deficient. Thus, the psychiatrically disabled helpee's problem, as seen from the rehabilitation perspective is that she or he has a deficit in skilled performance, that is, the psychiatrically disabled helpee does not possess the skills necessary to cope with certain living, learning, or working situations in her or his particular community. This lack of skills may cause the psychiatric symptoms, or the psychiatric symptoms may cause the deficit in skilled performance, or, an interaction effect may exist between the two causative factors. However, *the psychiatric rehabilitation practitioner's interest in the issue of causation is at this time more a theoretical than a practical concern* (Erikson, 1974). The critical issue for the psychiatric rehabilitation practitioner is, can the helpee, given her or his present level of symptomatic behavior, demonstrate the skill behaviors necessary to function in the community with a minimum amount of support from mental health workers. Thus, the general rehabilitation goal for the psychiatrically disabled helpee can be defined in the following manner:

The goal of the psychiatrically disabled helpee is to perform the physical, intellectual, and emotional skills needed to live, learn, and work in her or his particular community, given the least amount of support necessary from agents of the helping professions.

It is apparent from the preceding goal definition that the goals to be achieved by the psychiatric rehabilitation helpee dictate the rehabilitation process of the psychiatric rehabilitation practitioner. The **main activity** for the practitioner is to systematically diagnose and teach the disabled helpee the skills necessary to live, learn, and work, while the main activity for the helpee is to perform the skills necessary to live, learn, and work. The specific **conditions** under which these skills are to be performed are spelled out in terms of the amount of assistance still needed by the psychiatrically disabled helpee as he or she performs these skills. The **standards** toward which the rehabilitation practitioner's teaching is geared and the standards by which helpee's skilled performance is evaluated are determined by the requirements of the particular community in which the helpee is trying to function. For example, if the community in which the helpee is expected to work is a sheltered workshop, then the standards of performance demanded by sheltered workshops are the standards toward which the rehabilitation program is aimed and subsequently evaluated. If the community in which the helpee is expected to reside is at her or his home with spouse and offspring, then the skills must be taught and performed at a level equal to or above the level of skill needed for the helpee to live with her or his family.

Also, the conditions under which community living, learning, and working is achieved can be varied according to the legitimate goals of the rehabilitation program. For example, in examining the efficacy of the field of psychiatric rehabilitation (Chapter II), the overall goals of rehabilitation were defined in terms of recidivism and full-time employment, as this is the traditional manner in which research studies have defined these two particular goals. However, these two goals may be modified in terms of the conditions under which these behaviors are to be observed, resulting in a more detailed definition. Walker (1972) has considerably refined the measurement of recidivism and employment by defining a wide variety of conditions under which recidivism and employment can be measured.

Recidivism has been redefined as the degree of living independence and is categorized in terms of conditions into one of six levels, ranging from residing in an institution with no privileges, to residing in the community with no supervision. Likewise, the goal of employment has been redefined as the degree of employment restoration and is categorized in terms of conditions, into one of six levels, ranging from no work of any kind to regular work in the community. Table 3-1 (Walker, 1972) presents the goals of recidivism and employment as modified by Walker (1972). Depending on the psychiatrically disabled helpee's present level of skilled performance, any of levels 0-5 may be set as the immediate or ultimate goal for a particular helpee.

SPECIFIC REHABILITATION GOALS AS SKILLS

The overall observable goal for the psychiatrically disabled helpee can and must be broken down into the specific subgoals necessary for each helpee to achieve the overall goal of living, learning, and working in the community with a minimum amount of assistance. The subgoals which need to be defined are the individual skills which the helpee must have in order to function as independently as possible in his or her community.

The term *skill* is used to describe a behavior which is *observable*, *measurable*, and *teachable*. Once the goal is achieved, we speak of the behavior which achieves that goal as a skill. The goal-definition process is essentially the first step in a skill learning process and the achievement of a goal is in actuality the objective of a particular skill. Once a program to achieve that particular goal has been developed, the process of achieving the goal could also correctly be called the process of learning a skill. For example, while we say we have achieved the goal of landing a man on the moon, what we have actually done has been to develop the necessary skills to do it. Thus, while we may define the psychiatrically disabled helpee's goal as working full-time in competitive employment, what we are really saying is that the psychiatrically disabled helpee must develop the necessary skills to be able to work full time. When we refer to the psychiatrically disabled helpee's goals, we must eventually spell out the unique skills needed to achieve each particular goal.

Obviously, the specific goals necessary to achieve the overall goal of rehabilitation vary from individual to individual and flow out of the rehabilitation diagnosis (discussed extensively in Chapter IV). The individualization of these goals is typically carried out by identifying what conditions and at what level a certain skilled activity needs to be performed in the community. Without going into the specifics of the rehabilitation diagnostic process, it is possible to give examples of some typical physical, emotional, and intellectual skills.

SOME EXAMPLES OF REHABILITATION SKILLS

The definition of the overall goal of psychiatric rehabilitation contains the categorization of the psychiatrically disabled helpee's skilled behavior into physical, emotional, and intellectual skills. This categorization process is designed to facilitate a complete analysis of the helpee's skills. The lack of such a distinction has in part resulted in the ignoring of the psychiatrically disabled helpee's physical functioning. By neglecting the physical areas of functioning, practitioners in psychiatric rehabilitation have ignored an area in which psychiatrically disabled helpees perform poorly, an area which affects the intellectual and emotional areas of functioning, and an area which by virtue of its concreteness can provide valuable skill generalizations to other areas of functioning. (The physical functioning of the psychiatric patient is examined in Chapter VI.) This categorization process helps to make the analysis of the helpee's skills more comprehensive in relation to community demands. The research reviewed in Chapter II pertaining to the efficacy of psychiatric rehabilitation procedures clearly indicates that the psychiatrically disabled helpee must be treated comprehensively in order to have an effect on his or her community functioning.

One of the principles developed from the research reviewed in Chapter II alludes to the fact that the behavior of the psychiatrically disabled helpee is to a large extent situationally determined. The client's level of functioning in any one of these living, learning, and working environments is not consistently correlated with the client's functioning in any one of the other environments. For example, some psychiatrically disabled clients who are working successfully have to return to the hospital because of problems at home; others who are adjusting well to a living environment cannot find or hold a job; still other clients might perform adequately in a learning or school environment but are unable to hold a part-time job or relate well to family and friends. Thus, the rehabilitation practitioner must identify which specific living, learning, and working environments and which specific client skills will be the focus of the rehabilitation program. Success or failure in one environmental area does not assume success or failure in another environmental area.

The tactic of providing skill acquisition experiences for the psychiatrically disabled helpee is designed to make him or her increasingly less dependent upon the mental health caretakers. Rather than just solving his or her problem or assisting him or her through a crisis, the rehabilitation goal is to ultimately teach the psychiatrically disabled helpee the skills necessary to prevent future problems. (The skills needed by the psychiatric rehabilitation practitioner to maximize the probability that the helpee achieves these skills are discussed in Chapter XI.)

The examples of psychiatric rehabilitation skills presented in Table 3-2 are summary descriptions of some of the observable skills which various psychiatrically disabled helpees must demonstrate in order to function effectively in the community. Many other necessary skills become apparent to the rehabilitation practitioner as she or he begins to rehabilitate psychiatrically disabled helpees toward observable goals. Each skill activity can be individualized for each helpee by further

defining under what conditions and at what level the behavior must occur. For example, the skill of "using community resources" could be broken down in an infinite number of ways depending upon the psychiatrically disabled helpee's specific needs:

Using community resources: (1) The psychiatrically disabled helpee can identify from a phonebook the three community resources which can help him with financial problems. (2) The psychiatrically disabled helpee can travel from her residence to the Social Security office in one hour or less. (3) The psychiatrically disabled helpee can telephone the U. S. Employment Service and make an appointment with a counselor within seven days.

Other examples of possible definitions for various skilled activities follow:

Stigma reduction skill: The psychiatrically disabled helpee can orally respond to questions about prior hospitalization by describing the outcome of hospitalization in two or more sentences using positive terms only.

Selective reward skill: The psychiatrically disabled helpee can role play real-life situations with a coached actor and demonstrate at least one instance of a verbal positive reward response in each role playing situation.

Job qualifying skill: The psychiatrically disabled helpee can perform the job skills at the level demanded by the job requirements.

Each of these observable skills may consist of subskills. For example, to be skilled in job interviewing demands a number of even more specific skills, such as the skills involved in explaining job skills, turning noticeable liabilities into assets and terminating the job interview. For each of these subgoals systematic programs must be developed.

Expert diagnosis of the helpee's present and needed skill level leads directly into developing an effective rehabilitation program (discussed further in Chapter V). The rehabilitation diagnostic process determines the unique way the particular skilled activity is defined and the present skill level of the achiever. It is this individualized rehabilitation diagnosis that determines the characteristics of the helpee's individual rehabilitation program. However, it may often be possible to use all or part of a previously developed program on more than one psychiatrically disabled helpee. Many of the skilled activities given as examples in Table 3-2 have already been programmed. Many of the physical living skills have been programmed by nurses, physical therapists, and occupational therapists in a variety of physical rehabilitation settings.

Facilities for the mentally retarded also have programs to teach some of these activities of daily living skills. Carkhuff and his associates (Carkhuff, 1972; 1973; 1974; Carkhuff & Friel, 1974; Carkhuff, Pierce, Friel & Willis, 1975) have developed programs to teach human relations skills, problem solving skills, program development skills, program implementation skills, and career development and placement skills. Educators in most any school system have a variety of different reading, writing, and arithmetic programs. Swanson and Woolson. (1972) have reported a program which teaches psychiatric patients to use the skill of selective reward in interpersonal interactions. Many investigators, including Mahoney (1973), have reported on issues related to self control programs. Physical educators have developed numerous physical fitness and sports education programs. Study skills programs have existed for quite some time, as have programs in job interviewing skills (Carkhuff, Pierce, Friel, & Willis, 1975; Prazak, 1969).

The level to which a psychiatrically disabled helpee can reach is to a certain extent a function of the psychiatric rehabilitation practitioner's expertise in diagnosis and subsequent program development. Rehabilitation failure can not always be attributed to the pre-treatment level of functioning of the helpee or to the poor conditions in which the psychiatrically disabled helpee resides (Gurel & Lorei, 1973).

However, individualized goals cannot be set and programs constructed without a systematic rehabilitation diagnosis. It is the rehabilitation diagnosis which identifies the specific demands of the helpee's community and the helpee's present level of skilled behavior.

As the next chapter indicates, once the rehabilitation diagnosis is made, the individual's rehabilitation goals have then been defined in observable measurable terms.

THE IMPORTANCE OF INDIVIDUALIZING THE CLIENT'S SKILL GOALS

(Case Illustration 3-3) ━━

"Looking Efficient"

Bob Johnson was a therapist in a large community mental health center. Many demands were placed on his time, especially his rather heavy caseload. As a result, Bob's assessment skills were rather slipshod. Since assessment was a rather time-consuming process, Bob decided to cut some corners in this area and never really measured in an observable way his client's present and needed level of functioning. Rather, Bob would consider the rehabilitation diagnostic plan complete when he and the client had identified strengths and deficits in certain environmental areas.

Thus, Bob Johnson's clients were started on their rehabilitation treatment programs when they had identified such deficits as, for example — lack of self-control in the living area and lack of job interviewing skills in the working area. Unfortunately, Bob's inability to observably assess such client deficits set the stage for several problems to occur in later phases of the rehabilitation treatment process. For example, when Johnson attempted to develop systematic treatment programs he found that, without an observable goal, it became difficult to accurately sequence some of the steps to the goal. Difficulties also occurred when he tried to explain the client's goals to significant others in the client's life, as the concept of "self control" meant different things to different people. Even his clients had difficulties staying goal-directed when the goal was so abstract. And worst of all, when it came time to evaluate the outcome for each of his clients, it was very difficult to really know if his clients had actually reached their goals.

So for Bob Johnson and his clients, cutting corners in the assessment phases of the diagnostic planning process led to later difficulties, which in the long run consumed more time than was saved by eliminating the assessment steps. Never really knowing *exactly* what the client needed to overcome helped create more problems than it solved.

Compare Bob Johnson's attempts, which "look efficient," to Ruth Johnson's attempt to "be efficient."

"Being Efficient"

Ruth Johnson was always looking for places to cut corners. As a therapist in a large community mental health center, she saw many clients each day. She was always looking for ways to do things more efficiently, but she knew that taking shortcuts in the assessment phase would only backfire.

Thus, she made sure that before any rehabilitation programming occurred, both she and the client knew exactly the client's present and needed level of functioning for each skill area. For example, a client deficit was not just categorized as a lack of self-control in the living area, but for a specific client the deficit might be observably assessed as, "client presently raises voice to spouse five times a week during mealtime conversations and needs to reduce the frequency to zero times per week."

Having assessed her clients in such an observable, measurable way, several advantages immediately accrue to Johnson and her clients. First, systematic rehabilitation programs can be more easily developed when the program goal is so observable. Second, significant others in the client's life know exactly what the treatment programs are trying to accomplish. More importantly, the clients themselves can become more involved in the treatment program when the goal is less esoteric and more understandable. Third, the rehabilitation outcome of each rehabilitation client can be specifically assessed, so that specific types of treatment intervention programs can be evaluated and improved.

So Ruth Johnson, by performing her assessment skills, was in actuality cutting corners. By observably measuring each skill deficit, she was more effective in her program development, more efficient in explaining the rehabilitation goals to her clients and significant others, and more equipped to eventually evaluate the rehabilitation outcome of her clients.

TABLE 3-1

GOAL DEFINITIONS FOR THE GOALS OF LIVING INDEPENDENCE (RECIDIVISM) AND EMPLOYMENT RESTORATION (POST-HOSPITAL EMPLOYMENT)

Degree of Living Independence

5. The psychiatrically disabled helpee resides in the community without scheduled, regular on-site visits to or from a staff member of an agency supervising his community living adjustment.

4. The psychiatrically disabled helpee resides in the community but is scheduled for regular on-site visits to or from a staff member of an agency supervising his community living adjustment.

3. The psychiatrically disabled helpee resides in a full-care institution, but has been approved within the past two weeks for an absence from the institutional grounds on his *own* custody and has full ground privileges at the present time.

2. The psychiatrically disabled helpee resides in a full-care institution, but has not been approved for an absence from the institutional grounds in his *own* custody during the past two weeks but has full ground privileges.

1. The psychiatrically disabled helpee resides in a full-care institution, but his ground privileges have been partially restricted.

0. The psychiatrically disabled helpee resides in a full-care institution, with no freedom of the institutional grounds in his *own* custody.

Degree of Employment Restoration

5. The psychiatrically disabled helpee works in regular (non-sheltered) employment in the community for at least three days during the month.

4. The psychiatrically disabled helpee works in sheltered employment off the institutional grounds with total dollar (or cash equivalent) earnings at a rate of $30 or more per week.

3. The psychiatrically disabled helpee works in sheltered employment on the institutional grounds with total dollar (or cash equivalent) earnings at a rate of $30 or more per week.

2. The psychiatrically disabled helpee works on or off the institutional grounds whether or not under supervision with total dollar (or cash equivalent) earnings at a rate of $10-$29 per week.

1. The psychiatrically disabled helpee works on or off the institutional grounds whether or not under supervision with total dollar (or cash equivalent) earnings at a rate of $1-$9 per week.

0. The psychiatrically disabled helpee does not work for pay on or off institutional grounds.

TABLE 3-2
SOME EXAMPLES OF POTENTIAL SKILLED ACTIVITIES NEEDED TO ACHIEVE THE GOAL OF PSYCHIATRIC REHABILITATION

Living Skills

Physical	Emotional	Intellectual
personal hygiene	human relations	money management
physical fitness	self control	use of community resources
use of public transportation	selective reward	goal setting
cooking	stigma reduction	problem development
shopping	problem solving	
cleaning	conversational skills	
sports participation		
using recreational facilities		

Learning Skills

Physical	Emotional	Intellectual
being quiet	speech making	reading
paying attention	question asking	writing
staying seated	volunteering answers	arithmetic
observing	following directions	study skills
punctuality	asking for directions	hobby activities
	listening	typing

Working Skills

Physical	Emotional	Intellectual
punctuality	job interviewing	job qualifying
use of job tools	job decision-making	job seeking
job strength	human relations	specific job tasks
job endurance	self control	
job transportation	job keeping	
specific job tasks	specific job tasks	

REFERENCES

Angrist, S. The mental hospital: its history and destiny. **Perspectives in Psychiatric Care,** 1963, December, 20-26.

Carkhuff, R. R. **The art of helping.** Amherst, Ma.: Human Resource Development Press, 1972.

Carkhuff, R. R. **The art of problem solving.** Amherst, Ma.: Human Resource Development Press, 1973.

Carkhuff, R. R. **How to help yourself: The art of program development.** Amherst, Ma.: Human Resource Development Press, 1974.

Carkhuff, R. R. and Friel, T. W. **The art of developing a career: A student's guide.** Amherst, Ma.: Human Resource Development Press, 1974.

Carkhuff, R. R., Pierce, R. M., Friel, T. W. and Willis, D. G. Get a job. Amherst, Ma.: Human Resource Development Press, 1975.

Cole, J. D. and Davis, J. M. Antipsychotic drugs. In **The Schizophrenic Syndrome.** L. Bellak and L. Loeb, eds. New York: Grune & Stratton, 1969, 478-568.

Deutsch, A. **The mentally ill in America.** New York: Columbia University Press, 1949.

Erikson, R. Outcome studies in mental hospitals: A review. **Psychological Bulletin,** 1975, *82*: 519-540.

Eysenck, H. J. The effects of psychotherapy: An evaluation. **Journal of Consulting Psychology,** 1952, *16*: 319-324.

Eysenck, H. J. The effects of psychotherapy. In **Handbook of Abnormal Psychology,** H. J. Eysenck, ed. London: Pitmans, 1960.

Eysenck, H. J. New approaches to mental illness: The failure of a tradition. In **The Critical Issues of Community Mental Health,** H. Gottesfeld, ed. New York: Behavioral Publications, 1972.

Felix, R. H. **Mental Illness: progress and prospect.** New York: Columbia University Press, 1967.

Gurel, L. and Lorei, T. W. The labor market and posthospital employment. **Journal of Counseling Psychology,** 1973, *20*: 450-453.

Ivey, A. **Microcounseling: Innovations in interviewing training.** Springfield, Ill.: Charles Thomas, 1971.

Joint Commission on Mental Illness and Health. **Action for mental health.** New York: Basic Books, 1961.

Kennedy, J. F. Message from the President of the United States relative to mental illness and mental retardation. Washington, D. C.: U. S. Government Printing Office, 1963.

Leitner, L. A. and Drasgow, J. Battling recidivism. **Journal of Rehabilitation**, July-August, 1972: 29-31.

Levitt, E. E. The results of psychotherapy with children. **Journal of Consulting Psychology**, 1957, *21*: 189-196.

Mahoney, M. J. Research issues in self management. **Behavior Therapy**, 1973, *3*: 45-63.

Martin, H. R. A philosophy of rehabilitation. In **Rehabilitation of the mentally ill**. M. Greenblatt and B. Simon, eds. Washington, D. C.: American Association for the Advancement of Science, 1959.

Prazak, J. A. Learning job seeking interview skills. In **Behavioral Counseling**. J. D. Krumboltz and C. E. Thoreson, eds. New York: Holt, Rinehart and Winston, 1969.

Swanson, M. G. and Woolson, A. M. A new approach to the use of learning theory with psychiatric patients. **Perspectives in Psychiatric Care**, 1972, *10*: 55-68.

U. S. House of Representatives #3688, 88th Congress, First Session, 1963. A bill to provide for assistance in the construction and initial operation of community mental health centers and for other purposes.

Walker, R. The Brockton Social Adjustment (BSA) Scale. **Diseases of the Nervous System**, 1972, *33*: 542-545.

CHAPTER IV

The Rehabilitation Diagnosis

As developed in this chapter, a rehabilitation diagnosis is completely different from a psychiatric diagnosis, both in terms of the diagnostic process itself and the type of information obtained by the diagnostic process. As evidence presented later in this chapter indicates, the traditional psychiatric diagnosis provides the rehabilitation practitioner with little meaningful information relevant to the goal of rehabilitation. In addition, the debate over whether the psychiatric diagnostic process itself is reliable or valid for psychiatric treatment goals (Beck, Ward, Mendelson, Mock & Erbaugh, 1962; Rosenhan, 1973; Schmidt & Fonda, 1956; Thaler, 1973; Ward, Beck, Mendelson, Mock & Erbaugh, 1962; Zubin, 1967), although not a controversy to be thoroughly examined within the scope of this book, suggests further problems if psychiatric rehabilitation practitioners had to rely on the traditional psychiatric diagnostic process for diagnostic information relevant to rehabilitation outcome. Thus, it is incumbent upon the field of psychiatric rehabilitation to develop, use, and research a rehabilitation diagnostic process which is relevant to the rehabilitation goals of living, learning, and working in the community.

In order for the rehabilitation diagnosis to be of value to the psychiatric rehabilitation practitioner, the rehabilitation diagnosis must be functional, that is, the information gathered must possess either empirical validity or face validity with the overall rehabilitation goals. Empirically valid diagnostic information means that the diagnostic information collected by the psychiatric rehabilitation practitioner has been shown to significantly relate to psychiatric rehabilitation outcome in a variety of research studies. Diagnositc information which possesses face validity means that the information appears relevant to the rehabilitation goal of increased living, learning, and working skills. Thus, face valid diagnositc information appears at "face

value" to be very relevant to the rehabilitation goal of increasing the helpee's skilled behavior. If the goal of rehabilitation is the achievement by the psychiatrically disabled helpee of a higher level of skilled performance, then a face valid rehabilitation diagnosis should indicate her or his present level of skilled performance so that the psychiatric rehabilitation practitioner will be able to determine in what area the helpee has specific skill strengths and deficits. In addition, the diagnosis must obtain relevant information about the skill demands of the helpee's community so that the rehabilitation practitioner can determine the level to which specific helpee skills need to be developed.

The rehabilitation diagnostic process of obtaining information about the psychiatrically disabled helpee's skills and the skill demands of the community in which he or she wants (or ought) to function, is essentially the first step in the rehabilitation treatment process. The rehabilitation programs for each psychiatrically disabled helpee flow directly from the rehabilitation diagnostic process. That is, once the psychiatric rehabilitation practitioner has identified the helpee's strengths and deficits, a rehabilitation program is then developed to enable the helpee to achieve the needed level of skill in these particular areas which are essential to effective community functioning.

In brief, the present chapter focuses on the following two types of information needed to make a rehabilitation diagnosis: 1) information which research investigations have shown to relate to community functioning and 2) information pertaining both to the psychiatrically disabled helpee's present level of skilled performance and the particular level of skilled performance demanded by the community in which the psychiatrically disabled helpee is expected to function. In the final section of this chapter, the rehabilitation diagnostic process is also analyzed.

EMPIRICALLY RELEVANT DIAGNOSTIC INFORMATION

The following section examines a variety of research studies which have examined the relationship between various types of information and rehabilitation outcome. For reasons of consistency and ease of interpretation, almost all the studies reviewed in this section have used measures of recidivism and post-hospital employment as criteria of rehabilitation outcome. By examining these studies, it is possible to determine what information is valuable for the psychiatric rehabilitation practitioner to obtain as well as what is useless or redundant. This information is not a description of the helpee's skills, but rather an analysis of various helpee characteristics which have been empirically related to rehabilitation outcome.

The results of these research studies are useful in the rehabilitation diagnostic process as well as being valuable to the field of psychiatric rehabilitation in general. First, the research studies which have investigated the relationship between rehabilitation outcome and various types of rehabilitation information have provided practitioners with the means by which they may quickly identify "high risk helpees," those psychiatrically disabled helpees who are most likely to experience difficulty in the community and thus most in need of specific rehabilitation programs. Secondly, by identifying those "high risk helpees," evaluative studies of rehabilitation programs have an empirical basis upon which to assign subjects to various treatment and control groups. As a result, outcome studies can more effectively rule out helpee characteristics as a source of variance in treatment outcome.

A third contribution of the research designed to develop a meaningful rehabilitation diagnosis is the practitioner's understanding of the psychiatric rehabilitation process in general. Based on the data generated from these studies, tentative principles can be advanced which describe the relationship between the diagnostic information and psychiatric rehabilitation practice. The conclusion of each section identifies some of these tentative psychiatric rehabilitation principles.

The research studies which have evaluated the relationship between various types of diagnostic information and rehabilitation outcome can be divided into three categories on the basis of the type of diagnostic information obtained. These categories include: 1) demographic charac-

teristics; 2) ratings of the psychiatrically disabled helpee by professionals, significant others, or by the psychiatrically disabled helpee himself; and 3) psychological test scores.

DEMOGRAPHIC CHARACTERISTICS

The demographic characteristics which are reviewed in this chapter are those which are used most frequently to describe psychiatrically disabled helpees. Most of these demographic characteristics are biographical in nature and are routinely obtained by most psychiatric hospitals within the first few days of admission. The issue to be addressed in this section concerns whether or not the psychiatric rehabilitation practitioner's knowledge of any of these demographic characteristics will help him identify those psychiatrically disabled helpees most in need of rehabilitation programming.

The recent use of multiple regression analysis provides the psychiatric rehabilitation practitioner with suggestions as to the minimum amount of information necessary to achieve the maximum amount of relevant diagnostic information. Most of these research studies have reported their data in terms of correlations between the demographic characteristics and the rehabilitation outcome criteria of recidivism and post-hospital employment. However, several of the most recent investigations (Anthony & Buell, 1973, 1974; Buell & Anthony, 1973; Lorei & Gurel, 1972, 1973) have analyzed this same relationship by means of multiple linear regression. The multiple linear regression analysis provides evidence of the unique variance contributed by each predictor; in contrast, correlations obtained by the multiple correlation approach may provide redundant sources of information in that findings of significant correlations may be due to variance common to many characteristics rather than variance specific to one particular demographic characteristic.

The relationship between rehabilitation outcome and the following helpee demographic characteristics is reviewed in this section. These demographic characteristics have been selected for this review primarily on the basis of their frequent occurrence in the research literature. They include: age, sex, race, educational level, marital status, number of previous hospitalizations, length of previous hospitalizations, diagnosis, employment history, and occupational level.

The research to be reviewed will be analyzed separately based on whether or not the researchers used a multiple linear regression analysis. Those research investigations which did not use multiple linear regression techniques typically examined the correlations between several demographic characteristics and rehabilitation outcomes. A few of these studies used other statistical techniques to compare the demographic differences between those helpees who were successfully rehabilitated and those helpees who were not. In using primarily a correlational approach, none of these studies were able to ascertain the redundant contributions of each demographic characteristic to the prediction of rehabilitation outcome. These correlational studies will be reviewed first, followed by a review of the findings of the more recent multiple linear regression studies.

DEMOGRAPHIC CHARACTERISTICS AND REHABILITATION OUTCOME: A REVIEW[1]

The literature which has specifically evaluated the relationship between demographic variables and recidivism will be examined first. The findings will be presented in sequence from the most convincing evidence for a relationship between demographic characteristics and recidivism to findings where no relationship or conflicting evidence has been found. A summary of the results for both recidivism and employment are presented in Table 4-1.

Generally, a high number of previous hospitalizations have been related to high probability of recidivism (Arthur et al. 1968; Gregory & Downie, 1968). Lorei (1967) found that not being hospitalized in the two years prior to the last hospitalization differentiated between recidivists and non-recidivists. Likewise, Wessler and Iven (1970) report that readmissions

accounted for 58% of their total admissions during a three-year period, an amount they considered to be significantly disproportionate. Similar results have been obtained for the closely related variable of length of hospitalization. The data consistently suggest that the longer a patient is hospitalized prior to current treatment and discharge, the more likely he or she is to return to the hospital (Fairweather et al. 1960; Fairweather, 1964; Freeman & Simmons, 1963; Arthur et al. 1968).

Unlike these researchers, Lewinsohn (1967) found no relationship between number of hospitalizations and ability to stay in the community. This apparent contradiction is quite possibly due to Lewinsohn's sample, which included an unusually large number of first admissions (82%) resulting in a rather homogeneous sample.

In contrast, diagnosis has been found to be ineffective at differentiating those who return to the hospital from those who remain (Freeman & Simmons, 1963; Lorei, 1967; Wessler & Iven, 1970). It is only when measures of chronicity (typically defined by length of hospitalization) are included in the diagnosis that a relationship is found (Fairweather, 1964; Freeman & Simmons, 1963). Fairweather (1964) reports that acute psychotics (0-2 years prior hospitalization) stay out significantly more than neurotics or psychotics with more than two years prior hospitalization. Other studies have supported this interaction between diagnosis and chronicity with short-term psychotics staying in the community better than neurotics and chronic psychotics. (Fairweather et al. 1960; Fairweather & Simon, 1963). Thus, it would appear that when diagnosis has been found to be related to recidivism, it is the dimension of chronicity rather than the particular diagnosis which accounts for the results.

The findings with respect to both educational level and occupational level have also been quite consistent. Investigations of educational level have concluded that level of education and recidivism are unrelated (Gregory & Downie, 1968; Lewinsohn, 1967; Lorei, 1967). Concerning occupational level, although Gregory and Downie (1968) found that significantly more unskilled workers fail to ever be released from the hospital, there was no relationship between recidivism and occupational level for those who were released. Similarly, Lewinsohn (1967) reports no relationship between occupational level and ability to remain in the community.

Little work has been done relating either employment history or race to recidivism. Forsyth and Fairweather (1961) report in a factor analytic study that ten-year work history prior to hospitalization is not a factor in remaining in the community. Investigations of race and recidivism have likewise found no relationship between these two variables (Forsyth & Fairweather, 1961; Lorei, 1967).

No male-female differences in recidivism have been found (Freeman & Simmons, 1963), unless sex of the patient is combined with living arrangements. Miller (1966, 1967) found that adult sons discharged to parental homes return at the rate of 54%, while adult daughters at only a 31% rate. Males living with offspring return at 33%, while females return at a 52% rate. Male isolates return at the rate of 48% while female isolates only at a 38% rate. Spouses did not differ significantly, as wives returned at a 30% rate and husbands at a rate of 25%.

The research is notably inconsistent for marital status. Some researchers have reported that married patients are more likely than single patients to remain in the community after discharge (Freeman & Simmons, 1963; Gregory & Downie, 1968). Miller (1967) concluded that spouses have the lowest return rate of any other living arrangement (i.e., parent-child, brother-sister, isolate, etc.). Lewinsohn (1967) found a non-significant trend for married ex-patients to remain in the community to a greater extent than unmarried ex-patients. In contrast, other researchers have found marital status to be unrelated to recidivism (Lorei, 1967; Forsyth & Fairweather, 1961; Wessler & Iven, 1970).

The research with respect to age appears to be equally as conflicting. Some researchers have found that recidivists tend to be older than non-recidivists (Gregory & Downie, 1968; Wessler & Iven, 1970). However, others have found that age is unrelated to recidivism (Lewinsohn, 1967; Lorei, 1967; Freeman & Simmons, 1963). It should be noted that the former two studies had longer follow-up periods (1 to 3 years) than the latter three (6 months to 1 year).

POST-HOSPITAL EMPLOYMENT

The review for post-hospital employment is likewise presented in sequence from the most convincing results to the more conflicting findings.

With respect to marital status, the data is quite uniform. Ex-patients who are married obtain and hold jobs significantly better than their single or divorced counterparts (Goss & Pate, 1967; Hall, Smith & Shimkunas, 1966; Lorei, 1967; Olshansky, Grob & Ekdahl, 1960; Wilson, Berry & Miskimins, 1969). Only Knowlton and Samuelson (1968) report that marital status does not significantly distinguish the employed from the unemployed, although they did find a trend in the expected direction.

Similarly, the number of previous hospitalizations has been found to relate to securing employment after discharge. The patients who become gainfully employed tend to have had less previous psychiatric help (Goss & Pate, 1967; Green, Miskimins, & Keil, 1968; Wilson et al. 1969). More specifically, Lorei (1967) found that employed ex-patients had significantly fewer hospitalizations in the two-year period prior to the last hospitalization.

Closely related to post-hospital employment is the area of length of hospitalization. The data suggest that employed ex-patients tend to have had shorter stays in the hospital than the unemployed (Ellsworth et al. 1968; Olshansky et al. 1960). Likewise, Lorei (1967) reports that the employed have spent significantly less of their adult lives in the hospital than the unemployed. In contrast, Knowlton and Samuelson (1968) concluded that length of hospitalization did not distinguish those who become employed from the unemployed, although a trend in the expected direction was reported. A caution must be added to studies of length of hospitalization, however, now that deinstitutionalization has become a matter of public policy rather than a reflection of patient functioning, it would be expected that the "revolving door" type of treatment approach will render length-of-stay-data irrelevant.

With respect to diagnosis, the tendency is for psychotics to do worse than those in other diagnostic categories in obtaining employment after discharge. Results have indicated that patients diagnosed as having anxiety or depressive reactions (Goss & Pate, 1967), neurotics (Knowlton & Samuelson, 1968), neurotics or personality disorders (Wilson et al. 1969), or non-psychotics (Fairweather, 1964) have a greater tendency to be employed than do psychotics. Furthermore, when comparing the re-employed or stably employed with the marginally or unemployed, the finding was that the latter groups had significantly more psychotics than the former groups (Olshansky et al. 1960). Unlike the above studies, Hall et al. (1966) examined diagnostic subcategories within the primary diagnosis of schizophrenia, i.e., catatonic, paranoid, and simple undifferentiated and found diagnostic subcategories unrelated to employment.

The data on employment history suggests that pre-hospital work behavior is related to post-hospital work behavior. Some researchers have found that post-hospital employment is related to having worked on a single job for one year (Hall et al. 1966) or three years prior to hospitalization (Olshansky et al. 1960). Another study found that the unemployed held fewer jobs in the two years prior to hospitalization and had been unemployed for longer periods of time than the employed (Green et al. 1968). Likewise, Lorei (1967) reported that success in obtaining and holding a job for six months after discharge is related to having had a recent job prior to hospitalization.

Similarly, occupational level does appear to be related to post-hospital employment. Hall et al. (1966) found that being a skilled worker, rather than un-skilled, was a significant predictor when considering success in returning to a job. Similarly, Lipton and Kaden (1965) report that amount of income during the year prior to hospitalization is directly related to the level of income during the year following discharge. It appears that many ex-patients are able to return to their old jobs or to jobs similar to them. However, Perkins and Miller (1969) attempted to predict from files which patients would become employed after discharge, and found that occupational level did not add significantly to their prediction equation at twelve-month follow-up.

With respect to age, the findings have been inconsistent. There is some evidence to support the notion that those patients that eventually obtain employment are significantly younger than the patients who fail to obtain work (Green et al. 1968; Knowlton & Samuelson, 1968). Hall et al. (1966) found that patients in the age range 30-45 are best able to obtain employment. Contrary to these findings are those of Perkins and Miller (1969), who found that age is not a factor in distinguishing between employed and unemployed ex-patients.

Concerning race, Lorei (1967) reported that being white is related to obtaining and holding a job for six months after hospital release. Another investigation also found a greater percentage of black ex-patients unemployed, but concluded that this discrepancy is consistent with current general unemployment trends and not specific to ex-psychiatric patients (Hall et al. 1966).

Generally, the findings with respect to educational level have been consistent. The typical result has been that level of education does not differentiate the employed from the unemployed (Knowlton & Samuelson, 1968; Perkins & Miller, 1969). Hall et al. (1966) found that educational level below high school was unrelated to being employed, although they did report that having obtained some college credit enhances the ex-patient's chances of being employed.

The relationship between sex of the released patient and post-hospital employment has rarely been studied. The data which are available have reported neither employment differences between the sexes (Knowlton & Samuelson, 1968) nor that males find work more readily than females (Hall et al. 1966).

MULTIPLE LINEAR REGRESSION STUDIES OF DEMOGRAPHIC CHARACTERISTICS AND REHABILITATION OUTCOME

As graphically illustrated by Table 4-1, two demographic characteristics have been found to significantly relate to recidivism, and eight demographic characteristics have been found to significantly or tentatively relate to post-hospital employment. However, because of the manner in which the data were analyzed, there is no way of determining how much redundant information is provided by using all eight demographic characteristics. Multiple linear regression analysis overcomes this difficulty by identifying a nonredundant set of demographic variables which includes only those demographic characteristics that contribute unique variance to the rehabilitation outcome criteria.

TABLE 4-1

RESEARCH FINDINGS ON THE RELATIONSHIP BETWEEN HELPEE DEMOGRAPHIC CHARACTERISTICS AND POST-HOSPITAL ADJUSTMENT

Demographic characteristic	Recidivism	Post-hospital employment
Number of previous hospitalizations	Significant	Significant
Length of last hospitalization	Significant	Significant
Employment history	Non-significant	Significant
Marital status	Conflicting	Significant
Diagnosis	Non-significant	Significant
Race	Non-significant	Tentative
Occupational level	Non-significant	Tentative
Age	Conflicting	Tentative
Educational level	Non-significant	Non-significant
Sex	Non-significant	Non-significant

Significant	= positive results in 3 or more studies.
Tentative	= positive results in 1 or 2 studies or minor contradictions.
Non-significant	= no positive results.
Conflicting	= approximately equal number of significant and non-significant results.

Basically, the recent research studies which have analyzed their data by using multiple linear regression have investigated a large number of demographic characteristics simultaneously. The multiple linear regression analysis automatically selects that one demographic characteristic which correlates the highest with the rehabilitation outcome criterion. Depending on the particular multiple linear regression analysis used, the remaining demographic charac- teristics are then analyzed as to their ability to contribute any more predictive information about the criterion.

The results of the three recent multiple linear regressions which have examined the relationship between demographic characteristics and the rehabilitation outcome criteria of recidivism and post-hospital employment have been remarkably consistent (Anthony & Buell, 1974; Buell & Anthony, 1973; Lorei & Gurel, 1973).

Concerning the post-hospital employment criterion, all three of the previous studies found that the overwhelming amount of outcome variance accounted for by the demographic data could be attributed to one piece of demographic information — previous employment history. In two of the studies (Anthony & Buell, 1974; Buell & Anthony, 1973), length of follow-up was six months and employment history was categorized as either stable or unstable depending on whether the helpee had steady employment for at least one year in the same job prior to hospitalization. In the other study (Lorei & Gurel, 1973), the follow-up period was nine months and employment history was defined as months of full-time work in the last five years.

All the different demographic variables analyzed in these three studies accounted for between 27% - 53% of the variance in post-hospital employment with employment history, accounting for the overwhelming bulk of the variance. Of the eight demographic characteristics which previous research has found to be related to post-hospital employment (Table 4-1), the psychiatric rehabilitation practitioner should be concerned primarily with only employment history. The other seven demographic variables provide information which is redundant, i.e., information that tells us little more about the helpee's post-hospital employment prospects than can be ascertained by assessing the helpee's past employment history.

Concerning recidivism, these same three studies reported that all the demographic variables which were investigated accounted for a relatively smaller amount of the variance in recidivism, i.e., between 5% - 29%. Typically, the research indicates that the variable which accounts for the major amount of recidivism variance at follow-up periods of six months (Buell & Anthony, 1973), nine months (Lorei & Gurel, 1973) and twelve months (Anthony & Buell, 1974) has been the number of previous hospitalizations. However, at one six-month follow-up period, the demographic characteristic of marital status was found to account for more recidivism vari-

ance than the number of previous hospitalizations.

This discrepancy in the findings for recidivism, combined with the fact that the number of previous hospitalizations has accounted for a relatively minor amount of recidivism outcome variance, raises questions about the utility of predicting recidivism based on the number of previous hospitalizations or any other demographic variable. In general, the results of multiple linear regression analyses uniformly indicate that the attempts to predict recidivism from demographic variables have been less consistent and account for notably less outcome variance than similar attempts which have used demographic data to predict post-hospital employment.

DEMOGRAPHIC CHARACTERISTICS: PRINCIPLES FOR PSYCHIATRIC REHABILITATION

It is obvious that a significant amount of research has attempted to examine the relationship between helpee demographic characteristics and psychiatric rehabilitation outcome. Based on these research investigations, some tentative psychiatric rehabilitation principles are advanced which can serve as useful guidelines for the psychiatric rehabilitation practitioner:

1. **One of the best predictors of future helpee behavior is past helpee behavior.**

Those psychiatrically disabled helpees with a better pre-hospitalization employment history are more likely to become employed after hospital release; and to a lesser degree, future recidivists have been past recidivists. In operating from this principle, it would appear that the rehabilitation diagnostic process should assess the psychiatrically disabled helpee's past and present levels of skilled behavior, because these affect his ability to develop more skills. In some respects, the principle of past behavior predicting future behavior can be viewed as a rather pessimistic principle for a field whose goal is to change behavior. The fact that two pieces of demographic information can account for more rehabilitation outcome variance than almost any type of psychiatric treatment is certainly disturbing (Buell & Anthony, 1973). Rehabilitation programs must obviously devote more of their efforts to those psychiatrically disabled helpees whose past behavior indicates that they will have future rehabilitation difficulties.

2. **The characteristics of the psychiatrically disabled helpee who obtains employment reflect the biases of the job market.**

At one level, it is not really surprising that the psychiatrically disabled helpee who obtains employment has a better employment history. After all, employers prefer to hire persons with a more stable employment history, regardless of whether the person has been psychiatrically disabled or not. Similarly, the studies summarized in Table 4-1 emphasize traits which, in the past, many employers preferred in the typical worker who had no history of psychiatric disability, i.e., being married, white, young, and possessing job skills.

3. **The traditional psychiatric diagnostic system is not relevant to the goals of psychiatric rehabilitation.**

Research support for this principle continues to be reported (Cumming & Markson, 1975; Franklin, Kittredge & Thrasher, 1975); it would be reasonable to conclude that this principle is one of the most consistently supported in the research literature. The value of psychiatric labeling, as presently defined and practiced, has been debated extensively. The critical issues of disagreement most often revolve around whether the psychiatric diagnostic system is reliable and valid, or whether the label may do more harm to the psychiatric helpee than it might benefit him or her. However, independent of this controversy surrounding the whole issue of psychiatric labeling, there are other reasons why the psychiatric diagnostic system has so little to offer the rehabilitation diagnosis. As the research reviewed suggests, the psychiatric diagnosis does not provide any uniquely relevant information about the helpee's rehabilitation potential. This finding is really not that surprising as the psychiatric diagnostic system was developed to categorize symptom patterns, not to provide information about a psychi-

atrically disabled helpee's rehabilitation prospects. Independent of the debate over whether the psychiatric diagnostic system does what it was developed to do, it can be said, with considerable research support, that the psychiatric classification system is unable to provide information about the helpee's rehabilitation potential. The psychiatric diagnostic system consumes staff and helpee time that could be spent in rehabilitation programs. The amount of training time spent in developing the psychiatric rehabilitation practitioner's expertise in the use of the psychiatric diagnostic system might better be spent teaching the more relevant rehabilitation diagnostic procedures outlined in this chapter. These results do not mean, however, that rehabilitation practitioners cannot use the information collected by traditional psychiatric diagnosticians in their attempts to diagnose the psychiatrically disabled helpee. Rehabilitation practitioners must educate the traditional diagnosticians as to the information relevant to rehabilitation outcome. Specifically, rehabilitation practitioners should ask the traditional diagnostician for any information which they might have uncovered with respect to the helpee's skills, skill deficits, interests, and interactions with significant others. Some of this information might well be collected during a psychiatric diagnostic interview. The rehabilitation practitioner must be assertive in asking for this information and not settle merely for information about symptoms and labels.

4. **The success rates of various psychiatric rehabilitation programs may be more a function of the helpee's demographic characteristics than the rehabilitation program itself.**

Differences between rehabilitation programs in terms of percentage employed, or the percentage of recidivists, may be due to the characteristics that the helpee brings to the program rather than characteristics of the particular rehabilitation program itself. Psychiatric rehabilitation researchers must be especially aware of the possible confounding of their outcome statistics by the demographic characteristic variable. One recent outcome study attempted to overcome this possible confounding by first determining whether there were important demographic differences between helpees who were using rehabilitation services and those who were not (Anthony & Buell, 1973).

BEHAVIORAL RATINGS

The critical issue examined in this section concerns whether ratings of the psyciatrically disabled helpee's functioning made by helping professionals, significant others, or by the helpee her/himself can provide the psychiatric rehabilitation practitioner with relevant information about the helpee's chances of rehabilitation success. In the case of professionals, their ratings of the helpee are typically made after an interview with the helpee, who may be either an inpatient or outpatient. Ratings made by significant others in the helpee's life or by the helpee her or himself typically occur several weeks after the psychiatrically disabled helpee's discharge from the hospital.

Professional Ratings

In general it appears that professionals' ratings of the psychiatrically disabled helpee's behavior are related to post-hospital employment (Distefano & Pryer, 1970; Ethridge, 1968; Green, Miskimins & Keil, 1968; Gurel & Lorei, 1972; Lorei, 1967; Sturm & Lipton, 1967; Wilson, Berry & Miskimins, 1969) but not to recidivism (Gurel & Lorei, 1972, Lewinsohn, 1967; Marks, Stauffacher & Lyle, 1963; Williams & Walker, 1961). Only one study (Lorei, 1967) has reported statistically significant but small correlations between professional ratings and recidivism.

The type of ratings which are related to post-hospital employment are primarily ratings of social effectiveness and work skills rather than ratings of psychiatric symptoms. Examples of the types of behavior which have been found to correlate with employment are: ratings of job motivation, the ability to get along well with others, ability to work with others, a preference for social activity as opposed to social isolation, etc. A recent study using

multiple regression analysis (Gurel & Lorei, 1972) developed two rating items which accounted for 25% of the variance in post-hospital employment. These items referred to the rater's assessment that the helpee either lacked goals or a method to obtain these goals and the rater's prognosis that the helpee's future psychosocial functioning would be restricted.

In contrast to the studies of professional ratings of helpee characteristics and their relationship to post-hospital employment are the lack of studies which have found a substantial relationship between recidivism and professionals' ratings of helpee behavior. Somewhat surprising is the finding that the psychiatrically disabled helpee's symptoms, as rated by the professional, do not relate to recidivism. The recidivist does not seem to be characterized by any pattern of symptoms discernible to the professional (Gurel & Lorei, 1972).

Significant Other Ratings

There is a dearth of studies examining the relationship between ratings by significant others and recidivism and employment outcome. The few studies which do exist, however, seem to suggest that ratings by significant others, made shortly after the helpee's hospital discharge, are significantly related to recidivism but not to employment (Freeman & Simmons, 1963; Michaux, Katx, Kurland & Gansereit, 1969). Ratings by significant others of the psychiatrically disabled helpee's symptoms (Freeman & Simmons, 1963), as well as ratings of their satisfaction with the helpee's social and free-time activities (Michaux et al. 1969), have been found to correlate significantly with recidivism.

Helpee Self-Ratings

Well-controlled studies of the relationship between helpee self-ratings and rehabilitation outcome are practically nonexistent. One study has investigated this relationship and found significant correlations between the helpee's ratings of his or her own behavior made one month after discharge and the helpee's future recidivism (Michaux et al. 1969). In particular, psychiatrically disabled helpees destined to be rehospitalized were not satisfied with their performance of social activities.

The most valuable study of the relationship between the helpee's ratings of his or her own behavior and recidivism was carried out by Miller & Willer (1976). In this investigation, a self-assessment measure was administered to psychiatrically disabled helpees three months after discharge. At six-month follow-up, non-recidivists were characterized by higher self-ratings on such social factors as "ability to handle money, source of financial support, work behavior, job seeking behavior, and ability to deal effectively with anger." Of particular note in this study is that these social measures accounted for a much greater amount of the variance than the demographic characteristic of the number of previous hospitalizations.

BEHAVIORAL RATINGS: PRINCIPLES FOR PSYCHIATRIC REHABILITATION

1. **Professional ratings of helpee behavior and symptoms made from a hospital base cannot predict future recidivism.**

The implications of this principle for rehabilitation programming are several. First, any discharge decisions which are based in part on the professional's estimate of such things as behavior improvement strong enough to be maintained outside the hospital (Katz & Wooley, 1975) are based on an assessment which will be wrong as many times as it is right. The several studies which have found that ratings made by the psychiatrically disabled helpee and his family were correlated with recidivism would suggest that *any predictive efforts of the professional must take into account the helpee's interactions with significant others*. It appears that increased accuracy in both predicting and understanding recidivism may be obtained through various assessments of the helpee's behavior once he or she is functioning in the community (Anthony & Buell, 1974; Gurel & Lorei, 1972; Michaux et al. 1969). Results of one study indicated rather conclusively that complaints by significant others about the patient's inability to care for him or herself or to do what was ex-

pected in the community setting were strongly correlated with recidivism (Cumming & Markson, 1975). Obviously, if significant other interaction is critical to continued helpee functioning in the community, then the psychiatric rehabilitation practitioner must assess the demands which significant others may be placing on the helpee.

2. **The helpee characteristics which are related to employment are more observable and less variable than the helpee characteristics which are related to recidivism.**

It would seem that there is much less variability in the behavior an employer will tolerate from a psychiatrically disabled employee as compared to the behavior significant others will tolerate from a psychiatrically disabled family member. Likewise, it would seem that adequate employee behaviors are more obvious than those behaviors which are needed to reside in a community. Professionals appear to be on much more solid ground when they make an assessment of the helpee's work-related characteristics than when they attempt to ascertain characteristics related to recidivism.

3. **The employment of a psychiatrically disabled helpee is related to ratings of the helpee's skills and interests rather than ratings of the helpee's symptoms.**

This principle is certainly consistent with the previously stated principle concerning the irrelevance of psychiatric labels to rehabilitation outcome. The implications of this principle for the field of psychiatric rehabilitation are fairly straightforward — psychiatric rehabilitation practitioners must be trained in a manner which enables them to help the psychiatrically disabled helpee to develop his or her skills and interests. For example, psychiatrically disabled helpees who lack the skills to set goals and to develop a program to achieve these goals (Gurel & Lorei, 1972) can be taught these needed skills. Similarly, many other skills in which the psychiatrically disabled helpee is diagnosed as deficient can also be taught by the psychiatric rehabilitation practitioner.

4. The best predictor of future recidivism appears to be helpee and significant other ratings of the helpee's social skills made within three months of hospital release.

The direct implication is that the helpee must be followed up after hospital discharge if one wants to judge the helpee's chances of recidivism. Inpatient facilities must either reach out themselves or arrange for outpatient contact in order to obtain more input about possible recidivism. It appears that, at the present state of our knowledge, high probability recidivists can be most accurately identified shortly after hospital discharge rather than during his or her inpatient stay.

5. Neither recidivism nor post-hospital employment can be predicted accurately by professionals.

At first impression, this principle may seem contradictory to the research evidence presented earlier which indicates that professional's ratings of psychiatrically disabled helpee's behavior correlate significantly with post-hospital employment. However, although professionals may fill out rating forms which correlate with post-hospital employment, there is really no evidence to suggest that they know how to use these ratings to make an accurate prediction (Miles, 1967). If one's only interest was increased predictive accuracy, long-term (3-5 years) prediction could be improved by simply predicting that every psychiatrically disabled helpee will become a recidivist or unemployed; based upon the base rate figures presented in Chapter II, these predictions would be correct approximately 75% of the time. Obviously, the psychiatric rehabilitation practitioner's diagnostic system must become more refined than predicting failure for everyone. The principles of psychiatric rehabilitation outlined thus far would suggest a tentative direction for the refinement of the rehabilitation diagnosis, i.e., a sharper focus on indices of the psychiatrically disabled helpee's present skilled behavior and the level of skilled behavior expected of the helpee, either by significant others or by the helpee.

PSYCHOLOGICAL TEST SCORES: PRINCIPLES FOR PSYCHIATRIC REHABILITATION

1. Traditional measures of personality and intelligence are not very useful in predicting rehabilitation outcome.

A concluding phrase to this principle might be — and why should they be? These traditional measures were developed to describe personality dynamics, categorize symptom patterns, etc. These tests were not developed to predict rehabilitation outcome. This principle is similar to the principle pertaining to the irrelevance of the psychiatric diagnostic system to rehabilitation outcome. It appears that the techniques developed for psychiatric treatment cannot be borrowed by psychiatric rehabilitation practitioners. The practitioners of psychiatric rehabilitation must research and develop new procedures for the field of psychiatric rehabilitation.

2. Newly developed measures of ego strength and self-concept do relate to indices of post-hospital employment.

Some psychiatric rehabilitation practitioners have begun the research. These investigators successfully developed new tests, in part because they included in these tests measures of strengths and assets rather than primarily assessing weaknesses and symptoms. As indicated by the previously presented evidence concerning the relationship between behavioral ratings and post-hospital employment, it would seem that it is measures of skills rather than symptom patterns which relate to employability.

3. The use of psychological testing to predict rehabilitation outcome is more complex than first believed and may not be worth the effort.

In spite of the positive evidence upon which the preceding principle is based, psychological tests have still not demonstrated their unique worth. What is not yet known is whether the information provided by psychological tests accounts for any variance in post-hospital employment over and above that accounted for by demographic characteristics and behavioral ratings. As the latter two predictors are more simply and inexpensively obtained, psychological tests must be able to demonstrate that they contribute unique variance to the prediction of post-hospital employment. Future research, using multiple linear regression analysis, could determine whether psychological tests contribute any unique variance to the prediction of psychiatric rehabilitation outcome.

Other investigators have indicated that the test prediction process might be much more complex than first thought. Pierce (1968) has suggested that test prediction can be improved by predicting success as well as failure, using multiple scale patterns and by operating on the assumption that individual scales do not measure bipolar concepts. Goss (1968) believes that psychological tests have heretofore been ineffective at predicting rehabilitation outcome because tests predict differently for helpees with different symptom patterns. However, as the testing and interpretation process becomes more complex, psychiatric rehabilitation practitioners must be increasingly certain that the predictive information obtained is not duplicative of the more easily obtainable information provided by demographic characteristics and behavioral ratings.

PSYCHOLOGICAL TEST SCORES

In many psychiatric treatment settings, psychological tests have been used extensively, particularly for psychiatric diagnostic purposes. Rarely have researchers investigated the relationship between psychological test results and the rehabilitation outcome criteria of recidivism and post-hospital employment. The few investigations which have been carried out have examined primarily two types of tests, the traditional personality and intelligence tests and more recently developed tests of self-concept or ego strength.

Recidivism

Very few studies have attempted to identify psychological test correlates of recidivism. Those that have examined the relationship have been notably unsuccessful in finding significant correlations between test scores and recidivism. Neither the Minnesota Multiphasic Personality Inventory, the 16 PF test, Rotter Level of Aspiration Test, a specially constructed Sentence Completion Test, nor the Shipley-Hartford, have been able to distinguish future recidivists from non-recidivists (Lewinsohn, 1967; Marks et al. 1963).

Post-hospital Employment

A relatively greater number of studies have investigated the psychological test correlates of post-hospital employment. The research has indicated consistently that measures of I.Q. do not correlate with the ability to become employed after hospital discharge (Drasgow & Dreher, 1965; Goss & Pate, 1967; Lipton & Kaden, 1965; Lowe, 1967; Sturm & Lipton, 1967). Likewise, traditional personality measures have not been very successful in predicting post-hospital employment. Various Rorschach signs have shown little or no relationship to post-hospital employment (Drasgow & Dreher, 1965; Lowe, 1967), while evidence concerning the Minnesota Multiphasic Personality Inventory has been conflicting (Drasgow & Dreher, 1965; Lowe, 1967). One study has reported a significant relationship between various scores of the Edward Personality Preference Inventory and post-hospital employment (Goss & Page, 1967).

In contrast, newly developed measures of ego strength or self-concept consistently have been found to relate to measures of post-hospital employment (Bidwell, 1969; Berry & Miskimins, 1969; Lesh, 1968; MacGuffie, Janzen, Samuelson & McPhee, 1969). These various studies developed unique tests to assess ego strength or self-concept; regardless of the kind of psychological test used, a positive relationship was found between ego strength or self-concept and various indices of post-hospital employment.

A SKILLS DIAGNOSIS

The research studies that have investigated the type of information which correlates with rehabilitation outcome have provided the psychiatric rehabilitation practitioner with important principles with which to guide her or his diagnostic efforts. However, the empirically valid diagnostic information represents only a very small amount of information needed to make a rehabilitation diagnosis. In contrast, the major effort involved in undertaking a rehabilitation diagnosis is the process of obtaining information about the psychiatrically disabled helpee's skills and the skill demands of the community in which he or she wants (or ought) to function. The rehabilitation diagnostic focus on the helpee's skills and the environmental skill demands placed on the helpee are logical extensions of the overall goal of psychiatric rehabilitation. As presented in Chapter III, the psychiatric rehabilitation practitioner's overall rehabilitation goal is to increase the psychiatrically disabled helpee's ability to perform the physical, intellectual, and emotional skills needed to live, learn, and work in his or her particular community, given the least amount of support necessary from agents of the helping professions. If the psychiatric rehabilitation practitioner's overall goal is to help provide the means by which the psychiatrically disabled helpees increase their skills to a particular level, or find an environment which better accommodates their present skill level, then the psychiatric rehabilitation practitioner must first diagnose both the helpee's present level of skilled performance and the level of skills which the helpee wants or needs. In order to obtain this information, the psychiatric rehabilitation practitioner must engage in a diagnostic process distinctly different from the traditional psychiatric diagnostic process.

The outcome achieved by the psychiatric rehabilitation diagnostic process is essentially twofold. A rehabilitation diagnosis should enable the practitioner to:

1. List and measure according to some observable standard the psychiatrically disabled helpee's present level of skills in the living, learning, and working environments.

2. List and measure according to some observable standard the level of skills demanded by either the helpee her or himself or the helpee's living, learning, and working environments.

Once the psychiatric rehabilitation practitioner has made a rehabilitation diagnosis, she or he has essentially identified the specific skill deficits which the psychiatrically disabled helpee must overcome in order to live, learn, and work in a particular environment. *In other words, she or he has identified the helpee's individual rehabilitation program goals.* The discrepancies which appear between the diagnosis of the helpee's present level of functioning and the diagnosis of the level of skill demands placed upon the helpee will then become the programmatic areas of concern for the psychiatric rehabilitation practitioner.

MAKING THE DIAGNOSIS OBSERVABLE (OPERATIONALIZING SKILLS)

Determining a helpee's specific rehabilitation goals by *observably* assessing the helpee's present and needed level of functioning is not an easy task for most mental health professionals. Historically, professional training programs in mental health have tended to emphasize the learning and application of theory and concepts rather than teaching the specific skills involved in making observable assessments and developing systematic programs based on these observable assessments.

As mentioned in the previous chapter, however, an assessment process which culminates in the setting of observable helpee goals is an important step in the growth of the field of psychiatric rehabilitation. Observable goals increase the likelihood of the development of systematic programs; for without an observable goal, it is difficult to determine the correct sequencing of steps within the program. In addition, setting observable goals maximizes the chances of meaningful program evaluation being undertaken, for without an observable goal, it is only rehabilitation process rather than rehabilitation outcome which can be evaluated. To learn the principles involved in making a rehabilitation diagnosis in observable terms, practitioners in psychiatric rehabilitation must learn from their colleagues in education; for it is the educational innovators who have recently developed the assessment process most systematically (Aspy, 1972; Baker & Schultz, 1971; Carkhuff, Berenson & Pierce, 1977).

WRITING AN OPERATIONALIZED ASSESSMENT STATEMENT

An accurate rehabilitation diagnosis identifies in what areas the helpee is not functioning at the needed level and in so doing specifies what the helpee's individual rehabilitation goals should be. However, in order to insure that the helpee's goals which flow out of the rehabilitation diagnosis are in fact observable, the actual diagnostic statements that are written by the psychiatric rehabilitation practitioner must include *four* specific elements:

First, the assessment statement must indicate *who* it is that needs to achieve something. This first step is relatively simple as it is typically the psychiatrically disabled helpee who is the subject of the assessment. Occasionally, the achievers may include significant others in the helpee's life. For example, if a conflict exists between the helpee and his or her spouse, both members of the marital couple may become the subjects of the assessment.

It is important to define exactly who the achiever is because several common types of errors can be made in this first operation. For example, the achiever may be incorrectly identified as the helper rather than the helpee, as in the following assessment statement:

"The helpee needs to be told how he may use a certain community resource."

In the preceding assessment the answer to the question of *who* would do the telling is another person and not the helpee. In other words, the helpee in this diagnostic statement is merely a passive recipient. Incorrect diagnosis can also occur when the assessment is stated in such a way that the subject of the assessment becomes an inanimate object, such as a rehabilitation facility. An example of this type of error is illustrated by the following assessment statement:

"The rehabilitation setting needs to be modified for the helpee so that it more closely approximates a normal living environment."

In making this diagnostic error, the facility was the achiever and not the helpee. The first operation of effective assessment is to specifically identify the psychiatrically disabled helpee as the achiever, and not the passive receiver of some activity. The goals for which the psychiatric rehabilitation practitioner and the facility in which she or he works must then flow out of this assessment of the helpee.

The second requirement of a rehabilitation diagnostic statement is that the action expected of the achiever be described in observable terms. This operation involves spelling out *what* the subject is *doing* or must *do* and is typically the most difficult operation of writing an assessment statement. Grammatically, it requires placing a verb after the subject of the sentence — the subject being the achiever. The verb must describe an observable action or a product of the action. Unfortunately, most of the words traditionally used to describe the activities of psychiatric treatment do not depict observable events. For example, professionals typically describe the helpee as needing to become more motivated, adjusted, actualized, self-accepting, understanding, fulfilled, congruent, etc. These words certainly do not describe an observable activity. Rather, these words describe what the achiever *is* or *is not*.

In contrast, verbs such as earn, spend, work, attend, say, operate, write, list, and reside, describe *what* the achiever *does* or needs to *do* in terms concrete enough so that witnesses to the achiever's actions could agree on whether the activity had occurred. Words such as demonstrate, perform, and exhibit, followed by an observable action are useful in a rehabilitation assessment statement. Thus, the first two assessment operations have essentially spelled out an answer to the question:

Who does *what?"*

Examples of rehabilitation diagnostic statements which include only these first two operations follow:

"The helpee is working."

"All discharged helpees will reside

in the community."

"Each patient admitted to the hospital within the last thirty days will perform calisthenics."

The third operation involved in writing a diagnostic statement requires that the conditions under which the achiever is acting be sufficiently described. The conditions under which psychiatrically disabled helpees act may be different from typical conditions, and thus the conditions under which the observable behaviors are to be performed must be specifically spelled out.

For example, within psychiatric rehabilitation the verb "work" could mean work in a transitional workshop, a sheltered workshop, in sheltered employment, or regular competitive employment. Therefore, the conditions under which the patient works must be described. The following examples illustrate diagnostic operations 1, 2, and 3:

"The helpee is working in competitive employment."

"All discharged helpees will reside in the community without assistance from any mental health worker or facility."

"Each patient admitted to the hospital within the last thirty days will perform calisthenics, given his physician's permission."

By making a rehabilitation diagnosis using these three operations, we have now essentially answered the question:

"Who does what, where and when?"
However, these first three operations are not sufficient to write an assessment statement in its entirety, for these three operations have not defined at what particular level the achiever is expected to act, given a certain set of conditions.

The final assessment operation consists of defining the quality and quantity of the achiever's actions. The assessment must contain some standard against which the achiever's actions can be compared. Similar to the first three assessment operations, the standards must be defined in a

concrete manner so that observers can agree upon the level of achievement obtained by the achiever. In psychiatric rehabilitation, quantitative standards are often measures of length of time, money, or frequency of a particular behavior. Qualitative standards are usually defined numerically by a rating scale which may have been developed specifically for a particular behavior and upon which observers can obtain a high degree of reliability.

The following examples illustrate all four goal defining operations:

"The helpee is working in competitive employment, at a minimum of thirty-five hours per week, six months after his hospital discharge."

"All discharged helpees will reside in the community without assistance from any mental health worker for at least one year after hospital discharge."

"Each patient admitted to the hospital within the last thirty days will perform calisthenics, given his physician's permission, for a period of twelve minutes a day in accordance with the Royal Canadian Air Force exercise program."

By using all four assessment operations, we have essentially answered the question:

"Who does what, where and/or when and how well?"
The actions of the achiever are defined by these assessment operations in an observable and measurable way, thus allowing for systematic program development and systematic evaluation of goal attainment. Effective psychiatric rehabilitation programming must be preceded by an assessment process culminating in assessment statements characterized by these four operations:

1. Identify the achiever.
2. Describe the action expected of the achiever in observable terms.
3. Specify the conditions under which the action is to occur.
4. Specify the standards against which the achiever's actions are to be measured.

OPERATIONALIZING GOALS

Case Illustration 4-1

Sheila looked over Bob's shoulder at

the list of specific deficits and assets which

they had spent the last several sessions developing.

"We're agreed, then," she said. "One major goal has got to be to get control of your temper. That's a problem that you have found in every area — living with your family, going to night school, working, everywhere."

Bob nodded. "Yeah, there's not much question about that." His eyes met Sheila's as she came around to sit facing him again. "I've told you how it is. I'm O.K. for a while. But then things start happening. Little things — like maybe my car won't start in the morning, or my sister used up the last of the cereal, or my boss says something to me that gets under my skin. And wham! I feel this pressure building up in me until — well, I guess I just fly off the handle!" He shook his head and looked away unhappily.

"You feel pretty helpless when you can't control your own temper," Sheila agreed. "I think the first thing we've got to do is decide exactly what 'keeping your temper' really means."

"What does this mean? Doesn't it just mean — well, not getting mad any more?"

Sheila nodded. "Sure. Except phrases like 'losing your temper' and 'getting mad' don't really tell you enough. What kinds of things do you *do* when you lose your temper?"

Bob thought about this. "Well, I guess what I almost always do is end up hitting someone or something . . ." He looked away sheepishly. "Like that last big blow-up, where I ended up hitting my foreman at work."

Sheila nodded. "Right. That's what I thought. Well, then, we might say that your goal is to keep your temper. And you'll know you've reached this goal when *you* can *avoid physically hitting anyone or anything, everytime you feel yourself getting mad.* This made sense to Bob. With a goal as simple to understand as that, I guess I'll really be able to tell when I'm getting there, huh? And when I've reached it, too!"

"Sure," Sheila agreed. "You feel a lot more confident when you've got a really clear target to aim at!"

Sheila knew that while developing and defining a goal in clear, sharp and tangible terms was the last stage of the diagnostic planning process, it was only the first stage of a longer process. She would have to help Bob develop an adequate number of equally clear and tangible steps leading to the goal. She'd have to make sure each step was supported by appropriate reinforcements that would help Bob stay on track. She'd have to outline specific ways to evaluate his progress.

The goal was just the first stage. But without a clearcut goal, Sheila knew that none of the subsequent stages could even be begun. And Sheila was a firm believer in the idea that things usually end well only if begun well!

Some skill areas lend themselves more easily to writing observable assessment statements. For example, in the area of working skills, if the helpee consistently shows up for appointments fifteen minutes late and his or her prospective job demands that the helpee arrive for work on time, then this part of the diagnosis would indicate that the helpee needs to arrive fifteen minutes earlier for appointments. Similarly, in the area of learning skills, if the helpee was not able to read at a fifth-grade level and the prospective job training program demanded fifth-grade reading ability, the rehabilitation diagnosis would indicate a need to improve reading skills to the fifth-grade level. Likewise in the area of living skills, if the helpee wanted to walk a mile a day to visit with friends but was not physically fit enough to do so, the rehabilitation diagnosis would indicate a need to be able to walk a minimum of one mile per day.

The above examples of possible rehabilitation diagnostic statements are all similar in that the instruments used to measure the particular behaviors are common and straightforward; punctuality, reading ability and measures of physical fitness are behaviors which can easily be scaled. However, many of the other skills needed by the psychiatrically disabled helpee to function in the community are not so easily measured. Skill activities such as job interviewing, self-control, stigma reduction, selective reward, etc., have no traditional means of observable measurement. Thus the rehabilitation practitioner may have to develop the method of measuring time, frequency, or amount. In rare instances, this measuring difficulty can be overcome by developing a new scale which can be reliably used.

An example of such a new scale is illustrated by the three-point rating scale for measuring job-interviewing skills in Table 4-2. Critical to the development of any new scale designed to rate psychiatric rehabilitation skill activities is that at a minimum the scale must attain the following two criteria: 1) ordinal measurement (Siegel, 1956) and 2) sufficient reliability. In essence, a rehabilitation-skills-rating scale which achieved ordinal measurement means that the higher the numerical rating which a particular skilled behavior receives, the more highly skilled (and more difficult) that particular behavior is. The numbers assigned to specific behaviors are able to indicate a greater than or less than relationship between the skill ratings. Thus, using a scale with ordinal measurement, the rehabilitation diagnostician can measure skilled behaviors in a meaningful and observable way in order to describe numerically the relationship between the helpee's present level of functioning and the functioning level demanded of him. For example, a psychiatrically disabled helpee's present ability to "explain his job skills in an employment interview" may be assessed at level 2, while his environment demands at least a level-3 performance. His rehabilitation diagnosis would therefore indicate a skill deficit in this particular job-interviewing skill.

TABLE 4-2

JOB-INTERVIEWING-SKILL RATING SCALE

1. Interviewee *presents* the skill but for one or more reasons (timing, clarity, brevity, etc.) the skill presentation is *inaccurate* and noticeably detracts from the effectiveness of the interview.

2. Interviewee *presents* the skill *accurately* at a minimally effective level so as not to detract from the interview's effectiveness. However, the skill presentation is mechanical and unspontaneous, possessing a rehearsed quality and thus not able to add to the effectiveness of the interview.

3. Interviewee *presents* the skill *accurately* and *spontaneously*. The interviewee's voice quality and other personal characteristics show him to be quite involved in the skill presentation, so that the presentation adds to the interview's effectiveness.

In addition to possessing ordinal measurement, newly developed scales of rehabilitation skills should possess high rate-rerate and inter-rater reliability. High rate-rerate reliability means that a rater using the particular skill-rating scale would assign approximately the same rating to the same behavior on two different rating occasions. The correlation between these two different ratings at two different times gives an index of the consistency of the rating scale over time. High inter-rater reliability indicates that two or more raters rating the same skilled behavior assign that behavior approximately the same numerical rating.

Undoubtedly one of the best examples of rating scales which have achieved reliable measurements of at least an ordinal level are the five-point rating scales of human relations skills (Carkhuff, 1969). Literally hundreds of research studies have used these scales to measure seemingly qualitative skills such as empathy, genuineness, etc. and have generally reported reliability coefficients in the .80s and .90s. Carkhuff's (1969) numerical rating scales, which are capable of reliably measuring a qualitative dimension such as human relations skills, can serve as a model for the development of additional rating scales for other skilled activities. By developing a new rating scale and determining its reliability, the rehabilitation practitioner can help approximate the rehabilitation diagnostic outcome of listing and measuring according to some observable standard the helpee's present level of living, learning, and working skills, as well as those skills needed by the helpee to function in the community.

THE PSYCHIATRIC REHABILITATION DIAGNOSTIC PROCESS

Because the outcome of the psychiatric rehabilitation diagnostic process is so different from the outcome of a traditional psychiatric diagnosis, the diagnostic processes themselves are vastly different. Unlike the psychiatric diagnostic process, the rehabilitation diagnosis does not try to label or categorize behavior into abstract conceptual classifications; nor does the rehabilitation diagnostic process ever infer causation. Instead, the psychiatric rehabilitation diagnostic process attempts to describe the psychiatrically disabled helpee's behavior in an observable and straightforward manner.

In contrast to the typical psychiatric diagnostician, the psychiatric rehabilitation diagnostician need not possess classification skills. Instead, the practitioner of psychiatric rehabilitation must, at a minimum, possess the two sets of basic skills crucial to the success of the psychiatric diagnostic process: *interpersonal* skills and *assessment* skills. The psychiatric rehabilitation practitioner's interpersonal skills provide her or him with the ability to obtain information relevant to both the helpee's present functioning as well as the level of functioning which the helpee needs or wants to have in order to live, learn, and work in the community. The psychiatric rehabilitation practitioner must then describe this diagnostic information in a meaningful and observable manner by means of the practitioner's assessment skills. A detailed description of the skills needed by the rehabilitation diagnostician has been provided elsewhere (Anthony, Pierce & Cohen, 1977). The purpose of this present section is to simply overview the rehabilitation diagnostic process. The interpersonal skills needed to make a rehabilitation diagnosis have been researched and developed by Carkhuff (1969, 1971, 1972; Carkhuff & Berenson, 1977). These interpersonal or human relations skills have most often been thought of as fundamental therapy skills. As illustrated in this chapter, these skills are in essence the same skills needed to help formulate a rehabilitation diagnosis. These particular interpersonal skills have been recently categorized as responsive and initiative skills (Carkhuff, 1972). Specifically, the responsive interpersonal skills include the ability to attend, observe, listen, and respond to another person's expressions. The initiative interpersonal skills involve the ability to go beyond (interpret) another person's expressions so as to be able to identify the basic skills needed by the helpee to achieve his or her goals. These initiative interpersonal skills include the ability to effectively make empathic interpretations.

It is critical to recognize that in building a rehabilitation diagnosis the client must *accept the diagnosis as valid*, because he or she will later be expected to take action, based upon an understanding of his or her present functioning. Traditional psychiatric diagnostic attempts have not emphasized procedures for getting the client to accept the diagnosis, nor for that matter even getting the client to understand the diagnosis. In contrast to psychiatric rehabilitation, meaningful psychiatric treatment may proceed without prior client acceptance and understanding of the diagnostic label.

The psychiatric rehabilitation practitioner must rely heavily on these responsive and initiative interpersonal skills in the rehabilitation diagnostic process. It is the knowledgeable application of the responsive interpersonal skills which enables the psychiatric rehabilitation practitioner to obtain information relevant to the helpee's present level of functioning and the level of functioning which he or she will need to live, learn, or work in the community. It is the knowledgeable application of the initiative interpersonal skills which enables the psychiatric rehabilitation practitioner to use this information to arrive at a complete picture of the helpee's skills and skill deficits.

PHASES OF THE REHABILITATION DIAGNOSTIC PROCESS

The rehabilitation diagnostic process involves three stages or phases: an exploration phase, an understanding phase, and an assessment phase (Table 4-3).

By proceeding through these three phases, the practitioner achieves the goal of rehabilitation diagnostic process, i.e., the presentation of an observable, objective picture of the client's strengths and deficits with respect to specific living, learning, and working environments in which the client is or will be functioning. These three diagnostic stages are developmental in nature; the earlier stages must be accomplished before the later stages can be successfully implemented.

TABLE 4-3
THE PSYCHIATRIC REHABILITATION DIAGNOSTIC PROCESS

Diagnostic Phase	Diagnostic Skills	Diagnostic Goal
1) Exploratory	Responsive interpersonal skills	Collect information from the helpee and significant others about the helpee's present rehabilitation situation.
2) Understanding	Responsive interpersonal skills Initiative interpersonal skills Information-gathering techniques a) Simulation b) Role playing c) In vivo observation	Identify the helpee's present level of skills in the living, learning, and working areas and the level of skills in the living, learning, and working areas which the helpee wants or needs in order to function as independently as possible in the community.
3) Assessment	Responsive interpersonal skills Initiative interpersonal skills Information-gathering techniques a) Simulation b) Role playing c) In vivo observation Operationalizing and quantifying skills.	Assess in quantifiable, observable terms the helpee's present skill level in the living, learning, and working areas and the level of skills in the living, learning and working areas which the helpee wants or needs in order to function as independently as possible in the community.

In the exploration stage, the rehabilitation practitioner attempts to involve the client in an exploration of the client's unique rehabilitation situation and the feelings which the client experiences in relation to her or his own environment. The second stage of diagnostic planning is characterized by the rehabilitation practitioner's attempt to get the client to focus on his or her own role in the rehabilitation process in order to facilitate an understanding of the client's own unique strengths and weaknesses and how these personal characteristics help or hinder the client's ability to function in specific environmental areas. In the final stage of the diagnostic planning process, the rehabilitation practitioner assesses in observable, measurable terms the client's present and needed level of skilled functioning with respect to environmental areas of interest.

Each of the three stages of the diagnostic planning process requires specific practitioner skills. In the exploration stage of diagnostic planning, the rehabilitation practitioner uses his or her responsive interpersonal skills in order to facilitate the client's exploration of his or her unique rehabilitation situation. First, the practitioner must get the client involved in the rehabilitation process by *informing* and *encouraging* the client to appear for rehabilitation services and by *being attentive* to the client when she or he does appear. In addition, the rehabilitation practitioner must be able to skillfully *observe* the client's non-verbal behavior and *listen* to the client's verbal expressions. By using these attending, observing, and listening skills, the rehabilitation practitioner will be more able to accurately *respond* to the client's verbal and non-verbal expression. The rehabilitation practitioner's ability to respond, that is, demonstrate to the client that the practitioner can understand the client's situation, will encourage the client to explore his or her situation in greater and more relevant detail.

In the understanding stage of diagnostic planning, the practitioner uses his or her initiative interpersonal skills to help the client move from exploring the situation to understanding his or her personal strengths and deficits. Once again, it takes specific practitioner skills in order to facilitate the client's understanding. First, the practitioner must *personalize the meaning* of the client's self-exploration, i.e., get the client to discuss the personal implications of the facts and content that the client has been exploring. The practitioner must also *personalize the client's specific strengths and deficits*, that is, help the client understand his or her unique personal assets and liabilities in relation to the personal meaning of the situation. In addition, the practitioner must organize the client's strengths and deficits into a comprehensive and understandable diagnostic picture *by categorizing the client's strengths and deficits by client skill area*, that is, by indicating whether the client skills identified are primarily physical, emotional, or intellectual. Lastly, the practitioner must be able to *categorize the client's strengths and deficits by environmental areas*, to determine which specific living, learning, and working environments will be affected by the previously identified client strengths and deficits. By performing

these specific skills, the rehabilitation practitioner can help bring about the client's understanding of his or her personal role in the rehabilitation effort.

In the assessment stage of the diagnostic planning process, the practitioner observably and objectively assesses the client's previously identified relevant strengths and deficits. In order to undertake this assessment, the practitioner must possess certain skills. First, the practitioner must be able to *operationalize each important skill area*, which means to write a descriptive statement of the skill in terms that will allow the skill to be observably measured. The practitioner must also possess the expertise necessary to *quantify the client's present level of skill functioning* as well as to *quantify the client's needed level of functioning* with respect to each environmental area of interest. The discrepancies between the client's present and needed level of functioning are suggestive of the type of rehabilitation treatment intervention which will be needed.

More specifically, in the exploration phase the psychiatric rehabilitation practitioner attempts to encourage the helpee to talk meaningfully about his or her present and potential level of functioning. Initially, by attending, observing, listening, and responding to the helpee without any attempts at interpreting, judging, or controlling the helpee's behavior, the psychiatric rehabilitation practitioner can begin to get an accurate assessment of just "where the helpee is" in relation to his or her rehabilitation.

The various practitioner responsive interpersonal skills are designed to develop a relationship with the helpee which he or she experiences as caring and trusting. The practitioner skills of informing and encouraging are necessary because so many rehabilitation clients avoid showing up for treatment (Wolkon, 1970). Rehabilitation practitioners must do more than simply make appointments with psychiatrically disabled helpees. The psychiatrically disabled helpee must be specifically informed and encouraged to appear for rehabilitation. "No shows" are not clients who no longer need or want rehabilitation services; in fact, some of the "no shows" may be the clients who are most in need of rehabilitation intervention. The rehabilitation practitioner need not rationalize a client's failure to appear with an argument similar to "... if they don't want my help, there are plenty of clients that can take their place." Specific efforts must go into reducing the number of "no shows."

In addition, these responsive skills are also designed to create an environment which reduces the number of premature dropouts. The practitioner must insure that the helpee feels enough care and support so that the client does in fact wish to continue in treatment. Once again, similar to the difficulties involved in getting clients to appear for help, many clients choose to terminate treatment prematurely. Garfield (1971) has summarized data which indicate that a large number of clients prematurely drop out of counseling and psychotherapy of their own volition. A recent study by Sue and McKinney (1976) of 13,450 clients seen in seventeen community mental health facilities found that 40% of these clients terminated treatment after only one session!

The psychiatric rehabilitation practitioner must also use these responsive skills to encourage significant others in the helpee's life to explore "where they are" in relation to the helpee. Once again, the psychiatric rehabilitation practitioner uses her or his responsive interpersonal skills to encourage significant others' exploration, and in the process, obtains more diagnostic information relevant to the helpee's rehabilitation efforts. This first or exploratory phase of the psychiatric rehabilitation diagnostic process is designed to obtain as much information as possible about the helpee's present level of functioning in relation to his or her potential rehabilitation. If the helpee is functioning at such a low level that she or he is unable to verbally explore these areas of concern, the psychiatric rehabilitation practitioner may obtain some of this diagnostic information by responding to people who know the helpee well.

The psychiatric rehabilitation practitioner's goal in the second diagnostic phase, the understanding phase, is to identify the skill level of the helpee and the skill level demanded by the helpee and the helpee's environment. The understanding phase demands that the psychiatric rehabilitation practitioner be able to interpret the information collected in the exploratory phase in such a way that the practitioner can identify the helpee's skills and the helpee's environment skill demands. The psychiatric rehabilitation practitioner must be able to organize the obtained diagnostic information so that a meaningful picture emerges of the helpee's level of skilled performance and how these skills may or may not differ from the level of skills which the helpee needs or wants.

The conceptual distinction between the exploration and understanding phase is a real and significant distinction. Obtaining information through exploration is not the same as understanding what the information *means* to the helpee's rehabilitation plan. Many individuals, both helpees and helpers alike, can explore the information but cannot understand what the information means in terms of rehabilitation goals. The psychiatric rehabilitation practitioner, on the basis of what she or he has learned from the exploration phase, tries to understand the entire diagnostic picture from the bits and pieces provided by the exploration phase. The psychiatric rehabilitation practitioner achieves this understanding by drawing increasingly upon his or her own analysis of the helpee's situation. In other words, the psychiatric rehabilitation practitioner first responds to the helpee's and significant others' frames of reference in order to obtain as much information as possible; next, the psychiatric rehabilitation practitioner uses his or her own experience to go beyond or interpret what the helpee and significant others have expressed in order to achieve an understanding of the basic helpee skills and skill demands. Thus, by using responsive and initiative interpersonal skills, the psychiatric rehabilitation practitioner can identify the basic skills which the helpee wants or needs.

For example, during the exploratory phase, a recently readmitted psychiatrically disabled helpee named Ted says to the psychiatric rehabilitation practitioner, "I really don't care if I ever do anything anymore." In exploring the same general theme with other staff members, the psychiatric rehabilitation practitioner learns that the helpee is "too demanding, not trying, unmotivated." By responding to the helpee's family, the psychiatric rehabilitation practitioner hears that the helpee's "lethargic, lazy behavior is very annoying." By observing the helpee, the psychiatric rehabilitation practitioner notes that Ted is in fairly good physical shape, does enjoy some leisure-time activities if prompted to participate and engages in these activities with a high energy level. Relevant background data indicate that this is his second psychiatric hospitalization this year, but that prior to this year, Ted had been stably employed for five years.

During the understanding phase, the psychiatric rehabilitation practitioner uses her or his initiative interpersonal skills to go beyond the exploration of this helpee and his significant others in an attempt to identify the relevant helpee skills and environmental skill demands. In essence, the psychiatric rehabilitation practitioner must integrate the collection of information that describes the helpee as "not caring, lazy, unmotivated, and demanding" into a meaningful picture. These personal characteristics may be due to a variety of deficits in skilled performance; it is the practitioner's task to ensure that the real skill deficits are identified. For example, in this case the psychiatrically disabled helpee may be:

a. confused because he can't figure out what is expected of him;

b. afraid because he does not have the skills to interview for a job;

c. lonely because he has no method of interacting with his family;

d. annoyed because he can't obtain praise from significant others for anything positive he does.

By using the initiative interpersonal skills described by Carkhuff (1972, 1977),

the psychiatric rehabilitation practitioner seeks to identify the particular areas in which the psychiatrically disabled helpee actually has skill deficits and strengths. During the exploratory stage, the practitioner skills are primarily *responsive* in nature; they reflect ways in which the practitioner can absorb information and give it back to the helpee in the form of responses that mirror the client's own state. In the understanding phase of the diagnostic planning process, however, the rehabilitation practitioner must shift the focus to skills which are primarily *initiative* in nature — skills which enable the practitioner to provide each client with new and more constructive direction. In particular, the practitioner must help the client to understand the *personal meaning* of his or her situation and the *personal deficits and strengths* which are related to the situation. In the process of interpreting the personal meaning of the client's situation, the rehabilitation practitioner helps the client to identify why the situation is important to the client. This understanding is critical to the diagnostic plan because the identical situation may mean different things to different people. For example, for one client losing a full-time job may mean that he or she cannot experience him/herself as a real adult. For another client, losing a full-time job may mean that for the first time he or she will have to depend on others. Personal meanings are critical for the practitioner to diagnose and for the client to understand, because they supply the "emotional steam" which helps the client become motivated to overcome his or her personal problems.

The process of understanding the client's personal strengths and deficits involves the rehabilitation practitioner helping the client to identify those specific client skill behaviors which will help or hinder the client's attainment of his or her rehabilitation goals. For example, clients who are attempting to find competitive employment often succeed or fail based on their unique pattern of strengths and weaknesses. The rehabilitation practitioner and the client must understand the unique pattern so that either skills-training programs may be designed to overcome the clients deficits or a job placement can be arranged to accommodate the client's present strengths and deficits. In either case, the efficacy of the eventual rehabilitation intervention may be maximized by an understanding of the client's specific strengths and deficits.

In this understanding phase of the diagnostic process, the practitioner must not only identify the personal meaning and strengths and deficits of the client, he or she must also facilitate the client's understanding or acceptance of the diagnosis as well. Since the client must ultimately be involved in carrying out the treatment plan, practitioner understanding is not enough. The client must also understand the diagnosis.

In order to facilitate the client's understanding of the diagnosed strengths and deficits, the practitioner must *categorize the client's strengths and deficits* so that a meaningful and organized picture of the client's functioning emerges. Simply possessing a list of the client's personal strengths and deficits is not a sufficient basis from which to get the client involved in a rehabilitation treatment plan. Rather, the rehabilitation practitioner must paint a comprehensive and understandable picture of the client by means of a two-step categorization process. In the first step, the rehabilitation practitioner and the client categorize the client's strengths and deficits into physical, emotional, or intellectual skills. In the second step, the practitioner recategorizes these client skill areas in terms of the particular environment in which these skills are relevant. Out of this two-step categorization process emerges a picture of the psychiatrically disabled client's unique pattern of strengths and deficits as well as the specific environmental areas which will be affected by these skill behaviors. The resulting diagnostic picture is both comprehensive in scope and comprehensible in meaning.

An initiative response brings fresh insight to the client as to why the rehabilitation process is necessary and important to the client's well-being. It may be that some psychiatrically disabled clients will move to this level of self-exploration by means of the responding skills of the rehabilitation practitioner. Provided with a respectful relationship and the opportunity to explore, they may become more motivated and open to discuss their personal role in the situation. A very few clients may even be able to start their self-exploration at this personalized level. Such clients do not need the practitioner to make interpretations; they will do it themselves.

Typically, however, the practitioner must guide the client in the development of these insights by using personalized meaning interpretations. It is important to recognize that those interpretations are based on the client's previous explorations *and not on any one theory of personality or psychotherapy.*

The existence of many theories of psychotherapy, with new theoretical constructs being developed every year, is perhaps the clearest indication that no one theory is capable of organizing and explaining all human behavior. The proliferation of psychotherapeutic theories is a direct reflection of the inability of any one theory to prove itself universally correct and useful. Thus, the use of interpretive skills is not a function of the theory that the practitioner espouses, but rather how skilled the practitioner is in understanding each client's situation and his or her knowledge and skills in the area that the client is experiencing difficulty.

It would certainly be premature for rehabilitation practitioners to make interpretations based exclusively on any one theory of psychotherapy. It would appear that at the present state of our research and theoretical knowledge it would be most effective to assume an eclectic theoretical stance, i.e., using the theory that is appropriate to the situation. The "appropriateness" of the theory is a function of how well the theoretical perspective allows the practitioner to make personalized interpretations to the client — a personalized statement which the helpee can understand and agree to. The goal of the personalized interpretation is not to prove a theoretical interpretation; rather the goal is to get the client to understand the personal importance of the client's unique rehabilitation situation. This interpretive outcome is dramatically different from most other therapeutic interpretations in that there is no attempt to interpret the meaning of the client's situation in terms of developmental factors, or to attempt massive personality reconstruction. While developmental factors and historical personality traits may have been introduced into the exploration process by the client, the rehabilitation practitioner's emphasis is on the implications of past events only in terms of why they are important *in the present* and in the *future*, in terms of client capabilities and abilities.

In essence, the rehabilitation practitioner's diagnostic skills guide the client from a victimized exploration of past events to an understanding of present meaning and future directions. The diagnostic process develops from an *external exploration* of the situation to an *internal understanding* of the *client's responsibility* for actively *doing* a specific *skill behavior*. The client is guided through this exploration and understanding process by means of the responding and initiative skills of the rehabilitation practitioner.

Psychiatric rehabilitation helpees have an infinite number of strategies which they use to refrain from understanding their personal strengths and deficits. Those strategies are considered defense mechanisms. Most textbooks of abnormal psychology list the most common defense mechanisms, e.g., displacement, projection, rationalization, denial, etc. In psychiatric rehabilitation, these various defense mechanisms are not seen in a psychoanalytic context but as purposive behaviors which prevent the client from taking active responsibility for changing one's behavior. Some examples are:

a) A client who *displaces* his anger at his boss to his co-workers and then ends up getting fired for failure to get along with his co-workers.

b) A client who *projects* his own disrespect and distrust of teachers to the teacher and then leaves school because the teachers don't communicate well with him.

c) A client who, lacking the skills to find employment, *rationalizes* that the economy is in bad shape and thus never tries to learn how to look for a good job.

d) A client who, learning that she doesn't relate well to her children, *denies* that she really wants to return home and thus resigns herself to a long stay in the institution.

In each of the preceding examples, the clients have managed to avoid a personalized understanding of their situation by means of their defensive strategies. Until a personalized understanding occurs, they will have little motivation to work towards learning the following skills:

a) Assertiveness skills

b) Communication skills

c) Job-seeking skills

d) Parenting skills

In psychiatric rehabilitation, it is not enough for the practitioner to possess an intellectual understanding of the client's defenses, one that permits the practitioner to analyze the client's defenses in the safety of a case conference. This difficult practitioner skill involves getting the client to openly explore in detail his or her situations (responding skills) and then guiding the client to an *understanding and acceptance* of the specific deficits and strengths which the client has heretofore been defending against (initiative skills).

In practice, the exploratory and understanding phases are not as separate as the preceding example might indicate. The psychiatric rehabilitation practitioner may achieve an understanding of the skills needed in one area while he or she is just beginning to explore another area. Also important to note is that the psychiatric rehabilitation practitioner and the helpee can work together towards a psychiatric rehabilitation diagnosis. The rehabilitation diagnostic goal is certainly not as esoteric as the traditional psychiatric diagnostic goal. Thus, many psychiatrically disabled helpees can understand the overall diagnostic goal and actively participate in an attempt to identify their present skills and skill level which they want or need to obtain.

In addition to the diagnostic information which may be obtained by the practitioner's interpersonal skills, the psychiatric rehabilitation practitioner can also use special techniques to identify the helpee's present and needed level of functioning. These diagnostic techniques include simulation techniques, role playing, and in vivo observations. Various work simulation techniques have been developed which place the psychiatrically disabled helpee in a simulated work environment in order to assess the helpee's level of functioning in the working area. These simulation techniques which are used to explore the helpee's working skills are called "work samples" (Salkind, 1971).

Simulation techniques used in conjunction with role-playing techniques may also be used to gather information about the helpee's functioning in other areas. For example, a helpee may be asked to role play a job interview; or a simulated problem-solving situation may be set up in which the helpee role-plays how he or she would solve a particular problem. If necessary, the rehabilitation diagnostician may explore almost any rehabilitation skill through a combination of simulation techniques and role playing.

USING THE ENVIRONMENT TO HELP MAKE DIAGNOSTIC OBSERVATIONS

Case Illustration 4-2

Diane O. is a nineteen-year-old girl who graduated from high school in 1976. The patient, who lives with her parents, had become increasingly depressed, withdrawn, and forgetful over the past year. Her parents report that she laughs inappropriately, is afraid to work, and acts "strange." There was no consensus as to Diane's problem, but her parents could no longer afford her almost weekly trips to the general hospital for somatic complaints. During a six-month evaluation period, when she was given a complete battery of psychological tests, intelligence tests, and cortical-neurological tests, the diagnosis was: mental retardation, inadequate personality, and minimal brain dysfunction. The treatment was to include no psychotherapy because it was felt that she could not form a therapeutic alliance, remember, or conceptualize enough in order for it to be useful. Medication was ruled out because of the unclear diagnosis. Vocational placement, it was felt, would bind her thinking at least at a minimal level.

The rehabilitation department undertook a "skills" evaluation. The result was that Diane: 1) was found to be unable to complete basic motor tasks; 2) was unable to remember directions (as measured by her ability to repeat them) and unable to perform a directed task; 3) was unable to persist in the task as measured by the number of times that she did not complete "mail sorting"; 4) was unable to cope with failure as measured by the number of times she began to scream and smash furniture when the task was not completed; and 5) was able to focus on physical tasks when in the presence of a responsive instructor as measured by the number of completed tasks in this environment. The rehabilitation counselor then included Diane in the "Listening Skills" training group and found that, contrary to the evidence of neurological tests which were also contrary to the psychological tests), Diane *could* learn new skills in a highly structured framework. She was able to increase her ability to remember verbal statements from five words over a fifteen-second delay to thirty-five words over a thirty-second delay. She was also able to learn the body positioning involved in being attentive to another and could conceptualize to the point of identifying the relevant elements that made up the behavior, and was able to give other participants feedback based upon those behaviors. She displayed no screaming fits or furniture-throwing episodes during the four months of meetings. Diane's goals could now be specified as: a) increasing her memory span to a level of remembering seven instructions; b) increasing her ability to listen to at least one other person for more than five minutes at a time; and c) to develop a regular pattern of eating and sleeping, etc. Vocational placement was considered inappropriate before progress had been made on the level of basic goals.

Treatment plans could then be drawn up in relation to each skill deficit and basic training could begin. In the meantime, further testing and outside consultations were requested by the clinical team to find out which diagnostic category had still not been resolved. Three weeks later, Diane's insurance funds ran out and she had to be transferred to a public facility in another town.

Traditional diagnosis is based upon the premise that clear labeling of symptoms and dynamics as revealed in the interview and testing batteries produces information necessary for both treatment and prognosis. In the case of Diane O., the labeling was unclear and did not lead to functional treatment plans. The evaluation took six months and her insurance could only be renewed once after ninety days. In a "skills evaluation" approach, the practitioner used Diane's behavior in her environment — during vocational workshops, at community meetings, and her participation in the "Listening Group" — in order to assess what she *actually* did or did not do. The skills *training* model of the "Listening Group" further allowed Diane to demonstrate her ability to learn physical movements, verbal behaviors, and increase her memory. Goals could then be set in relation to her skill strengths and deficits as displayed in a variety of situations, rather than what could be inferred from her responses to test situations and interviewer questions.

In contrast, in vivo observation refers to observing behavior in the environment in which the behavior is actually performed. It is particularly important for the psychiatric rehabilitation practitioner to observe the behavior of significant others in the environment in which the helpee will be expected to function effectively. In this way, the psychiatric rehabilitation practitioner can explore what will be demanded of the helpee. In vivo observation, combined with the information obtained from responding to significant others in the helpee's environment, can provide the psychiatric rehabilitation practitioner with the information necessary to identify the environmental demands and deficits which will affect the helpee's rehabilitation success.

Achievement of the goal of the third phase of the psychiatric rehabilitation diagnostic process completes the rehabilitation diagnosis. During this assessment phase the practitioner first writes assessment statements for each identified skill and then measures according to some standard the helpee's present level of learning, living, and working skills as well as the living, learning, and working skills demanded by either the helpee or the helpee's environment. The practitioner's ability to write an observable assessment statement paves the way for the psychiatric rehabilitation practitioner to then quantify in a numerical way the level of the helpee skills and environmental skill demands which have been identified in the understanding phase of the rehabilitation diagnostic process. Thus the practitioner's assessment skills are composed of an ability to write *operationalized* assessment statements and an ability to gather the necessary information so that the client's skill level can be numerically quantified. Note that Table 4-3 indicates that even in the assessment phase, the practitioner continues to use his or her interpersonal skills. Specific numerical estimates concerning the helpee's present and needed skill levels can be obtained through interviewing the helpee, relevant treatment personnel, and significant others, as well as by means of the information-gathering techniques discussed previously. Table 4-3 illustrates that the flow of the diagnostic process proceeds from a non-judgmental exploration of the helpee's perceptions of his or her situation, through a deeper understanding of the helpee's skilled behavior, to a culmination in a specific numerical assessment of the helpee's strengths and weaknesses.

Using as an example the psychiatrically disabled helpee named Ted, who was used as an example earlier for the exploratory and understanding diagnostic phase, the psychiatric rehabilitation practitioner might numerically assess the helpee's present skill level and the skill level which the helpee needs or wants in the following manner, based on the four identified deficits "a" through "d".

a) Helpee can list a certain percentage of those activities which spouse would like him to perform. (Present level of functioning = 50%; needed level = 100%)

b) Helpee can perform the job-interviewing skills at a specified modal level on the job-interviewing scale. (Present modal level of functioning = 1.0; needed level = 3.0)

c) Helpee can converse with other family members on a certain number of current topics, at a minimum of five minutes per topic. (Present level of functioning = one topic for five minutes; needed level = five topics for five minutes).

d) Significant others in helpee's environment can verbally praise the helpee a certain percentage of the time when he behaves in a manner that they and helpee agree is desirable. (Present level of functioning = 5% of the time; needed level = 50%.)

Note that goal "d" is really a goal to be achieved by significant others rather than the helpee, and that goal "c" is a goal to be achieved by the family and the helpee. The psychiatric rehabilitation practitioner must assess and develop rehabilitation programs not just for the psychiatrically disabled helpee but also for the environment in which the helpee seeks to function. Environmental change programs will be discussed further in Chapter VIII.

PSYCHIATRIC REHABILITATION DIAGNOSIS: ADDITIONAL CONSIDERATIONS

The main purpose of the psychiatric rehabilitation diagnostic process is to assess the helpee's present level of skilled performance and to ascertain the level of skilled performance which the helpee will need to function as independently as possible in the community. However, in addition to arriving at a diagnosis, the rehabilitation diagnostic process itself may have a positive effect on the psychiatrically disabled helpee's functioning due to the psychiatric rehabilitation practitioner's systematic application of her or his interpersonal skills.

As mentioned previously, these interpersonal diagnostic skills are essentially the same skills which account for some of the positive variance in counseling outcome (Carkhuff, 1969; Truax & Carkhuff, 1967). Thus the rehabilitation diagnostic process, by guiding the helpee through an exploration and understanding of his or her unique situation may be helpful by itself. The psychiatric rehabilitation practitioner, by entering the helpee's frame of reference to facilitate helpee self-exploration and then going beyond the helpee's self-exploration by drawing on his or her own experience of the helpee to interpret the meaning of the helpee's situation, is in fact aiding the helpee to develop insights about his or her unique difficulties. While new helpee insights are typically not enough to bring about overall constructive change, it may instigate minor changes and make the helpee more amenable to the rehabilitation programs which follow.

The various types of rehabilitation programs needed by each psychiatrically disabled helpee flow directly out of the diagnostic assessment of the helpee's present level of functioning and the level of functioning which the helpee needs in order to function in his or her particular community. The communities in which psychiatrically disabled helpees function vary greatly. For example, in terms of residences, the helpee may reside in his or her own home, a halfway house, family-care home, satellite housing, etc. In terms of the community in which the helpee spends a major portion of the day, a helpee may be competitively employed, work in various types of workshops, attend a day-care center, remain at home, etc. Although the overall rehabilitation goal is to approximate as closely as possible independent functioning (independent living and competitive employment), for many of the lowest level functioning helpees these are long-range goals. More immediate short-term goals would be for the helpee to achieve the skill level necessary to function in less independent community settings.

The particular community or setting in which the helpee is expected to function typically is determined by several factors.

In many instances, no real choice exists as to where the helpee will live. Often the family is forced to house the helpee because few other possibilities exist or are desirable. Because of the planned phase-out of many large mental hospitals, the shortened inpatient stay, and the development of community-based outpatient facilities, more psychiatrically disabled helpees will be required to reside in their original community settings. No longer will psychiatric treatment require that the psychiatrically disabled helpee be temporarily removed from his or her place of residence. Thus the goal of the rehabilitation programs may be to provide the helpee with the skills necessary to live more effectively in the community setting in which he or she is presently residing rather than the setting to which the helpee is going to return. In terms of employment, the psychiatrically disabled helpee's past employment record is often a major factor in influencing how the helpee will spend his or her day in the community. A very poor employment history and accompanying lack of job skills often precludes many opportunities for immediate competitive employment, thus greatly restricting the employment settings in which the helpee may work. Another factor determining the particular community in which the helpee must function are the desires of the helpee and the helpee's significant others. A final influential factor is the judgment of the psychiatric treatment and rehabilitation specialists as to the helpee's probability of succeeding in a particular setting.

Thus, there is often little choice regarding the setting in which the helpee must have the skills to function. Overriding factors such as time, money, lack of facilities, and strong demands by the helpee or significant others restrict the range of possible settings. However, when there is a decision to be made regarding the community in which the helpee will function, the rehabilitation diagnostic process can clearly indicate the skills which the helpee must possess to function in each potential community. Provided with the knowledge gained by the rehabilitation diagnosis, the psychiatric rehabilitation practitioner and the psychiatrically disabled helpee can make a more informed decision regarding the alternative settings in which the helpee might function.

When a decision needs to be made as to which setting would be appropriate, the actual decision-making process can be facilitated by a psychiatric rehabilitation practitioner who possesses community coordinating skills (Cohen, Anthony, Pierce & Cohen, 1977). These decision-making or coordinating skills provide the psychiatric rehabilitation practitioner with a systematic, concrete, and observable means of making decisions based on how satisfying the decision will be for the psychiatrically disabled helpee. The information on which the decisions are based is collected during the exploration and understanding phase of the diagnostic process. These decision-making skills are discussed further in the chapter on community rehabilitation programming (Chapter VIII).

Throughout this discussion of the psychiatric rehabilitation diagnosis, the focus has been on the psychiatrically disabled helpee's skilled behavior and in particular, the deficiencies in skilled performance which prevent the helpee from functioning in the community. This diagnostic emphasis on skill deficits may at first glance appear to be antithetical to the philosophy of those who believe the concern of rehabilitation to be the helpee's "strengths" and "assets." However, merely stating that the rehabilitation focus is on strengths and assets is only a partial description; in actuality, rehabilitation is concerned with *increasing* strengths and *developing* assets. It is the psychiatrically disabled helpee's skill deficits which are preventing rehabilitation, not his or her strengths or assets; thus it is the helpee's deficits which must be the diagnostic focus. The diagnostic process does assess a broad range of skills and in so doing does discover areas in which the psychiatrically disabled helpee is relatively strong. Successful rehabilitation programs can achieve rehabilitation goals by maximizing the opportunities for the expression of the helpee's assets or strengths through the manipulation of various environmental settings.

AN EXAMPLE OF
DIAGNOSTIC OUTCOME

In sum, the psychiatric rehabilitation diagnostician attempts to assess the psychiatrically disabled helpee's present and needed level of functioning by engaging in a systematic rehabilitation diagnostic process. Prior to involving the helpee and significant others in the psychiatric rehabilitation diagnostic process, the practitioner attempts to obtain the empirically relevant diagnostic information outlined in the first section of this chapter. By collecting the available information on demographic characteristics, behavioral ratings, and test scores which significantly relate to rehabilitation outcome, the psychiatric rehabilitation practitioner can obtain a quick assessment of the need for a rehabilitation intervention. A further estimate of the psychiatrically disabled helpee's rehabilitation potential may be obtained if the rehabilitation practitioner is guided by the psychiatric rehabilitation principle that past behavior is the best predictor of future behavior.

Having obtained this initial estimate of the psychiatrically disabled helpee's functioning, the practitioner uses his or her responsive interpersonal skills to enter the helpee's frame of reference so that he or she may obtain information about the helpee relevant to the rehabilitation goal. Following this exploratory phase the rehabilitation practitioner must use his or her responsive and initiative interpersonal skills and information gathering techniques to identify the basic skill deficits which need to be overcome in order that successful rehabilitation is achieved. The rehabilitation diagnostic process is culminated by the practitioner describing in observable, numerical terms the helpee's present and needed levels of functioning.

The psychiatric rehabilitation diagnostic assessment for each helpee can be organized on a chart similar to the rehabilitation diagnostic assessment chart illustrated in Table 4-4. The hypothetical example provided on the chart is Mr. Jones, a psychiatrically disabled helpee whose immediate rehabilitation goal is to continue residing with his wife and children and to find work as a sales clerk in a department store. Each particular skill listed on the diagnostic chart is defined in observable terms.

By examining the ·client assessment chart depicted in Table 4-4, we see that the diagnostic interviewing and assessment process has culminated in a specific focus on eleven skill activities. This is not to say that other skills were not explored, only that based on Mr. Jones' situation these were the most crucial to assess. In three skill activities (stigma reduction, punctuality, and job qualifying), Mr. Jones was already functioning at the needed level. Thus these behaviors may be considered strengths (+). The other eight behaviors evidence discrepancies between Mr. Jones' present and needed levels of functioning and must become the focus of rehabilitation treatment programs if Mr. Jones wishes to be successful in these environments. The specific numerical estimates of present and needed levels were developed from a number of potential sources, such as the client, the rehabilitation diagnostician, interviews with other treatment personnel and significant others, client testing, in vivo observations, role playing, and other simulation techniques.

The client assessment chart may also be useful if various types of community settings are under consideration. In this event, a client assessment chart may be developed for each potential community setting so that the different diagnostic charts clearly illustrate the skills that must be achieved in order for the helpee to function effectively in that particular community.

For example, if the hypothetical Mr. Jones were going to be placed in a sheltered workshop, he would not need job-interviewing skills nor job-seeking skills; therefore, skills in that particular area would not be of immediate concern, and these skill activities would not need to be recorded on the diagnostic chart. Similarly, if Mr. Jones were planning on living in a satellite-housing arrangement with other former psychiatrically disabled helpees.

TABLE 4-4
CLIENT ASSESSMENT CHART

Living Environment: Home, Wife & Two Children   Name: M. S. Jones

*P.E.I.	Skill Activity	Strength or Deficit	Skill Behavior	Present	Needed
P	Physical Fitness	-	Number of miles can travel in twelve-minute walk/run test	1.0	1.4
E	Stigma Reduction	+	Number of positive and negative statements about self can make in response to questions about past hospitalization	2 positive 0 negative	2 positive 0 negative
E	Self-Control	-	Number of non-violent methods can use to express anger to spouse	0	3
E	Relaxation	-	Number of minutes (average) it takes to fall asleep each night	1 hour	30 minutes
E	Selective Reward	-	Number of times per day verbally praise children when they behave in a way which pleases him	0	2

Learning Environment: YMCA Fitness Class

*P.E.I.	Skill Activity	Strength or Deficit	Skill Behavior	Present	Needed
P	Punctuality	+	Amount of time takes to get to exercise class dressed in appropriate attire	45 minutes	45 minutes
E	Conversation	-	Number of times client initiates conversation in class	0 per day	1 per day

Working Environment: Department Store Sales Clerk

*P.E.I.	Skill Activity	Strength or Deficit	Skill Behavior	Present	Needed
P	Job Endurance	-	Number of hours can stand consecutively without taking a break	1	2
E	Job Inventory	-	Rated level of interviewing skills on three point Job-Interviewing-Skill Rating Scale	1	3
I	Job Qualifying	+	Rated level of performance when performing functions of sales clerk as detailed by a presently employed sales clerk	Acceptable	Acceptable
I	Job Seeking	-	Number of positions per month can locate for which qualified	0	3

*P — Physical, E — Emotional, I — Intellectual

then Mr. Jones' present level of cooking and cleaning skills would have to be assessed. Also, the psychiatric rehabilitation practitioner must be prepared to diagnose and record the deficiencies of significant others in the helpee's environment if the practitioner believes these deficiencies will have a detrimental effect on the helpee's skill development.

In essence, the rehabilitation diagnostic process utilizes both the practitioner's *interpersonal* and *assessment* skills in order to explore the client's strengths and deficits, to understand how these strengths and deficits affect the client's ability to function in specific environments, and to assess in an objective and observable manner the skill performance level in relation to the functional level in these specific environments.

Two principles underlying the entire diagnostic process are *comprehensiveness* and *comprehensibility*. That is, the diagnostic process should be broad in scope and presented in a way that maximizes the client's understanding of the diagnosis. To the greatest extent possible, the client should be involved in developing the diagnostic picture as this will improve the

probability of client involvement in the rehabilitation treatment procedures which flow out of the diagnosis. Client understanding as well as diagnostic comprehensiveness are facilitated by using the simple categorization process of physical, intellectual, and emotional skills by living, learning, and working environments.

Based on the diagnostic assessment chart, the rehabilitation diagnostician can write an exceptionally detailed referral statement to other agencies or treatment personnel who might become involved in the rehabilitation program. For example, using the data depicted in Table 4-4, if Mr. Jones were going to receive the services of a day treatment center for assistance with his home situation, the rehabilitation practitioner could write a very detailed referral. Included in the referral would be the specific skill goals which the rehabilitation practitioners would expect the day treatment center to accomplish. This type of referral would not only encourage accountability in their rehabilitation programming efforts but also inform the personnel as to what exactly was needed, thus avoiding any vague or abstract diagnostic information.

MAKING THE REHABILITATION REFERRAL

Case Illustration 4-3

M. . . . .Hospital

Mrs. D. R.
Valley Mental Health Center
Plainsville, MA

Re: Joanne C.

Dear Mrs. R.:

As a follow-up to our telephone conversation of March 10, 1977, I am referring Ms. Joanne C. to your Center.

Joanne C. is a 40-year-old, divorced female who is being discharged from her second M. . . . .Hospital stay, but fifth psychiatric hospitalization. Please see the history charts for further information. Her present program at the Partial Hospital involved psychotherapy with a female social worker twice a week, participation in a "medication" group, participation in a "psychosomatic" group, and involvement with the Rehabilitation Department once a week for interviews related to her vocational and post-hospital goals. I have been both her rehabilitation counselor, on a conjoint basis, and her primary case manager.

The enclosed chart is an assessment of Joanne's skill assets and deficits in relation to her continued accommodation at a halfway house/shared apartment setting. These behaviors were identified through observation of the patient on the ward, at the halfway house, at the workshop (voc.), and in interviews with the patients. Joanne offered many of the measures and assessments of her present and needed levels of functioning.

As you can see, Joanne's main strengths lie in skills related to inter-personal functioning. She is a helpful listener, and makes people feel at home with her, as well as having a strong sense of responsibility. She is, thus, a reliable friend, unless she herself is in crisis.

Her main deficit is the inability to apply the skills that she has without a clear structure of reinforcement. The chart indicates that her lack is not as much a deficient *number* of skills in her repertoire, but the lack of frequency and persistence in their performance.

Our goals in referring Joanne to you are:

1. To provide structured programming for her, particularly in the area of self-care. The specific goals are identified on the client assessment chart.

2. To provide programming that involves Joanne's ability to develop meaningful reinforcers in the community — particularly for skills such as deficits 38, 40, 55, 56, 62, etc.

Should you have any questions regarding this referral, please contact me at ext. 321. Furthermore, I would be willing to meet with you to discuss any planning steps that you feel we should take in order to effect as smooth a transition as possible. Thank you for your cooperation.

Yours sincerely,

Besides informing the referral source what must be achieved if the helpee wishes to remain in his or her present environment, a referral based on a comprehensive rehabilitation diagnosis can also indicate what specific behaviors need to be treated if the helpee goal is to eventually move to a new environment. In Mr. Jones' situation, if he were presently functioning successfully in a sheltered workshop situation, the working environment data on the client assessment chart would suggest what skill behaviors should be treated in the workshop if the workshop personnel hope to move Mr. Jones towards a competitive employment setting. It should be obvious that in order to make a comprehensive rehabilitation diagnosis, the rehabilitation practitioner needs both time and skills. The amount of time varies with respect to the amount of change which must occur in the client's life. For example, a client may have been functioning well in the work environment but lost her job because of difficulties in the home environ-ment. Perhaps these problems have been treated successfully and the client has now been referred to the rehabilitation practitioner for help in re-entering the work environment. In this example the diagnostic outcome may be achieved in several sessions with the helpee and several phone calls to significant others.

In other situations, however, the rehabilitation diagnostic process might take much longer. For example, an inpatient might have a number of skill deficits in the living and working areas. The client may be very reluctant to explore and understand his or her own deficits, preferring instead to focus on how others are causing her or him problems. In this case, the diagnostic process will take considerably longer. As discussed previously, the diagnosis must be accepted and agreed to by the client, if client motivation is to be maximized. Without client understanding, the rehabilitation diagnosis is really not complete. Attempted interventions directed at any possible skill goals not agreed

EXCERPT FROM MS. JOANNE C.'S CLIENT ASSESSMENT CHART

M . . . . HOSPITAL
REHABILITATION SERVICES

Patient: Ms. Joanne C.
Date of Discharge: March 30, 1977

LIVING ENVIRONMENT SKILLS: In relation to the demands of halfway house or other type of shared accommodation.

PHYSICAL SKILLS (EXCERPT)

ACTIVITY	ASSET	DEFICIT	DESCRIPTION OF SKILL BEHAVIOR	PRESENT LEVEL OF FUNCTIONING	NEEDED LEVEL
(SELF-CARE)					
Hygiene			Amount of time patient is able to:		
1.		-	wash once a day	60% of time	100%
2.		-	put on clean clothes	40% of time	85%
3.		-	comb her hair	60% of time	100%
4.		-	clean teeth, nails	40% of time	100%
5.	+		Amount of time patient is able to do all of above and get hair done for a special occasion (job interview, social outing, etc.)	85%	85%
Health			Amount of time patient is able to sleep eight hours a night:		
6.		-	without medication	10%	80%
7.		-	with medication	75%	100%
			Amount of time patient is able to relax when upset, before sleeping:		
8.		-	without staff assistance	15%	80%
9.		-	with staff assistance	50%	100%

EMOTIONAL SKILLS (EXCERPT)

ACTIVITY	ASSET	DEFICIT	DESCRIPTION OF SKILL BEHAVIOR	PRESENT LEVEL OF FUNCTIONING	NEEDED LEVEL
38.		-	No. of reinforcers patient is able to list existing in community	0	5
Finances			No. of times patient deposits own funds at bank, when lawyer sends		
39.	+		them	as needed	as needed
40.		-	on own initiative	25%	100%
			No. of times patient draws up monthly budget when shown a step-by-		
41.	+		step program of how to do it	Yes	Yes
42.		-	on own initiative	No	Yes
Environmental Responsiveness					
			Amount of time patient responds to questions from staff/others when angry or panicky:		
53.		-	by repeating phrases like "I'm so spacy"	60%	40%
54.		-	without the above sentences	15%	50%
55.		-	Amount of time patient plans and follows through on week-end activities during holiday periods (anniversary, birthdays, etc.)	10%	90%
56.		-	Amount of time patient goes through Fridays, anniversaries, etc. without over-medication	20%	100%

to by the client are very difficult to achieve.

The completed chart illustrated in Table 4-4 reflects the culmination of the psychiatric rehabilitation diagnostic process. At this point, the psychiatric rehabilitation practitioner has achieved the two-fold diagnostic goal of being able to list and measure, according to some observable standard, the psychiatrically disabled helpee's present levels of skill in the living, learning, or working areas, as well as the levels of skills demanded by either the helpee or the helpee's living, learning, and working environments. In essence, once the diagnostic process has identified and described the skills which are facilitating or impeding the psychiatrically disabled helpee's community functioning, the helpee's individual rehabilitation goals likewise have been identified and described. Rehabilitation goals flow directly out of the rehabilitation diagnosis. Thus, the rehabilitation goal is either to teach the helpee to overcome these diagnosed skill deficiencies so that the helpee is able to independently perform these skills in living, learning, or working settings at a functional level, or to find an environmental setting which accommodates the helpee's present skilled behavior. The specific rehabilitation goals for each helpee are achieved by comprehensive rehabilitation programming. The following chapter describes the principles of psychiatric rehabilitation programming and the many techniques used by the psychiatric rehabilitation practitioner to assist the helpee in achieving the necessary level of skilled performance.

ENDNOTES

[1]Adapted in part from the **Community Mental Health Journal, 1976,** *11*: 208-214, where it first appeared as "The relationship between patient demographic characteristics and psychiatric rehabilitation outcome." by G. J. Buell and W. A. Anthony.

REFERENCES

Anthony, W. A. and Buell, G. J. Predicting aftercare clinic effectiveness as a function of patient demographic characteristics. **Journal of Consulting and Clinical Psychology,** 1973, *41*: 116-119.

Anthony, W. A. and Buell, G. J. Predicting psychiatric rehabilitation outcome using demographic characteristics: A replication. **Journal of Counseling Psychology,** 1974, *21*: 421-422.

Anthony, W. A., Buell, G. J., Sharratt, S. and Althoff, M. E. The efficacy of psychiatric rehabilitation. **Psychological Bulletin,** 1972, *78*: 447-456.

Anthony, W. A., Pierce, R. M. and Cohen, M. R. **Psychiatric rehabilitation practice: The skills of diagnostic planning.** Amherst, MA: Carkhuff Institute of Human Technology, 1977.

Arthur, G., Ellsworth, R. B. and Kroeker, D. Schizophrenic patient post-hospital community adjustment and readmission. **Social Work,** 1968, *13*: 78-84.

Aspy, D. N. **Toward a technology for humanizing education.** Champaign, Ill.: Research Press, 1972.

Baker, R. L. and Schultz, R. E. eds. **Instructional product development.** New York: Van Nostrand Reinhold, 1971. Beck, A. T., Ward, C. H., Mendelson, M., Mock, J. E. & Erbaugh, J. K. Reliability of psychiatric diagnosis. 2: A study of consistency of clinical judgments and ratings. **American Journal of Psychiatry,** 1962, *119*: 351-357.

Beck, A. T., Ward, C. H., Mendelson, M., Mock, J. E. & Erbaugh, J. K. Reliability of psychiatric diagnosis. 2: A study of consistency of clinical judgments and ratings. **American Journal of Psychiatry,** 1962, *119:* 351-357.

Buell, G. J. and Anthony, W. A. Demographic characteristics as predictors of recidivism and post-hospital employment. **Journal of Counseling Psychology,** 1973, *20*: 361-365.

Buell, G. and Anthony, W. A. The relationship between patient demographic characteristics and psychiatric rehabilitation outcome. **Community Mental Health Journal,** 1976, *11*: 208-214

Carkhuff, R. R. **Helping and human relations. Volumes 1 and 2.** New York: Holt, Rinehart & Winston, 1969.

Carkhuff, R. R. **The development of human resources.** New York: Holt, Rinehart & Winston, 1971.

Carkhuff, R. R. **The art of helping.** Amherst, MA: Human Resource Development Press, 1972 (Third Edition, 1977).

Carkhuff, R. R. **The art of problem solving.** Amherst, MA: Human Resource Development Press, 1973.

Carkhuff, R. R. **The art of helping trainer's guide.** Amherst, MA: Human Resource Development Press, 1977.

Carkhuff, R. R. and Berenson, B. G. **Beyond counseling and therapy.** New York: Holt, Rinehart & Winston, 1977.

Carkhuff, R. R., Berenson, D. H. & Pierce, R. M. **The skills of teaching: Interpersonal skills.** Amherst, MA: Human Resource Development Press, 1977.

Cohen, M. R., Anthony, W. A., Pierce, R. M. and Cohen, B. F. **Psychiatric rehabilitation practice: The skills of community coordinating.** Amherst, MA: Carkhuff Institute of Human Technology, 1977.

Cumming, J. and Markson, E. The impact of mass transfer on patient release. **Archives of General Psychiatry,** 1975, *32*: 804-809.

Destefano, M. K. and Pryer, M. W. Vocational evaluation and successful placement of psychiatric clients in a vocational rehabilitation program. **American Journal of Occupational Therapy,** 1970, *24*: 205-207.

Ethridge, D. A. Pre-vocational assessment of the rehabilitation potential of psychiatric patients. **American Journal of Occupational Therapy,** 1968, *22*: 161-167.

Fairweather, G. W. ed. **Social psychology in treating mental illness.** New York: Wiley and Sons, 1964.

Fairweather, G. W. and Simon, R. A further follow-up comparison of psychotherapeutic programs. **Journal of Consulting Psychology,** 1963, *27*: 186.

Fairweather, G. W., Simon, R., Gebhard, M. E., Weingarten, E., Holland, J. L., Sanders, R., Stone, G. B. and Reahl, J. E. Relative effectiveness of psychotherapeutic programs: A multicriteria comparison of four programs for three different patient groups. **Psychology Monographs,** 1960, *74*: No. 5 (whole No. 492).

Forsyth, R. P. and Fairweather, G. W. Psychotherapeutic and other hospital treatment criteria: The dilemma. **Journal of Abnormal and Social Psychology,** 1961, *62*: 598-604.

Franklin, J. L., Kittredge, L. D. and Thrasher, J. H. A survey of factors related to mental hospital readmissions. **Hospital and Community Psychiatry,** 1975, *26*: 749-751.

Freeman, H. E. and Simmons, O. G. **The mental patient comes home.** New York: Wiley and Sons, Inc., 1963.

Garfield, S. L. Research on client variables in psychotherapy. In A. E. Bergin and S. L. Garfield eds., **Handbook of psychotherapy and behavior change: An empirical analysis.** New York: Wiley & Sons, 1971.

Goss, A. M. and Pate, K. D. Predicting vocational rehabilitation success for psychiatric patients with psychological tests. **Psychological Reports**, 1967, *21*: 725-730.

Green, H. J., Miskimins, R. W., and Keil, E. C. Selection of psychiatric patients for vocational rehabilitation. **Rehabilitation Counseling Bulletin**, 1968, *11*: 297-302.

Gregory, C. C. and Downie, M. N. Prognostic study of patients who left, returned and stayed in a psychiatric hospital. **Journal of Counseling Psychology**, 1968, *15*: 232-236.

Gurel, L. and Lorei, T. W. Hospital and community ratings of psychopathology as predictors of employment and readmission. **Journal of Consulting and Clinical Psychology**, 1972, *34*: 286-291.

Hall, J. C., Smith, K. and Shimkunas, A. Employment problems of schizophrenic patients. **American Journal of Psychiatry**, 1966, *123*: 536-540.

Katz, R. C. and Wooley, F. R. Criteria for releasing patients from psychiatric hospitals. **Hospital and Community Psychiatry**, 1975, *26*: 33-36.

Knowlton, V. and Samuelson, C. O. The rehabilitation of former mental patients. **Rehabilitation Counseling Bulletin**, 1968, *11*: 164-166.

Lewinsohn, P. M. Factors related to improvement in mental hospital patients. **Journal of Consulting Psychology**, 1967, *31*: 588-594.

Lipton, H. and Kaden, S. E. Predicting the post-hospital work adjustment of married, male schizophrenics. **Journal of Consulting Psychology**, 1965, *29*: 93.

Lorei, T. W. Prediction of community stay and employment for released psychiatric patients. **Journal of Consulting Psychology**, 1967, *31*: 349-357.

Lorei, T. W. and Gurel, L. Use of biographical inventory to predict schizophrenics' post-hospital employment and readmission. **Journal of Consulting and Clinical Psychology**, 1972, *38*: 238-243.

Lorei, T. W. and Gurel, L. Demographic characteristics as predictors of post-hospital employment and readmission. **Journal of Consulting and Clinical Psychology**, 1973.

Marks, J., Stauffacher, J. C. and Lyle, C. Predicting outcome in schizophrenia. **Journal of Abnormal and Social Psychology**, 1963, *66*: 117-127.

Michaux, W. W., Katz, M. M., Kurland, A. A. and Gansereit, K. H. **The first year out.** Baltimore, Md.: Johns Hopkins Press, 1969.

Miles, D. G. A research-based approach to psychiatric rehabilitation. In L. M. Roberts ed. **The role of vocational rehabilitation in community mental health.** Washington, D. C.: Rehabilitation Services Administration, 1967.

Miller, D. Alternatives to mental patient rehospitalization. **Community Mental Health Journal**, 1966, *2*: 124-128.

Miller, D. Retrospective analysis of post-hospital mental patients' worlds. **Journal of Health & Social Behavior**, 1967, *8*: 136-140.

Miller, G. H. and Willer, B. Predictors of return to a psychiatric hospital. **Journal of Consulting and Clinical Psychology**, 1976, *44*: 898-900.

Olshansky, S., Grob, S. and Ekdahl, M. Survey of employment experiences of patients discharged from 3 state mental hospitals during period 1951-1953. **Mental Hygiene**, 1960, *44*: 510-521.

Perkins, E. D. and Miller, A. L. Using a modified NM2 Scale to predict the vocational outcomes of psychiatric patients. **Personnel and Guidance Journal**, 1969, *47*: 456-460.

Rosenhahn, D. L. On being sane in insane places. **Science**, January 19, 1973, *179*: 250-258.

Salkind, I. The rehabilitation workshop. In H. R. Lamb ed., **Rehabilitation in community mental health**. San Francisco: Jossey-Boss, 1971. Pp. 50-70.

Schmidt, H. O. and Fonda, C. P. The rehability of psychiatric diagnosis: A new look. **Journal of Abnormal and Social Psychology**, 1956, *52*: 262-267.

Siegel, S. **Nonparametic statistics for the behavioral sciences**. New York: McGraw-Hill, 1956.

Sturm, I. E. and Lipton, H. Some social and vocational predictors of psychiatric hospitalization outcome. **Journal of Clinical Psychology**, 1967, *23*: 301-307.

Sue, S., McKinney, H. and Allen, D. B. Predictors of the duration of therapy for clients in the community mental health center system. **Community Mental Health Journal**, 1976, *12*: 365-375.

Thaler, O. F. Pseudo-research? **Saturday Review of the Sciences**, 1973, 55.

Truax, C. B., and Carkhuff, R. R. **Toward effective counseling and psychotherapy**. Chicago, Ill: Aldine, 1967.

Ward, C. H., Beck, A. T., Mendelson, M., Mock, J. E. and Erbaugh, J. K. The psychiatric nomenclature. **Archives of General Psychiatry**, 1962, 7: 198-205.

Wessler, R. L. and Iven, D. Social characteristics of patients readmitted to a community mental health center. **Community Mental Health Journal**, 1970, *6*(1), 69-74.

Wilson, T. L., Berry, L. K. and Miskimins, W. R. An assessment of characteristics related to vocational success among restored psychiatric patients. **The Vocational Guidance Quarterly**, 1969, *18*: 110-114.

Wolkon, G. W. Characteristics of clients and continuity of care into the community. **Community Mental Health Journal**, 1970, *6*: 215-221.

Zubin, J. Classification of the behavior disorders. **Annual Review of Psychology**, 1967, *18*: 373-406.

CHAPTER V
Psychiatric Rehabilitation Programs

Once the psychiatric rehabilitation practitioner has achieved a rehabilitation diagnosis, the groundwork has been laid for the development and implementation of the necessary psychiatric rehabilitation programs. In essence, a rehabilitation program describes the means by which a psychiatrically disabled helpee can progress from his or her present level of skilled performance to a more advanced level of skilled performance. By developing and implementing psychiatric rehabilitation programs, the psychiatric rehabilitation practitioner can help the psychiatrically disabled helpee learn the skills necessary to take him or her from "where he or she is" to "where he or she needs or wants to be" (See Table 5-1).

More loosely defined, a psychiatric rehabilitation program is any means used to reach a rehabilitation goal. However, the more effective programs are the programs in which each step moves systematically toward the rehabilitation goal. Indeed, the more knowledgeable the psychiatric rehabilitation practitioner is about what should be accomplished, the more systematic the subsequently developed and implemented rehabilitation programs will be.

This chapter analyzes the current state of psychiatric rehabilitation programs and programming, and outlines the principles upon which psychiatric rehabilitation programs should be developed and implemented. Following the presentation of those psychiatric rehabilitation programming principles, an overview is provided of the various rehabilitation techniques which can become important components of systematic psychiatric rehabilitation programs. Lastly, the research investigations of psychiatric rehabilitation skills training programs will be examined.

TABLE 5-1

THE FUNCTION OF A PSYCHIATRIC REHABILITATION PROGRAM

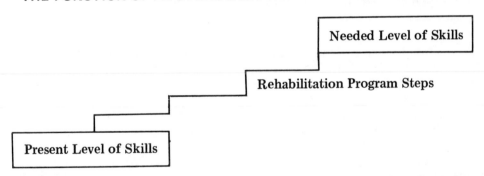

THE PRESENT STATE OF PSYCHIATRIC REHABILITATION PROGRAMMING

The typical psychiatric rehabilitation program has been designed to improve the psychiatrically disabled helpee's community functioning, or, at a minimum, to keep him or her functioning in the community. A number of psychiatric rehabilitation programs are currently run in such rehabilitation facilities as sheltered workshops, halfway houses, day-care centers, community mental health centers, family-care homes, etc. However, as mentioned in Chapter III, most of the rehabilitation programs are not as concerned with skill development as they are with attempting to maximize the health of the psychiatrically disabled helpee's environment; yet a more healthy environment does not automatically lead to increased helpee skills. The typical psychiatric rehabilitation program is not a systematic step-by-step program based on the program development principles outlined in this chapter but rather a maintenance program on which the psychiatrically disabled helpee can depend. Instead of teaching the psychiatrically disabled helpees the skills needed to function more independently in the community, the programs in many psychiatric rehabilitation facilities seem to encourage dependence on either the facility itself, or some employee of the facility. The typical psychiatric rehabilitation program's nonthreatening, comfortable environment, with only a minimum of demands made upon the psychiatrically disabled helpee, is a very ineffective way to develop the helpee's skills.

The most obvious difficulty with such maintenance programs, as opposed to skills training programs, is that once the helpee loses the support upon which he or she has come to depend, the helpee does not have the skills to function independently in the community. The clearest example of the deficiencies inherent in rehabilitation programs that lack a skills training component has been provided by the outstanding longitudinal research of Pasaminick (Davis, Dinitz & Pasaminick, 1972; Pasaminick, Scarpetti & Dinitz, 1967). In the initial project, Pasaminick and his associates clearly demonstrated that many psychiatrically disabled helpees who were supposed to have been hospitalized for psychiatric difficulties were able to be successfully maintained in the community without hospitalization for the duration of the two-year demonstration project (Pasaminick et al. 1967). The successful home-care maintenance program consisted of home visits by a nurse, and clinic conferences with a psychiatrist. Approximately one-half of the home-care group received chemotherapy while the other half received placebos.

Results of the two-year demonstration project indicated that a majority of the home-care drug group was able to continue to function in the community without ever requiring a psychiatric hospitalization. The one- and two-year hospitalization rate for the home-care drug group was 23% and 40%, while the one- and two-year hospitalization rate for the home-care placebo group was 67% and 78%. A group of control subjects who were initially permitted to be hospitalized, has a rehospitalization range of 46%. The results of the project were hailed by the director of the National Institute of Mental Health as "indisputable support for the validity of the concept of the community mental

health center ... (and) its constellation of community based mental health services" (Yolles, 1967). Yet what must be remembered is that all that the two-year demonstration project convincingly showed was that many psychiatrically disabled helpees could be maintained in the community without a psychiatric hospitalization experience. It provided no evidence to indicate that those individuals who successfully remained in the community were functioning any better than those control subjects who were permitted hospitalization. Because none of the helpees in any of the groups received any systematic rehabilitation skills training, it would be expected that once the helpees in the home-care group lost their community support they would exhibit a level of functioning no better than the initially hospitalized control group.

A five-year follow-up study confirmed these expectations (Davis et al. 1972). Five years after the demonstration project was concluded, new data was collected on 92% of the psychiatrically disabled helpees who had been involved in the original study. These follow-up results indicated that during the five-year follow-up period the rehospitalization rates for the home-care drug, home-care placebo, and hospitalized control group helpees were 61%, 57%, and 61%, respectively. In terms of an employment criterion the percentage of helpees in the same three groups who "had any occupation" was 27%, 26%, and 27%, respectively. Thus the results of the five-year follow-up indicate that the long-term rehabilitation goal of independent community functioning cannot be obtained by temporarily increasing the amount of community-based support which a helpee receives. These support services, regardless of whether they are in the community or in the hospital, must provide more than just support if they hope to provide a truly rehabilitative effect on the psychiatrically disabled helpee.

Unfortunately, most current psychiatric rehabilitation programs, except for some notable exceptions, appear more intent on changing certain conditions in the helpee's environment rather than on changing the helpee her/himself. Rather than operating on the psychiatric rehabilitation program principles advanced in this chapter, the typical rehabilitation program appears to operate on one or more of the following three principles: 1) principle of lessened demands, 2) principle of average expectations, 3) principle of normalization.

The psychiatric rehabilitation practitioner is guided by *the principle of lessened demands* in his or her attempts to develop sheltered work or living situations for the helpee. The rehabilitation environment is structured (sheltered) to minimize the pressure, threat or responsibility which the helpee experiences. The implicit assumption underlying this principle is that the reduced demands and increased environmental support are conducive to the psychiatrically disabled helpee's eventual rehabilitation. Many rehabilitation facilities guide their day-to-day functioning by the principle of lessened demands.

The principle of average expectations means that the psychiatric rehabilitation practitioner expects the psychiatrically disabled helpees to improve their functioning so that they will eventually be less dependent on the rehabilitation practitioners and the rehabilitation facilities. However, it is not enough to merely expect psychiatrically disabled helpees to achieve their maximum; they must also *learn* the skills which will help them realize their potential. A rehabilitation facility which operates on both principles, that is, minimizing the demands on the helpee yet expecting more of the helpee than is demanded, must of necessity develop systematic rehabilitation programs to take the helpee from the level where little is demanded to the level where much is expected. Without rehabilitation programs to teach the helpee how to perform at the expected level, such facilities would be considered inhumane and cruel. How could a rehabilitation facility justify refusing further service just because the helpee could not perform at the expected level of performance if the facility itself had not developed the rehabilitation programs capable of teaching the helpee the skills needed to function at the expected level

of skilled performance? Thus, once the rehabilitation facility has committed itself to operating on the principle of average expectations, it is ethically incumbent upon the facility to develop and implement the necessary rehabilitation programs which assist the helpee to meet these expectations. Most rehabilitation facilities only pay lip service to the principle of average expectations and have not demanded adherence to the principle primarily because the facilities lack systematic rehabilitation programs designed to get the helpees to perform at the expected level.

The principle of normalization first achieved widespread popularity in the field of mental retardation and was later extended into the field of psychiatric rehabilitation (Baker, Baker & McDaniel, 1975; Wolfensberger, 1970). The principle of normalization as applied to the field of psychiatric rehabilitation means that the psychiatrically disabled helpee should be exposed to experiences that are likely to elicit or maintain accepted (or normative) behavior. A psychiatric rehabilitation facility whose operations are based on the principle of normalization attempts to structure its services so as to provide the psychiatrically disabled helpee with the opportunity to live in a normal routine. Unless it is absolutely essential, the principle of normalization dictates that the psychiatrically disabled helpee should be as free and independent as the typical citizen. In essence, the psychiatrically disabled helpee should be treated as normally and as decently as possible.

In one respect, the necessity for a principle which indicates the need for psychiatrically disabled helpees to be treated normally and decently is an indictment of the field of psychiatric treatment and rehabilitation. There would be no need for a principle of normalization if mental health professionals had not been so inclined to treat the helpee as atypical. The indecent behavior toward psychiatrically disabled helpees in the past has necessitated the development of the principle of normalization. While the principle itself makes good sense, the field of psychiatric rehabilitation cannot pat itself on its back for directing its activities based on the principle of normalization; its time is long overdue.

In general, the present state of psychiatric rehabilitation programming is based upon principles which would appear to guide the field toward implementing unsystematic programs designed to keep the helpees in the community with a minimum of demands placed upon them, hoping that the helpees somehow improve to the level expected of them, while treating them as decently or normally as possible. However, if the goal of the psychiatric re-

habilitation practitioner is to assist the helpees in increasing their level of skilled performance, it is incumbent upon the psychiatric rehabilitation practitioner to develop new programs capable of achieving this rehabilitation goal. Although community support services and facilities are important components of a rehabilitation program, they need not be the whole program. The following section on psychiatric rehabilitation programming outlines how the psychiatric rehabilitation practitioner can develop more effective skills training programs.

A PROGRAM IS MORE THAN A PLACEMENT

Case Illustration 5-1

Up to now, Pam had worked carefully and effectively with Larry. Given his background and situation, she knew it would be bad news if he found himself involved in a program that didn't really fit his needs. For this reason, she had been particularly conscientious in gathering information about specific employment training programs and in helping Larry explore the alternatives and choose the best program for his purposes.

"This really sounds great." Larry's enthusiastic endorsement of the C.E.T.A. training program they had selected rewarded Pam for her time and effort. Larry obviously felt very good about the whole thing.

The particular program in which Larry would be involved was designed to give him the skills he would need to find full-time work as a hospital orderly. Larry found the possibility of working in this area very exciting. Larry was often moody and tense and his volatile temper had cost him a number of different jobs in the past. Now he yearned for employment that he could really count on, a job that would be steady and interesting. The C.E.T.A. program promised to move him quickly toward such a job.

Noting Larry's enthusiastic commitment to the program he had chosen, Pam allowed herself to relax. He would be fine, she felt. Now maybe she could shift her concentration to some of her other clients. Pam's secretary had already contacted the

C.E.T.A. people to arrange for Larry's initial visit. Having made sure that Larry knew when and where he should go on Monday to begin the program, and having scheduled a follow-up session with him, Pam saw him off.

Alas, she should not have abandoned Larry quite so soon. In particular, she should have explored the C.E.T.A. program a bit more and should have been careful to prepare both Larry and the program's instructor for Larry's involvement. The instructor, it turned out, was a gruff, ex-military type who made much of exercising his authority. And Larry, as Pam well knew, had a long history of difficulty in dealing with authoritative figures.

Unfortunately, Pam did not follow through in preparing either Larry or the instructor. She simply sent Larry off, assuming that all would be well. But all was most definitely not well.

Within ten minutes of Larry's entrance into the program the next Monday, he and the instructor had already locked horns over the matter of where Larry would sit. Losing this particular struggle, Larry was in a bad humor for the rest of the class. Still, he might have hung on if the instructor hadn't taken him aside as the first session was ending.

"Son, I've been keeping an eye on you," the older man said in the manner of a general addressing a rebellious soldier. "You're going to have to stay on the ball if you want to keep up in here. And that means you're going to have to have a positive attitude!"

"Oh yeah?" Larry's anger was evident. "What's wrong with my attitude?"

"Well, for one thing, you've done nothing but sneer at me from the back of the room since you came in." The instructor glared down at Larry. "I believe I heard you laugh several times as well."

"Is that right?" Larry was furious. "Well maybe it's because I thought you were a pretty funny old man!"

Things got worse after that. The argument ended by Larry stalking out of the room and slamming the door behind him. He simply could not deal with the crusty instructor.

But he could have dealt with him — and the instructor could have worked with Larry more effectively — if Pam had thought to prepare both of them in advance. Certainly, Larry was plagued by a lack of self-control, and the instructor was a man pre-occupied by his own authority; but the responsibility for the failure was Pam's. She could have developed programs for each of them. Failing to do so, she paved the way for Larry's inevitable departure.

PSYCHIATRIC REHABILITATION PROGRAMMING PRINCIPLES

Psychiatric rehabilitation skills training programs are designed to increase the psychiatrically disabled helpee's skills to a level at which he or she can actually perform the skills necessary to function as independently as possible. These rehabilitation skills training programs are constructed to enable the psychiatrically disabled helpee to perform the particular skill in the situations that it is needed.

The present section outlines the basic ingredients of rehabilitation program development and implementation. A more detailed analysis of rehabilitation programming can be found in Anthony, Pierce & Cohen (1977). The particular methods used to train psychiatric rehabilitation practitioners in these skills are presented in Chapter XI.

1. **Rehabilitation programming involves both program development and implementation.**

   Practitioners must be skilled in *writing* the necessary program as well as in *getting the client to act* on the program that has been developed.

2. **The ability to develop the specific program steps is a function of the rehabilitation practitioner's expertise in four basic program development skills.**

   First, the rehabilitation practitioner must be able to *develop the major program steps*, which, if implemented, will get the client from the client's present skill level to the client's needed skill level.

This development process usually occurs by brainstorming and writing down the steps that are brainstormed. The next skill which the rehabilitation practitioner must employ is the ability to *sequence the major program steps*. The steps that have been brainstormed must be ordered in a logical progression so that each subsequent step moves the client closer to her or his goal. The third practitioner skill is the ability to *develop and sequence the necessary secondary steps* that the client must perform in order to achieve each major step. Many clients might need help in performing some or all of the major steps. Secondary steps attached to each major step will enable the client to perform these major steps. The final practitioner skill of program development involves the practitioner's ability to *develop the necessary check steps*. Check steps are the questions the client should be mentally asking and answering before, during, and after the performance of each step. These "think steps" force the client to become aware of whether she or he is prepared to do the step (before), doing the step correctly (during), and has evaluated his or her performance of the step (after).

3. **The number of and need for major steps, secondary steps, and check steps varies as a function of the client's level of functioning and the complexity of the skill behavior.**

   The general principle is that the more simple and brief the program is, the better, so long as it gets the client to the goal. There are procedures within the program development process to assist the practitioner in adhering to the principle. The skilled practitioner, however, must be capable of writing a very lengthy and complex program if that is what the client needs in order to accomplish the rehabilitation goal.

4. **The prerequisite skill needed to develop the major program steps is the ability to define the client's present and needed functioning in observable terms.**

This goal setting should have occurred during the diagnostic planning process. Once the rehabilitation practitioner is equipped with this diagnostic assessment, she or he can brainstorm and sequence the steps that will get the client from where he or she is to where he or she needs to be.

5. **Each program step must be written in behavioral terms.**

This means that the helpee's behavior on each step is capable of being experienced by one of the five senses, most typically the senses of sight and hearing. Specifically, this may be accomplished by carefully selecting the verbs which are used to describe the behavior. Using behavioral verbs is not as simple as it might appear. If the practitioner is not careful, she or he will find her or himself inadvertently using such non-behavioral verbs as think, explore, imagine, understand, reflect, and so forth. To avoid this possibility, the practitioner should ask him or herself after the major steps have been brainstormed — "Can others experience (see or hear) these steps?" If the answer is no, then this step should be made observable. If this is not done, the step will be difficult for the client to perform and for the client and practitioner to evaluate.

6. **The ability to brainstorm the program steps depends upon the practitioner's ability to do this particular skill.**

If the practitioner him or herself cannot perform the skill, it would be difficult to see how the practitioner could develop a program for someone else. This principle may be seen most clearly in the extreme. If the client needed mountain climbing skills and the practitioner didn't know anything about mountain climbing, it would be impossible for the practitioner to develop a program without the assistance of an expert in mountain climbing. Thus the practitioner needs both the skills of program development and the skills in the subject area. A less extreme and more realistic example would be a practitioner trying to develop a job-interviewing-skills program, when the practitioner's own job-interviewing skills are poor. In situations such as these, the practitioner should either master the skills her or himself, bring in an expert in the area, or simply modify an already existing program to meet the unique needs of the client.

7. **The ability to get the client to implement the specific program steps is a function of the rehabilitation practitioner's expertise in four basic program implementation skills.**

First, the practitioner must *develop time lines* for the major steps, for example, the specific times by which the client needs to perform certain skill behaviors. Secondly, the practitioner must *develop specific reinforcements* which may be administered based on the client's ability to perform each step. If the client is acquiring a new skill or parts of a new skill, then the practitioner must *implement the necessary teaching steps* so that the client knows the skill before she or he attempts to apply the skill. When the skill is either being acquired or applied, the practitioner must *monitor the client's performance* so that the time lines can be adhered to, differential reinforcements can be administered, and program modifications made.

8. **Time limits should be set for the implementation of major program steps.**

In the historical development of rehabilitation techniques, time limits for the client's achievement of rehabilitation goals were neither set nor monitored. It seemed that demanding that the clients attain a certain level of behavior by a certain time was somehow antithetical to the traditional warm, supportive environment that was a part of many psychiatric rehabilitation settings. To a lesser extent, the lack of many systematic rehabilitation programs within these settings also contributed to the laissez-faire attitude toward time criteria. It would have seemed cruel to demand that clients perform a certain behavior by a certain time if the practitioners had not actually tried to teach clients these behaviors. Gradually, however, these routinely low expectations of client behavior began to be seen as detrimental to client functioning. Time limits were set which the client was expected to meet. Not surprisingly, it seemed that the practitioner's increased expectations that the client could in fact perform a certain behavior by a certain time had a therapeutic effect in and of itself (Lamb, 1971).

Thus the setting of time limits is now seen as advantageous for several reasons: first, it can exert a subtle effect on the client to increase the client's own expectations about him or herself; second, time limits give the client a target to shoot for and a guide to keep the client on the program; third, time limits set the criteria on which client performance may be evaluated and differential reinforcement administered.

As a general principle, time lines are set for the completion of each major step. Adding these time lines together establishes the time lines for the entire program. Sometimes time limits are also set for secondary steps.

9. **Clients should receive specific reinforcements with the completion of each major step.**

One of the major errors that is sometimes made by rehabilitation practitioners during the implementation stage is the failure to develop a specific reinforcement strategy. All too often, clients and practitioners believe that the goal of the program will be sufficiently rewarding to keep the client working on the program. Goals such as a job, a passing grade, and living at home, are often believed to be so sufficiently motivating that the practitioner believes that the client needs no other incentives. Or, perhaps the practitioner believes that the learning process itself will be so interesting that the stimulation of learning will be enough of an incentive.

Unfortunately most clients (and most everybody else for that matter) need more reinforcements than either the long-term goal itself or the reinforcements inherent in the process of learning and doing. Consider the working person's situation. Although the long-term goal of receiving a promotion, salary increase, and early retirement and incentives for continual employment, often the worker may not be able to remain motivated long enough to stay employed in order to receive these rewards. Fortunately workers are rewarded more often by accruing pay each week. Similarly, clients must be frequently rewarded, based on their performance in trying to achieve their rehabilitation goals.

An enormous number of books, speeches, and articles have been written about how to improve a person's learning by means of manipulating reinforcements. The professionals who have studied the reinforcement process in such great detail are often referred to as "behavior modifiers" or "behavior therapists." Out of their study of reinforcement has emerged a set of principles, complex theoretical constructs, and a new esoteric jargon. The practitioner who wishes to employ straightforward reinforcement strategies in rehabilitation programming may wonder if she or he need master this new language and theory before she or he is capable of employing a reinforcement strategy.

Although the mastery of new concepts and theories may be a viable learning experience, the practitioner who wishes to implement program steps need not be a knowledgeable learning theorist. There is, in fact, no one learning theory that can account for all the various behavior techniques which have emerged. Naive adherents to a learning-theory approach may not be aware of all the controversy generated by the inadequacy of learning theory to explain and predict why and how certain behavioral techniques work. Indeed, it has been the behaviorist's own commitment to ongoing research and technological development that has undermined the relevance and applicability of current learning theory.

London (1972) has written a provocative article which addresses the need for therapists to devote their energies toward developing new therapeutic techniques rather than trying to stretch learning theory to account for the effectiveness of each new technique that emerges. London maintains that all the theorems and principles espoused by the behaviorists of the 1960's can be ". . . reduced to one or one-and-a-half principles — namely, that learning depends on the connections in time, space, and attention between what you do and what happens to you subsequently." Armed with this principle and a modicum of common sense, the practitioner may devise various reinforcement strategies designed to encourage the client to implement his or her skills program.

10. **The particular behavior which is selected as the reinforcer must come from the client's frame of reference.**

Just because the practitioner perceives a certain behavior as reinforcing (eating dessert, buying new clothes, watching TV), does not mean the client considers these behaviors as reinforcing to him or her. To assist the practitioner in identifying all the possible activities that might possess reinforcement properties for individual clients, various reinforcement survey schedules have been developed (e.g., Cautela & Kastenbaum, 1967).

It must not be overlooked that the practitioner is often a potent reinforcer to the client. This is particularly true of practitioners who have demonstrated a high level of interpersonal skills with their clients. These interpersonal skills are essentially the same diagnostic interviewing skills discussed in the previous chapter. More specifically, these interpersonal or interviewing skills have been called attending, observing, listening, and responding skills. In popular vocabulary, these skills have often been summarized under the term "empathy"; in more professional writings, these skills have become known as responding skills, meaning the ability of the practitioner to communicate to the client that the practitioner accurately understands the client's unique situation and feelings. (A more detailed examination of these responding skills may be found in Anthony, Pierce & Cohen, 1977.) The practitioner who has used these responding skills to develop an understanding relationship with the client will be able to use him/herself as a reinforcer. That is, praise and attention from such a practitioner can serve to reinforce the client's performance.

In this regard, several experimental studies have demonstrated that the experimenters' responding skills may affect the outcome of a verbal-conditioning or-modeling verbal-reinforcement program. The power of a conditioning or modeling reinforcement program was found to be, in part, a function of the level of responding skills exhibited to the subject by the experimenter/helper (Dowling & Frantz, 1975; Mickelson & Stivic, 1971; Vitalo, 1970).

Undoubtedly, the most significant and meaningful finding with respect to the relationship between responding skills and skill development outcome has been made, not in the field of helping *per se*, but in the field of education. Over the past decade one finding has consistently emerged from educational research: Positive relationships exist between the teacher's responding skills and various measures of student achievement and educational outcome. Thus a teacher's ability to respond to her or his students will affect how well the students learn. More recent studies have shown that a teacher's responding skills are not only positively related to educational outcome criteria but also to criteria which have primarily been the goals of guidance counselors and other mental health professionals — criteria such as improved student self-concept and decreased student absenteeism (Aspy & Roebuck, 1977). Thus, the interpersonally skilled practitioner who is either teaching or monitoring the rehabilitation program can affect the client's performance by using him/herself as a differential reinforcer.

11. **Rehabilitation programs are of two basic types: a) application programs and b) acquisition programs.**

An application program is for the client who has demonstrated the skill, or a slight variation of it, in an environmental area different from the environment in which she or he is presently deficient. An acquisition program is for a client who cannot presently demonstrate the skill or a variation of it in any environment. Thus he or she no longer possesses the skill or never possessed the skill and therefore must be taught the skill. In contrast, the application program is written for the client who possesses the skill but is deficient in its application in the specific rehabilitation environment of concern.

The resulting programs that need to be developed for the two situations are vastly different. The application program usually will have much larger steps and focus more specifically on reinforcement and monitoring strategies. The acquisition program must, in addition to these foci, develop a program with much smaller steps and include a strategy for teaching the steps.

12. **In acquisition programs the skill-teaching process is essentially a tell-show-do process.**

Typically each major and secondary program step should include each of these three components. In this way, the practitioner has provided the client with auditory, visual, and kinesthetic learning stimuli in order to maximize the skill-learning outcome. In essence, the tell component comprises the instructions for performing the skill step. These instructions are given to the client before the skill step is demonstrated or shown. In this way, the client knows some of the behaviors to look for when she or he is presented with a demonstration of the skill.

The importance of the show steps or skill demonstration has achieved increasing recognition. Many studies, falling under the rubric of modeling, have investigated the importance of the show step before the client actually attempts the skill. By means of both the tell and show steps the practitioner will have maximized the possibility of success in the client's initial practice attempts.

The number of practice situations which are included is obviously a function of how well the client is able to perform the skill. For less skilled clients, the practitioner might arrange more and varied positive situations before the client actually attempts the skill in the appropriate community setting.

Appendices A and B contain two examples of rehabilitation programs. The program in Appendix A is for the skill of "using community resources." The specific community resource is the local aftercare clinic. In this case, the client is about to be discharged from the hospital. Past client behavior, after the last hospitalization, indicates that the client eventually obtained a clinic appointment (in about thirty days) but only with considerable prodding. The practitioner realizes that while the client possesses parts of the skill, past client behavior would suggest that the appointment will not be made within five days.

In the diagnostic process the practitioner and client operationalize the skill in the following way: number of days after hospital discharge that the client arrives for a scheduled appointment at the outpatient clinic. The client's present level was assessed at thirty days; the client's needed level was assessed at five days. The program in Appendix A is an application program; the client does not need to learn the skill, but needs to apply the skill in this specific context. The client is perfectly capable of using community resources in other situations, for example, making and keeping dental appointments and appointments to get his car repaired.

In contrast, the "stigma reduction" program in Appendix B is an acquisition program; the client does not seem to possess this skill in any setting. The client for whom this program is constructed is a thirty-five-year-old single female who has had a rather successful career as an executive secretary. Her psychiatric hospitalization was precipitated by several crises in her home and the promotion to a new position in a different city from that of the person with whom she had worked for the last ten years. The diagnostic planning process indicated that the client is terrified of being asked by an employment interviewer about her recent psychiatric hospitalization. She can think of nothing positive to say. In a simulated job interview she mumbled something about "being committed to the hospital and taking tranquilizers because I was very sick." Obviously, a response of this type does nothing to reduce the stigma associated with her hospitalization for psychiatric difficulties. It mentions nothing positive about herself and contains two negative comments ("being committed" and "very sick").

The practitioner and the client operationalized the stigma reduction skill in the following way: number of positive and negative comments that the client can make in response to questions about her psychiatric hospitalization when asked by an employment interviewer. The client's present level was assessed at 0 positive comments and 2 negative comments; the client's needed level was assessed at 2 positive and 0 negative comments.

AN ACQUISITION REHABILITATION PROGRAM

Case Illustration 5-2 ━━━

"What you really want then, is to find an apartment that fits all your requirements," John said. Ellie nodded shyly, her eyes fixed on his face. "You need a place that's under $185 a month; a place no more than one block from the main bus route; a place close enough to your new job so you can get there without having to transfer buses; and a place where you don't have to sign a lease in case this particular job doesn't work out."

Ellie nodded again. "Uh huh . . . Gee, but that's a lot of stuff I have to find out! How can I ever learn all that about each possible apartment on my list?"

"It's a little frightening to think about all the information you need to get," John agreed. "But I think by going over the questions you need to ask we can pretty much make sure that you'll learn everything you need to learn."

John meant what he said, too. One of Ellie's greatest problems was her shyness — a fact of which they were both acutely aware. For this reason, John had helped Ellie to develop an extremely detailed program to get her where she wanted to go — the point where she could make the best possible decision concerning her future living arrangement. But he knew that simply developing a program with Ellie wasn't going to be enough. She had to be able to put the program to use — and that meant she would have to go over every step until she was thoroughly comfortable with it.

Consequently, John began the next stage of things by *telling* Ellie once again

what each of the steps in her program involved. Since most of these steps involved questions she would have to ask landlords about different buildings, he made sure Ellie understood just what information each question was designed to elicit.

Next, John *showed* Ellie how she could phrase each question and take each step in her program. "Hello, my name is Ellie Saunders and I'd like to get some information about the apartment you're advertising for rent . . . "

After this, John got Ellie to actually *do* the things that each step required — which meant in most cases that Ellie had to practice asking the various questions herself. At the end of this phase, John role-played several different landlords and had Ellie go through her entire spiel while she sat with her back to him and spoke into the telephone as she would actually be doing.

"I'm — I'm really getting it, aren't I?" Ellie said as they finished this phase of activity. She sounded surprised at her own newly discovered capability. There was fresh eagerness in her subsequent efforts to work out a time frame for taking each step in her program and to come up with a set of positive and negative reinforcements to keep herself on track.

"I know!" she said at one point. "If I make all the calls I'm supposed to between now and Friday, and if I don't goof any of them up, I'll treat myself Friday night by going to see *The Sting* at the Art Cinema. That's one of my favorite movies!"

"Good," said John. "And if you don't make all the calls, you can administer a swift kick to yourself by not watching any T.V. for the next week."

In point of fact, however, John was beginning to doubt that Ellie would need to miss her movie that Friday. So long as her program had been no more than a set of intellectually understood steps. Ellie had remained quite apprehensive. Now that she had been able to rehearse all of the steps, however, they were becoming real to her.

"We learn not just by hearing or seeing, but by doing!" John had often appreciated the truth of this statement before — but never so much as he now did with Ellie. She could handle herself and her program. She *would* handle it.

And of course she did handle it.

Rehabilitation Skill Generalizability

It is meaningful to make distinctions between rehabilitation programs based on the extent to which the program has provided the helpee with the ability to generalize the particular skill. Although the minimum goal of any effective rehabilitation program is for the helpee to be able to *perform* the particular skill, rehabilitation programs do vary in terms of the expected *context* in which the psychiatrically disabled helpee must perform the skill. That is, will the helpee be expected to perform the skill independently, or will some type of support be present? The context in which the particular rehabilitation skill is performed can be meaningfully described as varying across two dimensions: an assistance dimension and an environmental dimension (See Table 5-2).

The assistance dimension recognizes the fact that some rehabilitation programs enable the helpee to perform the rehabilitation skill only in the presence of a person or device which assists the skilled performance; while other rehabilitation programs enable the helpee to perform the skill without assistance of any type. For example, in Chapter III, one of the skills mentioned for illustrative purposes was the skill of "using community resources," which was defined in this way: "The psychiatrically disabled helpee can travel from his residence to the Social Security Office." The goal of the rehabilitation program may be for the helpee to perform this activity independently or with the assistance of a device (such as a map especially drawn for the helpee, a volunteer to accompany the helpee, etc.).

TABLE 5-2
PROGRAM DISTINCTIONS BASED ON SKILL SUPPORTS

| | | Environmental Dimension | |
		Outside Training	Within Training
	Absent	A	C
Assistance Dimension	Present	B	D

In contrast, the environmental dimension recognizes the fact that some rehabilitation programs train the helpee to perform the skill only in the context of the training environment while other programs train the helpee to generalize the skill outside of the training situation. For example, in Chapter III, the skill of selective reward was defined in this way: "The psychiatrically disabled helpee can role play real-life situations with a coached actor and demonstrate at least one instance of selective reward technique in each role-playing situation." This particular goal definition indicates that this particular rehabilitation program taught by this rehabilitation practitioner will only develop the skill to the extent that it can be demonstrated within the training environment. Other practitioners in the community may then train the helpee to be able to perform the skill outside the training environment.

Other examples of rehabilitation programs which only train the helpee to perform the skill in the training situation might be various training programs run in sheltered work or living situations. Sometimes these training programs are concerned only with the helpee's ability to cook, clean, work, reside, etc., within the particular sheltered facility, and are not concerned with the helpee's ability to generalize his or her skills to less sheltered situations.

The ideal rehabilitation program is one that enables the helpee to perform the skill outside the training environment without any assistance (cell A, Table 5-2). However, an activity performed with assistance of some type (cell B) is certainly better than no activity at all. Cell B is often an appropriate programming level when the helpee's initial functioning is very low, or the skill to be learned is very complex. On the other hand, some rehabilitation programs may not even be designed to achieve skill learning beyond the training situation (cells C and D).

In many instances, however, these "training specific" rehabilitation programs may be part of a larger program designed to eventually enable the helpee to perform the skills beyond the training situation. It should be pointed out that regardless of the contextual distinctions between various rehabilitation programs, the skills needed to construct the rehabilitation program remain the same.

Undoubtedly, one of the most difficult tasks for the rehabilitation practitioner is to insure that the client actually uses (generalizes) the skills learned in the rehabilitation program in the community. The successful use of rehabilitation diagnostic and programming skills has attempted to maximize this occurrence in a number of ways.

1. The program steps are developed after the client has developed a personalized understanding of why he or she needs to acquire or apply these skills. The problem of "client motivation" to accomplish a program may be due, in part, to the fact that the client has never owned the need to learn the skills. Rather, the "unmotivated" client often has had the program imposed upon her or him.

2. The client is encouraged to assist in setting the program goals and in developing the program steps. Once again, the practitioner attempts to maximize the client's involvement in the program so that the client works harder to accomplish the program steps with which she or he is familiar and has some understanding.

3. The client can use the check steps as a way to monitor his or her own performance in order to help keep his or her behavior as goal directed as possible. These check steps or think steps provide a means by which the client can monitor and correct his or her own behavior on the spot.

4. The teaching process includes a variety of situations and settings in which all or parts of the skill are practiced. In this way, the client can approach the natural environment more skillfully and with more confidence.

5. If possible, parts of the teaching program should be conducted in the natural environment. In this way, the stimuli and reinforcers which occur during the actual skill performance are also present during the learning of the skills.

6. The program always contains reinforcers that come from the client's frame of reference. Many of these reinforcers can often be administered by the client him/herself.

7. Significant others are taught how to differentially reinforce the client's performance. In this way, the client is encouraged to continue to perform the skill in the natural environment. Besides serving as reinforcers, significant others might also be used to serve as models for the skill, to teach parts of the skill, and to monitor the skill. The research on psychiatric rehabilitation supports the notion that client skill behaviors may be increased by developing community support systems (Anthony, 1977).

8. The practitioner attempts to develop a relationship with the client which maximizes the practitioner's potential of becoming a significant reinforcer for the client.

Rehabilitation Skill Extendability

The issue of skill generalizability may be distinguished from the issue of skill extendability. Skill extendability refers to the helpee's ability to extend the trained skill to the extent that the helpee can make modifications and variations in the trained skill to increase its effectiveness.

A skill is considered to be extended if the helpee either modifies the skill or uses the skill in an environment for which the helpee has not been trained. For example, a helpee who has learned to apply a selective reward or differential reinforcement skill with her spouse may make modifications in the skill (i.e., change the rewards) and use the skill with her employees.

Skill extendability can occur in three ways. First, the skills training program can be designed to teach the helpee how to modify the skill or adapt the skill to different environments. The rehabilitation program need not be discontinued when the helpee is able to perform the specific skill in the needed environment; steps may be built into the program to enable the helpee to perform the skill in various ways in different situations. In such cases, the goal of the rehabilitation program would be defined so as to specifically indicate that the successful completion of the program would enable the helpee to perform at these various levels of skill functioning.

Second, on some occasions a psychiatrically disabled helpee may also learn to extend the skill without a specific rehabilitation program to assist him or her. Extensive practice of the trained skill may enable the helpee to gradually make modifications or to use the skill in situations for which he or she has received no specific training.

Third, the helpee may make useful modifications in the skill by integrating aspects of previously mastered skills into the trained skill. The skill integration occurs because the trained skill and another skill may be significantly correlated with one another in certain situations.

For example, a psychiatrically disabled helpee who has mastered stigma reduction skills may be able to "orally respond to questions about psychiatric hospitalization by using phrases which contain no apologies or references to present difficulties." The helpee can use variations of the skill in a variety of situations, as for example on a job interview when a question is asked about an extended period of unemployment. The helpee may obtain this skill level by learning the skill from a program designed to teach him or her this particular variant of the stigma reduction skill; or, the helpee may on his or her own practice the stigma reduction skill to such an extent that he or she attempts it successfully in situations for which he or she was not specifically trained. Also, the helpee may be skilled in job interviewing and be able to integrate job-interviewing skills with stigma reduction skills so that he or she may effectively respond to questions about past employment difficulties without having been specifically trained in this skill variant. Rehabilitation programs often reap unexpected and unplanned benefits because of the occurrence of rehabilitation skill extendability.

Rehabilitation Programming Techniques

In addition to possessing knowledge of the principles of program development and implementation, the psychiatric rehabilitation practitioner must be aware of specific rehabilitation techniques which the practitioner may use as part of the overall rehabilitation program. Historically, these techniques have mistakenly been considered to be complete rehabilitation programs. Unfortunately, when used singly these techniques represent a rather piecemeal approach to rehabilitation programming. However, it is important for the psychiatric rehabilitation practitioner to be aware of these techniques as they may be important components of various systematic rehabilitation programs. These techniques are best conceptualized as tools, which when used according to the principles of program development, and within the context of a more comprehensive rehabilitation program, may be instrumental in facilitating the psychiatrically disabled helpee's skill development.

1. Environmental Techniques

These techniques involve changing the environmental conditions under which skilled performance is required. The initial direction of change in the environment is typically toward reducing the pressures and demands upon the psychiatrically disabled helpee. Examples of techniques which change the conditions under which the helpee lives, learns, and works are: sheltered workshops, halfway houses, day-care centers, family-care homes, etc. To the extent that these environmental techniques are chiefly concerned with rehabilitation, the implicit assumption of these techniques is that the reduced environmental pressures, more supportive atmosphere, and the passage of time may eventually restore the helpee's ability to function in a less sheltered setting.

When these environmental techniques are used in accordance with the principles of program development, they provide a means by which the psychiatric rehabilitation practitioner can gradually increase the environmental demands placed upon the helpee as he or she develops increasingly higher levels of skilled performance. In this way, the helpee has an opportunity to practice his or her newly developing skills in an environment which is suitable to the helpee's present skill level.

It is simply not enough for the psychiatric rehabilitation practitioner to initially decrease the environmental demands placed upon the helpee; the psychiatric rehabilitation practitioner must also be prepared to systematically change these environmental demands in accordance with the helpee's developing skill level.

Some rehabilitation programs are not successful in generalizing the helpee's skills outside the training situation because these programs have not used environmental techniques to increase, as well as decrease the environmental demands made upon the helpee. One of the major difficulties encountered in rehabilitation programming is the fact that the ability of the helpee to perform the skill outside the training situation does not insure that the helpee will perform the skill in the most appropriate time and place. For example, a helpee may have mastered stigma reduction skills but uses these skills in situations where stigma reduction skills are not needed. Or, the helpee may be capable of skillful selective reward skills but does not remember to use them at the appropriate time.

The psychiatric rehabilitation practitioner's systematic use of environmental techniques provides a means of overcoming this particular generalizability problem. One possible solution is to have the helpee practice the skilled behavior in situations which systematically approximate the environment in which the helpee will be performing the skill. For example, a helpee who is learning a particular self-control skill to be used in the work environment, may first perform the self-control skill in the hospital work therapy program. This should be followed sequentially by a sheltered workshop environment, a sheltered placement experience, and finally competitive employment.

Another possible solution mentioned previously in the section on rehabilitation generalizability is to reprogram the natural environment to deliver reinforcement contingent upon the helpee's minimally effective skill performance. This procedure usually entails teaching selective reward skills to significant others in the helpee's life. The psychiatrically disabled helpee's newly developing skills must be reinforced by the helpee's environment or the skills will tend to dissipate. Indeed, it may be the previous lack of selected reward for appropriate skilled performance which has restricted the helpee's skill development in the first place.

Significant others can plan an important role in either encouraging or impeding the helpee's ability to develop and use these new skills appropriately. The psychiatric rehabilitation practitioner's involvement in the psychiatrically disabled helpee's environment is discussed further in the chapter on community rehabilitation programming.

A final environmental method of insuring that helpees use their skills in the appropriate time and place is to conduct at least part of the skills training program in the natural environment, so that the program allows for the skills to become influenced by natural reinforcers. For example, transportation skills may be taught in the transportation system, so that helpees who use the skills arrive at their destination whereas helpees who are less skillful experience delays, or within the limits of safety are allowed to become lost. The introduction of natural reinforcers into the training program can increase the future possibility of the skill being performed in the appropriate time and appropriate place.

It is certainly possible and desirable to use environmental techniques in combination with other rehabilitation programming techniques. What is most important is that the psychiatric rehabilitation practitioner conceptualize various environmental techniques as merely one aspect of the overall rehabilitation program. Historically, psychiatric rehabilitation practitioners have spent a major portion of their time successfully developing different environmental settings or techniques. As the effort of developing new environmental settings continues, rehabilitation practitioners must also concentrate on maximizing the effect of these environmental settings. They must conceptualize using these various environmental techniques as rehabilitation tools whose effectiveness may be increased by systematically integrating these techniques into overall rehabilitation programs.

2. Surrogate Techniques

The use of surrogate techniques can be an important component of many rehabilitation programs. Similar to environmental techniques, surrogate techniques can be useful in overcoming the generalizability

program mentioned previously, i.e., the ability of the helpee to perform a skill does not insure that the skill will be performed in the appropriate time and place.

This particular rehabilitation programming technique involves the use of an assistant to either supervise or assist in the helpee's performance of rehabilitation skills. The typical assistant is usually referred to as a paraprofessional, a volunteer, or an indigenous community member. The effective use of these assistants is discussed further in the chapter on psychiatric rehabilitation training (Chapter XI). The surrogate is essentially a paid or volunteer substitute for helpful significant others, which many psychiatrically disabled helpees unfortunately do not have. The effectiveness of surrogate techniques may be enhanced by ensuring that the assistant who is functioning in the surrogate role be well informed about the helpee's rehabilitation goals.

The surrogate can use his or her selective reward skills to reinforce the appropriate use of the skills and to extinguish inappropriate skilled performance. In addition, the individual functioning as a surrogate may check to make sure that the trained skills are actually being used in the community and that individuals in the helpee's environment are not hindering that helpee's skill. Information of this type relayed to the program developer may be useful in devising more effective programs for the particular helpee. If the surrogate is demographically similar to the psychiatrically disabled helpee (e.g., resides in the same community, the same socio-economic class, the same sex, etc.) the surrogate can serve as a model for the psychiatrically disabled helpee.

3. Engineering Techniques

Many psychiatrically disabled helpees achieve a specified level of skilled performance through use of a device or tool to assist their performance. As stated earlier in this chapter, distinctions may be made between programs based on whether the helpee can perform the skill with or without assistance. Engineering techniques involve the successful development and implementation of the tools or devices capable of facilitating the helpee's skilled performance. The previously discussed surrogate techniques represent the people component of the assistance dimension.

Similar to surrogate techniques, engineering techniques are useful when the skill to be performed is very complex, or the person performing the skill is functioning at a very low level. For illustrative purposes, the best example of the use of engineering techniques is a non-rehabilitation example — the manned exploration of the moon. In order to be able to explore the moon, the astronauts had to learn many skills, such as how to steer a rocket-propelled command module, how to drive a moon rover, and how to "walk" in space. Yet even equipped with many skills, the astronauts were still dependent upon many devices and tools to insure the successful completion of the moon mission.

Although the tools and devices presently engineered by psychiatric rehabilitation programmers are less complex than those used in space exploration, they are by no means less useful to the psychiatrically disabled helpee. Often these devices are needed because the helpee is functioning at such a low skill level rather than the complexity of the skill to be mastered.

An example of such an engineering technique would be a program designed to enable the helpee to arrive for a scheduled appointment at an aftercare clinic which uses a map depicting the helpee's route from his residence to the clinic. The map would be considered an engineering technique. Other examples of engineering techniques might be such things as: written directions of how to perform a particular skill, charts, graphs, pictures, and the like. Indeed, any device which the psychiatric rehabilitation practitioner can use to facilitate the helpee's skilled performance would be considered an engineering technique.

Depending on the overall rehabilitation goal, the helpee's reliance on the tool or device may or may not be eventually phased out. While the ideal goal would be for the helpee to perform the skill without the use of engineering techniques, the more realistic immediate goal may be to just get the helpee to *perform*. At a later date, it may be possible for the helpee to perform the skill without assistance. Thus, engineering techniques might be most important during the early stages of the rehabilitation program and then gradually phased out.

The use of chemotherapy is perhaps the best example of an engineering technique in psychiatric rehabilitation. Unfortunately, similar to some other rehabilitation techniques, drug therapy has often been considered to be the entire rehabilitation program rather than merely a supportive technique. As indicated in Chapter III, the innovation of chemotherapy was at first thought by some to preclude the need for psychiatric rehabilitation. Most simply stated, it was hypothesized that once the symptoms were contained by the drug intervention, the helpee would once again be able to function productively in her or his particular community. This optimistic hypothesis has simply not been born out by the facts.

The research results indicate that the presence or absence of drug therapy alone does not make a difference in terms of rehabilitation outcome (see Chapter III). There is little or no correlation between a chemotherapy regimen and the ability to live, learn, and work more independently in the community. Franklin, Kittredge, and Thrasher (1975) conducted a follow-up of a random number of patients discharged from a state mental hospital. These researchers reported ". . no significant difference between those readmitted or not readmitted in medications prescribed, users of medication, length of prescription, dosages, and current use of medication."

Such findings are really not that surprising as rehabilitation outcome is more closely related to skill level than to symptom level. As mentioned in Chapter II, drug treatment appears successful in reducing recidivism only when it is combined with monthly aftercare or outpatient contacts.

In terms of the helpee's vocational functioning, Engelhardt and Rosen (1976) concluded from their review: "Evidence for a direct effect of pharmacotherapy on the work performance of schizophrenic patients is so far lacking." They suggested that drug therapy plays an indirect role in vocational rehabilitation by modifying symptomatology and extending the period that the patient is able to remain in the community. Once again, the lack of a relationship between chemotherapy and productive community functioning should come as no surprise. In no way does drug therapy provide the psychiatrically disabled helpee with the skills, energy, and community opportunities necessary for seeking, obtaining, or retaining employment.

Another consideration relevant to drug therapy and rehabilitation is the controversy surrounding the issue of maintenance medication for chronically disabled helpees. A massive body of data exists in support of the conclusion that withdrawal leads to behavioral deterioration with long-term hospitalized patients. However, whether or not this data is methodologically sound and warrants such a conclusion has been questioned. Practitioners who desire to investigate this controversy in depth might wish to first examine the following reviews: Davis, Gosenfeld and Tsai, 1976; MacDonald and Tobias, 1976; Tobias and MacDonald, 1974.

Of interest to the practitioner of psychiatric rehabilitation is the rather consistent finding that approximately 20%-50% of the patients on placebo do *not* relapse and that 20%-50% on drugs eventually do relapse (Anthony, Cohen & Vitalo, 1978). These findings are consistent with the review of outpatient maintenance medication conducted by Gardos and Cole (1976). These authors concluded that ". . as many as 50% of such patients might *not* be worse off if their medications were withdrawn," either because they can do well without medication or because for a variety of reasons they do not do well on drugs. These findings are critical to the rehabilitation practitioner because the serious and often irreversible complications of prolonged maintenance medication can interfere with rehabilitation programs.

Particularly distressing are the side effects and the problems in drug-state learning and transfer of learning to the non-drug state (Tobias & MacDonald, 1974). It may be that although drug therapy can help support the rehabilitation intervention, long-term maintenance medication may do the opposite and actually hamper rehabilitation programming.

The relationship between drug therapy and rehabilitation may also be viewed in a slightly different way. It may be that a rehabilitation intervention could be conceived of as supportive to the withdrawal of drug therapy. That is, once drug therapy has prepared the helpee for rehabilitation, *a successful rehabilitation intervention might prepare the helpee for the removal of drug therapy.*

Another way in which rehabilitation programming may be supportive of drug therapy is by using the principles of rehabilitation programming to increase the probability of drug therapy compliance. A review of noncompliance data indicates an average noncompliance of 48% for phenothiazines, 49% for anti-anxiety or anti-depressant drugs and 32% for lithium (Barofsky, 1976). Following a drug regimen may be considered to be a skill and can be taught to a psychiatrically disabled helpee.

Providers of drug therapy might also wish to consider whether or not a rehabilitation diagnosis provides any additional information relevant to the need for drug therapy. It could be that client skill-level may partially predict the client's response to chemotherapy.

In summary, drug therapy may be considered as an often necessary but rarely sufficient component of rehabilitation programming. From a rehabilitation perspective, drug therapy must be considered to be a supportive technique, but hardly ever as an entire rehabilitation program. Likewise, practitioners of drug therapy may conceive of rehabilitation programming as supportive of their efforts at necessary drug compliance, determining the initial need for drug therapy or withdrawing (decreasing) drug dosage.

4. Counseling Techniques

On some occasions, counseling techniques may serve a useful function as part of an overall psychiatric rehabilitation program. Counseling techniques involve attempts to change the helpee's self-understanding.

At times, improved helpee self-understanding may be enough to affect the helpee's skilled performance. For example, the development of helpee insights may increase the frequency of helpee attempts at a particular skilled behavior. A concrete example of increased helpee insight, leading to changes in skilled performance, might be that of a helpee who refuses to work hard to improve his physical fitness skills until he or she first understands how the lack of physical fitness is restricting various aspects of his or her physical and emotional functioning.

The particular counseling skills needed to develop helpee insights are the same responsive and initiative skills discussed in the chapter on rehabilitation diagnosis (Carkhuff, 1972). Counseling techniques used in the context of a rehabilitation program are extremely goal directed, that is they are useful only to the extent that they affect the helpee's level of skills. In this regard, counseling techniques may be helpful when the psychiatrically disabled helpee is not attempting to perform a rehabilitation skill because he did not develop the necessary insight during the diagnostic process.

The inclusion of counseling techniques in a list of rehabilitation programmatic techniques is not meant as an attempt to encourage psychiatric rehabilitation practitioners to engage in the more traditional forms of counseling or psychotherapy. As noted earlier in Chapter II, research on psychiatric rehabilitation outcome has failed to support the belief that psychotherapeutic techniques alone can improve the helpee's community functioning.

5. Didactic Techniques

An important component of any rehabilitation program is that part of the program which tells the helpee exactly what type of skill he or she will be learning. The "tell" step is a fundamental step in any rehabilitation program. However, if the didactic step is mistakenly considered to be the entire program, skill learning rarely occurs.

Merely telling a person what to do does not insure that it will be done differently or better. This is especially true for a behavior which is well rehearsed or established. For example, telling a helpee to look for a job more frequently does not mean that his or her more frequent job-seeking behavior will be any more effective. In other words, increased frequency does not necessarily insure increased accuracy.

Unfortunately, much of the psychiatric rehabilitation practitioner's helping efforts in the past have revolved around advice giving or telling the psychiatrically disabled helpee what he or she should do. Yet the psychiatric rehabilitation practitioner's advice would be much more effective if it were part of an overall rehabilitation program which included opportunities for the helpee to be shown and to practice the desired behavior, as well as an observable standard against which the helpee could measure and receive feedback about his or her performance.

6. Modeling Techniques

Like didactic techniques, the efficacy of modeling techniques may be improved by incorporating these techniques into an overall rehabilitation program. Most simply, modeling techniques involve providing the helpee with the opportunity to observe other persons performing the skilled activity. This person is most often another helpee, a member of the helpee's community, or the person implementing the program. Effective models are often individuals with characteristics similar to the helpee; the major difference being that the model can effectively perform the skills which the helpee needs to develop. Pairing a psychiatrically disabled helpee with an effective community member may provide added incentive for the helpee to develop his or her own skills.

This opportunity to see the skilled activity performed, or the "show" step, is a fundamental part of any systematic rehabilitation program. Like all the rehabilitation programmatic techniques already mentioned, the value of the modeling technique may be increased by including the modeling technique in a systematic rehabilitation program developed and implemented on the principles of program development outlined in this chapter.

CONDUCTING REHABILITATION PROGRAMS IN A GROUP SETTING

Case Illustration 5-3

History

M is a 32-year-old, married man from a wealthy family in the Middle East. M's father is a successful businessman, who was also once a successful professor. M is the youngest child and has an older brother and sister, both relatively successful. M was sent to an English boarding school at the age of thirteen and reported that life was "a bit" difficult away from home, and that he had a hard time making friends. In the summers, while his father stayed at home, he, his mother, and his brother and sister would travel around Europe. During his university career, where he struggled with the high demands of his father's expectations, he received a minor electric shock when a coffee pot short-circuited. From this moment on, he began to deteriorate, hearing voices speaking to him from various appliances, fearing a conspiracy among his professors etc. He dropped out before completing his final year. At age twenty-five, he married a young Middle Eastern socialite who was fairly high-strung also. They had two children, who were aged two and three when M was first hospitalized. After his first hospital experience in Paris, M returned to the Middle East determined to make more money than his father, but failing at every business venture that he tried. By the time he arrived in America (brought by his now-frantic mother), he had ceased work of any kind. M appeared each day at ward meeting, exceedingly well dressed, and was often mistaken for one of the psychiatrists. He played the part of a businessman who had come to the United States to "investigate the market" rather than admit that he had been brought by a family who could no longer tolerate his erratic behavior and lack of communication with them.

Treatment

Because of his initial difficulty in separating his "voices" from those speaking to him in reality, and his cultural uneasiness in discussing any feelings, he was initially given Haldol, along with other medication, rather than psychotherapy right away. He was scheduled to participate in ward life: sports, community meetings, current affairs, etc., which he only did erratically. The medication seemed to help him participate in that he did arrive and could respond if directly questioned. He could not follow a conversation, however, and rambled so tangentially when spoken to that other patients seemed to avoid him.

Signs of tardive dyskinesia began to appear (dry mouth, fingers rolling, tongue flicking, etc). The Haldol had to be reduced and the confusion over the "voices" began to re-appear. As his decomposure increased, suggestions for the new strategies were requested of the treatment team by the psychiatrist. The rehabilitation counselor, supported by the team, approached M. The counselor wanted to see if M would be willing to participate in a training group that, it was explained, would help him to listen and respond to others. He became quite excited by the idea, and he confided that he often felt unable to give a "smart" answer when someone spoke to him because he had no idea what had been said. There was some concern on the part of the staff that M's paranoia might be so rampant as to possibly make training threatening for him.

M participated nonetheless in a step-by-step procedure that taught him to physically attend to others, reinforced his ability to maintain eye contact, increased his ability to hear what was said as measured by his ability to repeat the content verbatim, and his ability to repeat the essence of a statement to indicate to others that he had understood.

Feedback on M's behavior was directly solicited by both M and the rehabilitation counselor from other patients on the day ward, and particularly from those staff and patients attending the "team meetings," an arena identified by M as one in which he especially felt it important to be able to communicate. Patients reported that M seemed more "open" in that he looked at them more frequently. Staff reported that M spoke more in team meetings and was communicating more frequently in relation to the content of the meeting, rather than tangentially.

RESEARCH INVESTIGATIONS OF PSYCHIATRIC REHABILITATION PROGRAMMING

The present section divides the research investigations of psychiatric rehabilitation programming into two categories: 1) those investigations which demonstrate that psychiatrically disabled helpees can in fact learn skills and 2) those investigations which demonstrate that skill training for psychiatrically disabled helpees can have a positive effect on community functioning.

At first glance, investigations concerned with whether or not psychiatrically disabled helpees can learn skills seem superfluous. Our common sense tells us that, like anyone else, psychiatrically disabled helpees can learn skills. Yet skills training programs designed to increase various helpee skills have been far from the norm. Our common experience of psychiatric inpatient and outpatient facilities tells us that little of the psychiatrically disabled helpee's time is spent in systematic training designed to increase the helpee's level of skilled performance.

However, a great number of research studies have now been carried out which offer support for the belief that psychiatrically disabled helpees can learn skills. Analyzed as a group, these studies have used a variety of psychiatrically disabled populations (for example — inpatients and outpatients, chronically disabled and acute-

Discussion: Mental Health Practitioners

Mental health practitioners and rehabilitation practitioners must complement each other in the treatment process. In this case, the use of drugs to reduce symptoms had to be discontinued for a time. "Skill Training" was able to reduce the symptoms for the period of drug discontinuance.

The value of a group approach in this instance was to: 1) give the practitioner additional information about the client's learning and relationship skills; 2) use the members of the learning group as peer reinforcement; 3) give the client an experience of success both in terms of learning the skills presented and in helping other group members to learn those skills.

ly disabled) and have found that all psychiatrically disabled helpees studied were capable of increasing their levels of skilled performance. Particularly impressive is the fact that many of these studies successfully trained chronic long-term patients who had a lengthy history of symptomatic behavior. These findings, which demonstrate rather conclusively that psychiatrically disabled helpees who still possess severe symptoms are able to profit from rehabilitation skills training programs, are in direct contrast to the theory that rehabilitation begins only after psychiatric treatment ends. The psychiatrically disabled helpee's symptoms do *not have* to be overcome before rehabilitation programming can begin. It appears that the presence of severe psychiatric symptomatology does not preclude the effective utilization of rehabilitation skills training programs.

Specific research investigations have provided evidence of the fact that a variety of skills training programs for psychiatrically disabled helpees have either been developed or researched. Different programs have been developed and implemented to increase the psychiatrically disabled helpees physical, intellectual, and emotional functioning. In the physical area of functioning, training programs have been devised to extend the helpees' skills in a variety of areas, including the areas of: personal hygiene (Harrand, 1967; Retchless, 1967; Scoles & Fine, 1971; Weinman,

Sanders, Kleiner & Wilson, 1970), cooking (Scoles & Fine, 1971; Stein, Test & Marx, 1975; Weinman et al. 1970), use of public transportation (Harrand, 1967; Stein et al. 1975), use of recreational facilities (Harrand, 1967), use of particular job tools (Shean, 1973), and physical fitness (Dodsen & Mullens, 1969). In the emotional-interpersonal area of functioning, training programs have been designed to increase the psychiatrically disabled helpees' skills in such areas as: interpersonal skills (Hinterkopf & Brunswick, 1975; Ivey, 1973; Pierce & Drasgow, 1969; Vitalo, 1971), socialization skills (Bell, 1970; Goldsmith & McFall, 1975; Hersen & Bellack, 1976; Wood, Lenhard, Maggiani & Campbell, 1975; Weinman et al. 1970), self-control skills (Cheek & Mendelson, 1973; Rutner & Bugle, 1969), selective reward skills (Swanson & Woolson, 1972), problem-solving skills (Coche & Flick, 1975), and job-interviewing skills (McClure, 1972; Prazak, 1969). Lastly, in the area of intellectual functioning, training programs have increased the psychiatrically disabled helpees' abilities in such skill areas as: money management (Weinman et al. 1970), job seeking (McClure, 1972), and job applying (McClure, 1972; Safieri, 1970).

The research which has shown that psychiatrically disabled helpees can learn such an impressive variety of skills is an important finding within itself. The mere fact that psychiatrically disabled helpees can be trained to increase their skill levels may be a sufficient rationale for the use of rehabilitation skills training programs. However, if the skills training programs are truly rehabilitative in nature, they must also demonstrate that the helpees' improved physical, intellectual, and emotional functioning positively affects the helpees' ability to live, learn, and work in their community as independently as possible. The studies which have investigated whether or not skills training programs can have a positive effect on the helpees' community functioning are few in number but exhibit unanimity in their findings that effective skills training programs can translate into more effective community functioning.

The community-functioning criteria commonly used by these skills training outcome studies are the traditional rehabilitation outcome measures of recidivism and employment. Except for the study by Stein and Test (1975; 1976), similarities exist between many of these skills training outcome studies in that each used chronically disabled helpees, reinforced the skills generalization process through environmental or surrogate techniques, and used hospital recidivism rate as one of the criteria of success (Retchless, 1967; Scoles & Fine, 1971; Shean, 1973; Weinman et al. 1970; Wood et al. 1975). Each of these studies but one (Shean, 1973) provided training primarily in the living-skills area of functioning, including such skills as personal hygiene, other activities of daily living, and social or interaction skills. In contrast, Shean (1973) provided vocational skills training for a group of chronically disabled women.

Results of these studies have consistently indicated that skills training programs can have an effect on community functioning as measured by recidivism. Weinman et al. (1970) reported preliminary recidivism data which indicated that the group of helpees who received skills training combined with surrogate techniques had significantly outperformed the helpee group which had received traditional hospital treatment and aftercare. Although the remaining three studies did not make control-group comparisons, it is possible to obtain an estimate of their effectiveness by comparing their recidivism rates with the base-rate figures presented in Chapter II.

Retchless's (1967) skills training program combined with environmental techniques obtained a one-year recidivism rate of approximately 24%. Of the thirty-five psychiatrically disabled helpees who completed the eleven-week program, twenty-nine were released from the hospital and only seven returned. Scoles's and Fine's (1971) skills training program also utilized counseling, environmental, and surrogate techniques. Of the first one hundred helpees involved in this comprehensive program, the twelve- and eighteen-month recidivism rates were 6% and 9% respectively. Shean (1973) combined an inpatient vocational training program with outpatient environmental techniques and reported that the three-year recidivism rate for the sixteen psychiatrically disabled helpees discharged from the program was 12%. Wood et al. (1975) trained seventeen chronic female inpatients in interpersonal and assertive skills. After a two-month program (90 minutes, 3 times a week) sixteen of the seventeen patients were released from the hospital. At eight-month follow-up only one individual had returned to the hospital, a figure way below the base-rate percentages reported in Chapter II. The recidivism percentages for all of these studies are even more impressive due to the fact that recidivism rates for subgroups of chronically disabled helpees are typically higher than for an unselected population of psychiatrically disabled helpees.

Stein and Test (1976), in contrast to the aforementioned studies, trained their psychiatrically disabled helpees in the community instead of in the hospital. Subjects for this study consisted of helpees seeking admission to a state hospital. These helpees were randomly divided into an experimental and control group. The control subjects were treated in the hospital and then linked with appropriate community agencies. The experimental subjects were not hospitalized (except in rare instances) and instead received the authors' "Training in Community Living" approach. Results through the first year of the study indicated the experimental group hospitalization rate was significantly decreased and that these experimental group helpees spent significantly less time unemployed and earned more income through competitive employment than control group helpees.

A skills training program specifically designed to affect the outcome criterion of employment was undertaken by McClure (1972), who attempted to improve his rehabilitation clients' job-seeking and job-interviewing skills. It is not clear from McClure's (1972) description of the client population exactly what proportion of his skill learners were psychiatrically disabled helpees. However, what is clear from McClure's (1972) account is that the skills training program had a pronounced effect on the employment criterion of "employed for thirty days or more" at nine-week follow-up. Fifty percent of the helpees who received complete or partial training met the employment criterion, in contrast to only 24% of an untrained group.

Undoubtedly the most comprehensive skills training program to date is the program conducted by Carkhuff (1974). Although not concerned with adult psychiatrically disabled helpees, the reorganization of a training school for delinquent boys from a custodial orientation to a skills training orientation can serve as a model for the psychiatric rehabilitation field. The results of the program evidence further support for the concept of skills training. After one year of skills training programs, the training school's recidivism rate had decreased 30%, the runaway rate had decreased 57%, and the crime rate in the surrounding community had decreased 34%. In addition, the adolescents' physical fitness scores had increased 50% and reading ability had increased 157%.

Summarily, it would seem that the research investigations of psychiatric rehabilitation programming have successfully demonstrated that psychiatrically disabled helpees can in fact learn skills, and that these skills, when properly integrated into a comprehensive rehabilitation program, can have an effect on the helpee's community functioning. However, this is not to imply that there are not methodological shortcomings in the skills training research. The same methodological problems that plague all psychiatric rehabilitation research are also present in the rehabilitation skills training research. Among the shortcomings of some of the studies is a very small number of subjects, incomplete follow-up, lack of legitimate control groups, an inadequate description of the helpees studied or the specific skills upon which they were trained, a propensity to report the data on only those who have completed the program rather than data on all who have entered the program, and a superficial presentation of the outcome data.

It is rather easy (and meaningless) to state critically that more and better research is needed. What is not so easy is to actually conduct the research. Indeed, the field of psychiatric rehabilitation is fortunate that a few program developers and researchers have braved the ever-present research pitfalls, and have provided psychiatric rehabilitation practitioners with a foundation upon which to develop better rehabilitation skills training programs and more efficient ways to evaluate and report on the efficacy of these programs.

PSYCHIATRIC REHABILITATION PROGRAMMING – FUTURE NEEDS

In addition to more comprehensive research investigations of our psychiatric rehabilitation programming efforts, there are a series of other interdependent rehabilitation programming needs. A pressing need exists for the dissemination of information about those psychiatric rehabilitation programs which have been successfully developed and implemented. Because the field of psychiatric rehabilitation cuts across various disciplines, it is extremely difficult to remain knowledgeable about the various rehabilitation programming innovations. It would seem that a definite need exists for the development of a series of books or a specific journal devoted to providing detailed descriptions of effective psychiatric rehabilitation programming.

A related rehabilitation programming requirement, which would make the dissemination of programming information more valuable, is the need for the descriptions of present and future programs to be reported more systematically. If the psychiatric rehabilitation program is not written in a systematic observable manner, it cannot be used by other psychiatric rehabilitation practitioners. It is therefore imperative that the words used to describe the program are concrete and understandable to a psychiatric rehabilitation practitioner who is initially unfamiliar with the program.

This detailed dissemination of information can be improved if another related programming need is met, that is, the specific training of psychiatric rehabilitation practitioners in the skills of program development. Indeed, program development skills should be a requirement for all personnel engaged in the practice of psychiatric rehabilitation (Chapter XI provides a further discussion of psychiatric rehabilitation training). The psychiatric rehabilitation practitioner trained in programming skills would be better able to describe his or her program in an observable systematic manner. Also, because the practitioner possesses the necessary reporting ability, she or he might be much more likely to insure that the programming information is disseminated.

Thus, the key to the future needs in the field of psychiatric rehabilitation programming would appear to be best met through program development training. A psychiatric rehabilitation practitioner trained in program development skills, as well as some of the other rehabilitation practitioner skills outlined in Chapter XI, would have the ability to develop and implement rehabilitation programs, evaluate the effectiveness of these programs, and describe these programs in detail to other psychiatric rehabilitation practitioners.

OPERATIONALIZING THE TEAM APPROACH

Case Illustration 5-4

One of the advantages of training rehabilitation practitioners in program development skills is that the responsibility for different programming tasks can be specifically determined. For example, John and Elaine were young parents (both in their early 20's); they came to the attention of the mental health facility because they had physically abused their children and were frightened that this would continue. The eldest child was already a "school problem" and had been suspended

97

a number of times.

A diagnostic planning chart was developed with the parents, focusing on their emotional problems in the "living" area, and specifically in those in relation to George, their eldest child. It soon became clear that the programs that had to be developed would involve a number of persons, from a number of different sectors. The following chart was drawn up with the treatment team and the parents together. A copy was given to each, in order to be clear on who was responsible for what. The parents reported that just having the chart made them feel more hopeful — "If it is all down on paper, and we know who is doing what, it just doesn't seem so impossible to do!"

As illustrated by the Program Planning Chart, it is possible to indicate who will be ultimately responsible for developing the program, teaching the program (in the care of acquisition programs), and monitoring the program. Basically, the person who *develops* the program is the person responsible for writing and sequencing the necessary program steps. The person who *teaches* the program is the person who devises and implements the teaching strategy to insure that the client actually acquires the skill.

The person who *monitors* the program assures that differential reinforcement and needed modifications are made as a result of the client's successful or unsuccessful program performance. Often, but not always, one person performs the same three functions for each skill behavior.

Note that there are a number of people involved in the development, instruction, and monitoring processes. Although initially this may look unduly complicated, essentially this program planning chart operationalizes what has heretofore euphemistically been called the rehabilitation "team approach." The problem with the historical use of the team approach has been an inability of the team members to understand what the other members are specifically responsible for, with the result often being confusion of the client and conflict between the team members.

Psychiatric rehabilitation cannot have a team approach without a game plan.

However, the team must be a team in more than name only. *Each member must have observable goals for each client and other team members.* Without this there is no team. Obviously the complexity of the program plan that develops is a function of the number and kind of client skill deficits, as well as the number of rehabilitation environments under consideration. If there is one lesson that psychiatric rehabilitation must learn, it is that low-level-functioning clients require complex and detailed program plans.

It is obvious that a number of psychiatric rehabilitation programs still need to be developed in a variety of physical, intellectual, and emotional areas of functioning. The next chapter highlights one area of functioning that has been almost devoid of rehabilitation programming — the psychiatrically disabled helpee's physical area of functioning. The emphasis on the physical area of functioning is of much greater importance than the intellectual and emotional areas of functioning. Rather, the emphasis of the next chapter on the psychiatrically disabled helpee's physical functioning is due to the seemingly systematic avoidance of this area in our current attempts at both psychiatric treatment and rehabilitation.

REFERENCES

Anthony, W. A. Psychological rehabilitation: A concept in need of a method. **American Psychologist**, 1977, *32*: 658-662.

Anthony, W. A., Buell, G. J., Sharratt, S. and Althoff, M. E. Efficacy of psychiatric rehabilitation. **Psychological Bulletin**, 1972, 78: 447-456.

Program Planning Chart

Environment	Person	Skill	Program Type	Program Development	Instructor	Monitor	Begin	End
Living	John Elaine	Discipline Children	Acquisition	Rehabilitation Center	PET Leader	S.W.	Sept. 76	April 77
	John	Making Verbal Feeling Statements	Application	Therapist	—	Elaine S.W.	Sept. 76	1 Month
	Elaine	Assertiveness Skills	Acquisition	Rehabilitation Center	Women's Center	John W.C. Lr.	August 76	1 Month
Learning	George	Attendance	Application	Child-Care Worker	—	Grade Teacher	Sept. 76	June 77
		"Learning to Learn Skills"	Acquisition	Rehabilitation Center	Child-Care Worker	Grade Teacher	August 76	Oct. 76

Anthony, W. A., Cohen, M. R. and Vitalo, R. The measurement of rehabilitation outcome. **Schizophrenia Bulletin**, 1978, in press.

Anthony, W. A. and Margules, A. Toward improving the efficacy of psychiatric rehabilitation. A skills training approach. **Rehabilitation Psychology**, 1974, *21*: 101-105.

Anthony, W. A., Pierce, R. M. and Cohen, M. R. **Psychiatric rehabilitation practice: The skills of diagnostic planning.** Amherst, Mass.: Carkhuff Institute of Human Technology, 1977.(a)

Anthony, W. A., Pierce, R. M. and Cohen, M. R. **Psychiatric rehabilitation practice: The skills of rehabilitation programming.** Amherst, Mass.: Carkhuff Institute of Human Technology, 1977. (b)

Aspy, D. N. and Roebuck, F. N. **KIDS don't learn from people they don't like.** Amherst, Mass.: Human Resource Development Press, 1977.

Baker, F. M., Baker, R. J. and McDaniel, R. S. Denormalizing practices in rehabilitation facilities. **Rehabilitation Literature**, 1975, *36*: 112-115.

Barofsky, I. Therapeutic noncompliance by the psychiatric patient. Paper presented at the New England Conference on the Chronic Psychiatric Patient in the Community, Boston, Mass., Nov., 1976.

Bell, R. L. Practical applications of psychodrama: Systematic role-playing teaches social skills. **Hospital and Community Psychiatry**, 1970, *21*: 189-191.

Carkhuff, R. R. **Cry twice! From custody to treatment — The story of institutional change.** Amherst, Mass.: Human Resource Development Press, 1974.

Cautela, J. R. and Kastenbaum, R. A reinforcement survey schedule for use in therapy, training and research. **Psychological Reports**, 1967, *20*: 115-130.

Cheek, F. E. and Mendelson, M. Developing behavior modification programs with an emphasis on self-control. **Hospital and Community Psychiatry**, 1973, *24*: 410-416.

Coche, E. and Flick, A. Problem solving training groups for hospitalized psychiatric patients. **The Journal of Psychology**, 1975, *91*: 19-29.

Davis, A. E., Dinitz, S. and Pasaminick, B. The prevention of hospitalization in schizophrenia: Five years after an experimental program. **American Journal of Orthopsychiatry**, 1972, *42*: 375-378.

Davis, J. M., Gosenfeld, L. and Tsai, C. C. Maintenance antipsychotic drugs do prevent relapse: A reply to Tobias and MacDonald. **Psychological Bulletin**, 1976, *83*: 431-447.

Dodson, L. C. and Mullens, W. R. Some effects of jogging on psychiatric hospital patients. **American Corrective Therapy Journal**, 1969, *23*: 130-134.

Dowling, T. H. and Frantz, T. T. The influence of a facilitative relationship on imitative learning. **Journal of Counseling Psychology**, 1975, *22*: 254-263.

Engelhardt, D. M. and Rosen, B. Implications of drug treatment for the social rehabilitation of schizophrenia patients. **Schizophrenia Bulletin**, 1976, *2*: 454-462.

Franklin, J., Kittredge, L. and Thrasher, J. A survey of factors related to mental hospital readmissions. **Hospital and Community Psychiatry**, 1975, *26*: 749-751.

Gardos, G. and Cole, J. O. Maintenance antipsychotic therapy: Is the cure worse than the disease? **American Journal of Psychiatry**, 1976, *133:1*, 32-36.

Goldsmith, J. B. and McFall, R. M. Development and evaluation of an interpersonal skill training program for psychiatric inpatients. **Journal of Abnormal Psychology**, 1975, *84*: 51-58.

Harrand, G. Rehabilitation programs for chronic patients: Testing the potential for independence. **Hospital and Community Psychiatry**, 1967, *18*: 376-377.

Hersen, M. and Bellack, A. S. Social skills training for chronic psychiatric patients: Rationale, research findings and future directions. **Comprehensive Psychiatry**, 1976, *17*: 559-580.

Hinterkopf, E. and Brunswick, L. K. Teaching therapeutic skills to mental patients. **Psychotherapy: Theory, Research and Practice**, 1975, *12*: 8-12.

Ivey, A. E. Media therapy: Educational change planning for psychiatric patients. **Journal of Counseling Psychology**, 1973, *20*: 338-343.

Lamb, H. R. **Rehabilitation in community mental health.** San Francisco: Jossey-Bass, 1971.

London, P. The end of ideology in behavior modification. **American Psychologist**, 1972, *27*: 913-920.

MacDonald, M. L. and Tobias, L. L. Withdrawal causes relapse? Our response. **Psychological Bulletin**, 1976, *83*: 448-451.

McClure, D. P. Placement through improvement of client's job-seeking skills. **Journal of Applied Rehabilitation Counseling**, 1973, *3*: 188-196.

Mickelson, D. J. and Stivic, R. R. Differential effects of facilitative and nonfacilitative behavioral counselors. **Journal of Counseling Psychology**, 1971, *18*: 314-317.

Mosher, L. R., Feinsilver, D., Katz, M. M. and Weinckowski, L. A. **Special report on schizophrenia.** Bethesda, Md.: National Institute of Mental Health, 1970.

Pasaminick, B., Scarpetti, F. R. and Dinitz, S. **Schizophrenics in the community.** New York: Appleton-Century-Crofts, 1967.

Pierce, R. M. and Drasgow, J. Teaching facilitative interpersonal functioning to psychiatric inpatients. **Journal of Counseling Psychology**, 1969, *16*: 295-298.

Prazak, J. A. Learning job-seeking interview skills. In Krumboltz and Thoreson eds. **Behavioral Counseling.** New York: Holt, Rinehart & Winston, Inc., 1979, 414-424.

Retchless, M. H. Rehabilitation programs for chronic patients: Stepping stones to the community. **Hospital and Community Psychiatry,** 1967, *18*: 377-378.

Rutner, I. T. and Bugle, G. An experimental procedure for the modification of psychotic behavior, **Journal of Consulting & Clinical Psychology,** 1969, *33*: 651-653.

Safieri, D. Using an education model in a sheltered workshop program. **Mental Hygiene,** 1970, *54*: 140-143.

Scoles, P. and Fine, E. Aftercare and rehabilitation in a community mental health center. **Social Work,** 1971, *16*: 75-82.

Shean, G. An effective and self-supporting program of community living for chronic patients. **Hospital and Community Psychiatry,** 1973, *24*: 97-99.

Stein, L. A., Test, M. A. and Marx, A. J. Alternative to the hospital: A controlled study. **American Journal of Psychiatry,** 1975, *132*: 517-522.

Stein, L. A. and Test, M. A. Training in community living: An alternative to mental hospital treatment. Paper presented at the New England Conference on the Chronic Psychiatric Patient in the Community, Boston, Mass., Nov., 1976.

Swanson, M. G. and Woolson, A. M. A new approach to the use of learning theory with psychiatric patients. **Perspectives in Psychiatric Care,** 1972, *10*: 55-68.

Tobias, L. L. and MacDonald, M. L. Withdrawal of maintenance drugs with long term hospitalized mental patients: A critical review. **Psychological Bulletin,** 1974, *81*: 107-125.

Vitalo, R. The effects of facilitative interpersonal functioning in a conditioning paradigm. **Journal of Counseling Psychology,** 1970, *17*: 141-144.

Vitalo, R. L. Teaching improved interpersonal functioning as a preferred model of treatment. **Journal of Clinical Psychology,** 1971, *27*: 166-171.

Weinman, B., Sanders, R., Kleiner, R. and Wilson, S. Community based treatment of the chronic psychotic. **Community Mental Health Journal,** 1970, *6*: 12-21.

Wolfensberger, W. The principle of normalization and its implications to psychiatric services. **American Journal of Psychiatry,** 1970, *127*: 291-297.

Wood, D., Lenhard S., Maggiani, M. and Campbell, M. Assertive training of the chronic mental patient. **Journal of Psychiatric Nursing and Mental Health Services,** 1975, *13*: 42-46.

Yolles, S. F. In foreword to **Schizophrenia in the community** by B. Pasaminick, F. R. Scarpetti and S. Dinitz. New York: Appleton-Century-Crofts, 1967.

CHAPTER VI
Physical Fitness as a Component in Psychiatric Rehabilitation

The concept of physical fitness has achieved significant visibility over the past decade. Where once a person jogging along a road or neighborhood street was greeted by astonished stares — today, that same phenomenon rarely evokes an attending response from passers-by. Indeed, as evidenced by the increase in sales of jogging equipment, in the numbers and memberships of local exercise classes for adults, and even in the growing popularity of marathon running (10,000 - 20,000 participants yearly, Consumer Reports, 1977), the concept of physical fitness has clearly emerged in popular awareness. To a large extent, this popularity may be attributed to the highly readable and widely disseminated works of Cooper (1972, 1972a).

Notwithstanding the emergence of popular concern for the issue of physical fitness, the topic has achieved little attention in the fields of psychology and rehabilitation. This judgment sustains despite the emergence of the corrective therapy movement of the 1940's (Knudson & Davis, 1949; Layman, 1960) which initiated the introduction of physical activity into psychiatric inpatient treatment programming, but which failed to significantly penetrate the fields of psychology, psychiatry, or social work and enter the general arena of therapeutic intervention outside inpatient care. The failure of the issue of physical fitness to penetrate the attention of the fields of psychiatry, psychology, and social work may, in part, be due to the little importance the dimension of physical fitness has had in psychological theory, especially in the areas of personality and therapy (Currie & Harris, 1971). Indeed, until recently, few theorists have given even passing attention to the contribution of the fitness dimension to the overall effective functioning of people. Process theorists such as Rogers, Maslow, and Allport place no stress on this dimension, although Maslow (1954) does state that the self-actualizing person evidences a high energy level, an unusual capacity for work, and an unusually high level of productivity. Rogers (1959), however, does not include the dimension of physical energy and fitness in his definition of the fully functioning person, nor does Allport (1961) in his definition of the "mature personality."

Trait and factor theorists such as Cattell (1957) and typologists such as Sheldon and Kretchmer (Hall & Lindsey, 1957) include reference to physiological factors of a constitutional nature in determining personality functioning. Functional and behaviorally modifiable criteria such as fitness are not referred to. Similarly, while dynamic theorists such as Freud and Jung do refer to energy level and energy resources, they too appear to be talking about constitutional and behaviorally unmodifiable capacities. This maintains despite the Freudian hypothesis that reduction of energy resources due to illness may be a precipitating cause for the onset of neurosis (Fenechel, 1945).

The only significant exception to this apparent indifference to the concept of physical fitness is in the work of Carkhuff (1969). He reintroduces the physical dimension as a critical dimension in the effective functioning of the healthy person. Indeed, success in the physical area of living is seen as a prerequisite for success in the emotional-interpersonal and intellectual areas (Carkhuff, 1969). Relatedly, this author posits that effective educational and therapeutic processes must incorporate the enhancement of students and clients on physical dimensions.

With the significant exception of the work of Carkhuff (1969), then, the question of the relevance of physical fitness for the therapeutic and rehabilitative process has not received significant professional exploration. Indeed, with the exception of several unpublished papers (Vitalo, 1973; 1973a), the existing findings relating physical fitness to areas of concern in the field of psychology do not appear to have been integrated and professionally reviewed. Thus, even the existing professional efforts to explore the relationship of elements in this concept of physical fitness to processes of therapeutic rehabilitation has not achieved wide visibility. Thus, the full range of implications of physical fitness for therapeutic and rehabilitative processes has not been explored, nor have guidelines for integrating physical fitness into the rehabilitative treatment process been offered (Vitalo, 1973b). This chapter addresses the need for expanding the awareness of professionals to the relevance of physical fitness in the rehabilitative process, and some fundamental guidelines to assist in introducing fitness as a component of psychiatric rehabilitation. As a prerequisite to this objective, it is first necessary to form a common understanding of the concept of physical fitness and, as well, the concept of psychiatric rehabilitation. From this base, we can make some initial formulation concerning the mutual relatedness of these two realms. This base of initial understanding will serve as a starting point for a more detailed analysis of the relevance of physical fitness to psychiatric rehabilitation.

PHYSICAL FITNESS

Physical fitness has a variety of conceptual identifications. For some, fitness is understood as an athletic ability or participation. For others, fitness is identified with one or another type of exercise — as for example, jogging or cycling. Still further, for some, it is identified with body building.

Paralleling this variety of conceptual identifications has been a wide variety of empirical definitions for physical fitness. Empirically, fitness has been equated with athletic participation, especially with varsity team membership. It has also been assessed and therefore operationally defined by indices of balance and coordination, speed, strength, muscular endurance, and cardiovascular endurance. Specific indices of assessment have included: length of time for balancing on one foot, dynometer measures of strength of hand grip, time for 60-yard dash, number of push-ups or length of time for arm-hang, step test, and 12-minute run test. In general, these diverse measures may be divided into two classes: (a) measurements of skill and (b) measurements of capacity. Measurements of skill evaluate balance and coordination. Measurements of capacity evaluate such dimensions as speed, strength, muscular endurance, and cardiovascular endurance.

Factor analytic studies (McCloy, 1938; Fleishman, 1964) suggest that there are six basic factor groupings or measures of fitness (speed, agility, strength, balance/coordination, muscular endurance, and cardiovascular endurance) which should be assessed if a complete picture of physical fitness is to be obtained. It is important to note that athletic participation does not appear to be a good predictor of physical fitness as measured by these dimensions (Olree, 1961; Fleishman, 1964).

While much detailed work on specific measures of "physical fitness" and their inter-relatedness has been done in the field of sports medicine and sports physiology, no integrated functional definition of physical fitness has been provided. It is as though the field began with the analysis of the elemental parts of fitness and has never been able to regroup those elemental parts to rediscover the experiential whole from which their initial research efforts evolved. Thus, the confusion as to just what the concept of physical fitness means has persisted. Integrative research has only produced statements of intercorrelation between measures and identification of factor loadings. While such discoveries facilitate more efficient research design, they do not facilitate the applied scientist's efforts to translate research findings into human applications and benefits. This failure in turn compromises the pure researcher's ability to recycle his or her initial efforts and deepen their significance.

What has been lacking — and what is essential for exploring the relevance of physical fitness to rehabilitation — is the perspective that physical fitness is a statement of functional capacity. In essence, it is a statement of the functional capacity of the body to produce sufficient energy, strength, and flexibility in order to support the effective performance of one's living-, learning-, and working-role functions. In essence, the question that has not been asked is simply: fitness for what? With this perspective it is clear that fitness is not any specific exercise nor is it the process of exercising. It is, in fact, a statement of vital capacity. Minimal fitness simply denotes the presence of sufficient energy, strength, and flexibility such that physical functioning does not detract from the quantity and quality of expected role performance across the variety of responsibilities a person assumes in the course of his or her living.

This perspective on physical fitness derives from two fundamental understandings. First, people are physical beings. Second, while the focus of people is usually on the activities they are engaged in and the responsibilities they are executing — each of a person's behavioral operations depends on some requisite level of physical resources in order to be implemented. The relevance of physical fitness for human functioning, then, becomes self-evident. In essence, no activity engaged in and no objective that might be pursued is at all achievable without some specific requirement of energy, strength, and movement (flexibility). Relatedly, any activity or pursued objective which is not supported by sufficient energy, strength, and adequacy of movement will fail.

This functional perspective on physical fitness generates three additional important implications. First, it becomes clear that physical fitness as a qualitative statement of adequacy of physical resources will denote *different levels* of energy, strength, and flexibility for different people, since the quantity and quality demand of roles and goals maintained and pursued by people in their living, learning, and working endeavors varies widely. This is not to say that there may not be some absolute level of production of energy, strength, and movement (flexibility) necessary to ensure adequate health or prolongation of life. It is to say that any general standard defining a specific level of energy production, strength development, and

movement capacity as a criteria for minimal fitness is useless unless it also specifies the quantity and nature of life's responsibilities and role performances which it will sustain. Furthermore, it is clear that the level of fitness a person will need at one point in his or her life may differ from the level needed at another point as roles or personal objectives are added or relinquished.

A second significant implication emanating from this perspective on physical fitness is that the selection of an exercise is determined by its functional relationship to the capacity which is required in order to better support one's life-role functioning. Thus, although all of the measures suggested earlier have relevance for one's physical fitness, the particular exercise one chooses depends upon its ability to develop the capacity (energy production, strength development or movement) which is currently insufficient to support effective and efficient role performance. Thus, no particular exercise has *a priori* eminence.

A third important implication is that the value of any particular exercise regimen is in its capacity for increasing energy production, strength development, and movement capacity in order to better support effective goal functioning.

In summary, the perspective on physical fitness offered is pragmatically determined. It answers the question of "fitness for what?" by defining fitness as a vital capacity of the body to produce energy, develop strength, and facilitate movement. It assigns the standards of fitness individualistically and functionally as that level of energy production, strength development, and movement capacity which is necessary to support the effective and efficient performance of role functions determined by the responsibilities and objectives one has assumed in his or her living, learning, and working activities.

REHABILITATION

Previous chapters have distinguished rehabilitation from traditional psychotherapy. Rehabilitation requires a competency-based understanding of problems in living in terms of "skill deficits." The skill

deficits undermine effective role performance and a successful implementation of role functions (Anthony, Cohen and Vitalo, 1978; Carkhuff, 1969, 1971, 1976).

Rehabilitation, then, is a process of teaching an individual to function effectively in his or her life. Although it shares with traditional psychotherapy the mission of helping someone who has been identified as emotionally disabled or mentally ill terminate that status of impairment, it distinguishes itself from traditional psychotherapy by singularly emphasizing the delivery of real skills to clients which they can then competently apply to real-life situations. In this regard, the process of rehabilitation can be understood as steps of exploring and understanding the areas of the client's negative life outcome, exploring and understanding the specific skill deficiencies producing these negative life outcomes, teaching clients the skills needed to remedy their skill deficiencies, supervising the application of these newly learned skills to achieve the reversal of the negative life outcomes and, indeed, the achievement of positive life outcomes (Anthony, Cohen and Vitalo, 1978; Carkhuff, 1976; Vitalo, Cohen and Walker, 1974). The efficacy of the rehabilitation process is assessed at two levels. First, at the process level, the efficacy of the rehabilitation process is assessed by the level of success in skill acquisition evidenced by the client. Second, at the outcome level, the rehabilitation process is assessed by the level of positive outcomes achieved in the client's life through his or her successful application of the newly learned skill(s).

TENTATIVE LINKAGE BETWEEN PHYSICAL FITNESS AND PSYCHIATRIC REHABILITATION

By definition, physical fitness relates to success in living. It refers to the level of vital capacity requisite for successful role performance. In essence, it is the underlying physical resources required for the successful achievement of any personal life outcome. The rehabilitation process relates also to success in living. Indeed, the rehabilitation process is the re-establishment of successful life process and, even more specifically, it enables a person to achieve positive life outcomes which, in the past, have been sources of failure. Thus, the concepts intercept in mutual

support of personal achievements and success. Logically, one might suspect that inadequate fitness might in fact be an area of breakdown in role performance and a source of problem in living. Indeed, supporting this logic is the repeated research finding of a significant relationship between fitness levels and the presence of psychiatrically diagnosed disorders, severity of disorders, and length of hospitalization (Hodgdon and Reimer, 1960, 1962; Linton, Hamelink and Hoskins, 1934; McFarland and Huddelson, 1936; McKinney, 1947; Morgan, 1968, 1970a; Nadel and Horvath, 1967). The absence of the skill of fitness in the repertoire of the distressed client may be a significant contributor to failures in living. Since rehabilitation is itself a life process with role functions defined for both the rehabilitation counselor and the client, it too presumably requires a certain level of fitness for successful fulfillment.

Although the question remains as to the relevance of physical fitness for the rehabilitation process, an empirically based answer could potentially open up an area of understanding which might significantly enhance rehabilitation outcomes. To generate that answer, research will be reviewed relating physical fitness to effective living and learning, including learning as manifested in the therapeutic and rehabilitative process. Implications for the area of rehabilitation will be drawn and principles or guidelines for the introduction of physical fitness to rehabilitative process will be provided.

PHYSICAL FITNESS AND EFFECTIVE LIVING

Although the rehabilitation process may be freely defined as the elimination of skill deficiencies which undermine a person's ability to achieve personally valued life outcomes, it remains essentially an empirical question as to whether physical fitness does indeed relate to personal achievement. Although a considerable body of research has investigated the relationship of fitness to a variety of indices of effective living, few studies have incorporated a comprehensive evaluation of fitness itself.

Most studies assessed the dimensions of speed, strength, and muscular endurance. Some studies have assessed skill type measures such as balance and coordination, while still others have used indices of cardiovascular fitness. The strongest research emphasis has been in the areas of speed, strength, and muscular endurance. Since most studies have not included measures of cardiovascular endurance, a negative bias in the research may have been introduced. Cardiovascular fitness or the capacity of the body to generate and sustain high energy levels is considered the most critical component of functional fitness (Collingwood, 1972; Cooper, 1972).

In reviewing research investigating the relationship of fitness to areas of effective living, studies incorporating athletic participation as an index of fitness were eliminated. As indicated above, athletic participation is not a good predictor of other indices of physical fitness. Finally, for the purpose of communication, research findings relating fitness to areas of effective living will be organized in terms of realistic results relating fitness to performance of living functions, learning functions, and working functions.

Physical Fitness and Success in Living Area Role Functions

The living area of activity refers to those personal, family, and community roles which an individual assumes. Research relating fitness to this arena of roles has predominantly focused on the contribution of physical fitness to characteristics of personal well-being and social effectiveness.

A repeated finding has been the relationship of physical fitness to the presence, severity, and duration of diagnosed psychiatric disorders. Generally, schizophrenic patients have demonstrated significantly poorer cardiovascular and muscular strength fitness than normal subjects (Hodgdon & Reimer, 1962; Linton, Hamelink & Hoskins, 1934; McFarland & Huddelson, 1936; Nadel & Horvath, 1967). Diagnosed male depressives show similar poor fitness levels (Morgan, 1968) and emotionally disturbed students report in-

ferior levels of physical fitness in comparison to normal students (McKinney, 1947). Furthermore, although fitness does not appear to decrease through the course of psychiatric hospitalization (Rice, Rosenberg, and Radzyminski, 1961), levels of fitness appear related to the severity of psychiatric diagnosis (Hodgon and Reimer, 1960) and to the length of hospitalization (Morgan, 1970a). Finally, at least one factor analytic study found support for the conclusion that lack of fitness related to emotional instability (Ismail and Young, 1976). Generally then, despite Reid's (1955) failure to find differences in fitness levels between normal and deviant scoring students on the MMPI, and Morgan's (1970) finding of no difference between fitness levels of diagnosed female depressives and normal controls, the positive findings of nine out of eleven studies do suggest an inverse relationship between fitness and the presence of psychiatric diagnosis.

A related area of research investigation has studied the relationship between fitness levels and performance on written tests of personality and adjustment. One highly consistent finding has been that fitness negatively relates to scores on tests assessing anxiety, tension, and cynicism (Breen, 1959; Harris, 1963; Ismail, Kane and Kirkendall, 1969). The finding of a negative relationship between physical fitness and anxiety is reinforced by the findings of Wood (1977) and Folkins (1976). Both researchers observed significant decreases in anxiety in initially high anxious subjects following a fitness-enhancing training program.

Mixed results, however, are reported for the relationship of fitness to written measures of overall adjustment. Weber (1954) found no relationship between fitness scores and MMPI scales scores. Keogh (1959) reports similar findings for personal adjustment scores as measured by the California Personality Inventory. Similarly, Clarke and Clarke (1960) report no difference in fitness levels between high- and low-scoring subjects on the Mental Health Adjustment Index, and Clarke and Greene (1964) found only twelve significant correlations out of one hundred twenty-one between fitness and indices of low adjustment. Even more recently, Carron and Witzel (1975) found no relationship between fitness measures and personality scores as measured by the Cattell High School Personality Questionnaire. Yet, Morgan, Roberts, Brand, and Feinermain (1970) report a significant multiple correlation between physical variables and depression scores, and Bossung (Cowell and Ismail, 1962) reports a significant relationship between scores on the Cowell Social Adjustment Scale and fitness. Further, in contrast to Keogh's results, Biddulph (1954) reports a significant relationship between fitness and self-adjustment scores on the California Personality Inventory. In contrast to the Carron and Witzel's (1975) findings, a review of Werner and Gottheil's (1966) apparent negative findings reveal that significant changes in personality as measured by Cattell's 16 PF did follow a four year program of physical education for a group of college age students without prior athletic experience. Also in contrast to Weber's findings Sharp and Reilly (1975) find that physical fitness scores correlate significantly and negatively with seven out of twelve indices drawn from the MMPI. Still further Folkins (1976), Morgan et al. (1970), Hellerstein et al. (1967) each reported significant reduction in scores on written tests assessing depression in initially high scoring subjects following systematic fitness training. Morgan et al. (1970) and Naughton et al. (1968) found no change in depression scores following fitness training for subjects whose initial scores were in the normal range. Thus, of fourteen findings relating fitness to scores on written tests of emotional adjustment, eight report significant inverse findings and six report no significant results. Finally, studies by Harris (1963), Tillman (1965), and Wells (1969) provide a profile of individual personality characteristics significantly related to levels of fitness. High levels of fitness were found positively related to such preferred indices of functioning as: social confidence, social acceptance, social initiative, calm, composure, competent assertiveness, critical ex-

actness, high motivation, persistence, greater group dependence, greater insight into others, adventurousness, good appearance, leadership, and greater self awareness. Typically, the physically fit person is depicted on written tests as resourceful and independent yet group oriented, uninhibited yet able to control feelings, adventurous yet dependable, calm, assertive, socially esteemed, and competent.

Another area of research also involving written assessments has related fitness levels to positive self-concept. Findings in this area have been more consistent. With the exception of the study by Bolton and Milligan (1976), research supports a positive relationship between levels of fitness and levels of positive self-concept (Leonardson, 1977), and improvement in levels of fitness with significant improvement in reported self-concept (Collingwood, 1972a; Collingwood and Stockwell, 1973; Collingwood and Willett, 1971; Johnson et al. 1968). Relatedly, significant improvement in fitness levels has also been related to increased positive body image (Dodson and Mullens, 1969; Johnson et al. 1968).

Other studies relating physical fitness to different objective indices of emotional adjustment and social achievement have produced even more consistent findings. Eleven studies have investigated the relationship between fitness levels and its interpersonal effectiveness using peer sociograms. In extreme group comparisons of subjects scoring most fit and least fit, Biddulph (1954) and Clarke and Clarke (1960) report that high fitness groups are significantly more frequently chosen as friends by peers than low fitness groups. Approaching the issue from the opposite direction, Hardy (1937) found a significant difference in fitness levels for most popular and least popular students. Correlational analysis reported by Cowell and Ismail (1962), Huey (1949), McGraw and Tolbert (1953), Oliver (1960), Raven (1951), and Shaw (1960) all indicated significant relationships between levels of fitness and social success. Reported coefficients range from a low of .24 to a high of .78. Furthermore, a trend emerges in which the strength of the relationship between fitness and social success increases with the age groups of the subjects being studied. Thus, and contrary to intuitive expectation, physical fitness appears to be a more critical component of effective social adjustment in older groups than in younger groups.

Additional studies have investigated a relationship of fitness with still other objective measures of interpersonal adjustment and social effectiveness. Lindsey (1970) researched the effects of two years of fitness training on normal subjects and found significant improvement in personal and social adjustment as evaluated by objective ratings. Kratochvil, Carkhuff, and Berenson (1969) report finding a significant relationship between level of fitness in elementary school children and level of social skills. Two studies using teacher ratings of students (Rarick and McKee, 1949; Smart and Smart, 1963) find significant relationships between fitness and achievement in the areas of popularity, leadership, happiness, dependability, calm, freedom from tension, resourcefulness, group orientation and overall emotional adjustment. Still another study (Alexander, 1956) found significant differences in fitness levels for a group of grade school children rated well adjusted (n = 486) and a second group of children rated non-well adjusted (n = 228). Finally, Smith and Hurst (1961) report that motor ability accounts for 76% of the variance in social initiative (frequency of initiating social contacts) and social acceptance (frequency of receiving initiated contacts) in educable mental retardees, and 55% of the variance in trainable mental retardees. In an earlier review of the research, Vitalo (1973a) estimated that fitness accounted for between 25% to 30% of outcome variance in emotional adjustment and social achievement among intellectually normal subjects based on correlational and factor analytic research reported to that date.

Physical Fitness and Performance in the Learning Area

A number of studies have investigated the relationship of physical fitness and academic success. In general, findings strongly support a significant relationship between fitness and learning performance. The relationship between fitness and intelligence tests scores, however, has received more modest support.

Hart and Shay (1964) report a Product-Moment correlation of .49 between first-year college grades and physical fitness for female students. The relationship between fitness and academic success rose to .66 when the effects of Scholastic Aptitude Tests scores were removed. Using a much larger sample of women freshmen, Arnet (1968) obtained similar results (r = .560). Weber (1954) reported a coefficient of .410 between fitness and grades for freshmen males, and a multiple correlation coefficient of .666 for the prediction of grades by fitness level and scholastic aptitude scores. While Johnson (1942), using a single skill type test to assess fitness, found a zero-order correlation between fitness and grades, Carkhuff, Banks et al. (1971), using a more comprehensive fitness assessment, reported a significant correlation of .63 between fitness and intellectual performance as measured by an essay type exam.

Collingwood (1973) explored the relationship between students functioning on six different indices of fitness and their final level of performance as measured by behavioral ratings in a course teaching social and problem-solving skills. Correlational matrix showed eleven out of twelve significant relationships between initial fitness scores and final levels of skill performance with coefficients of correlation ranging from .41 to .92. Williams, Collingwood, and Vitalo (1974) report three separate studies exploring the relationship of initial fitness levels to final level of course achievement for three different student groups (master-level students in psychology, master-level students in guidance and counseling, and police academy trainees). Significant correlations were found in each instance, and physical fitness was identified as accounting for 24% to 48% of the variance in student learning outcome.

Using a factorial design, Williams and Collingwood (1974) found a significant difference in the levels of learning achievement for three groups of students representing three different levels of physical fitness. The greatest learning gain was achieved by the highest-level-of-fitness group. Other investigators have researched the relationship of fitness and scholastic performance using extreme group comparisons. Biddulph (1954), Clarke, and Jarmon (1960) and Rarick and McKee (1949) each found significant differences between high- and low-fitness students on such indices as grades, reading ability, and writing achievement.

Still other investigators have looked at the augmenting effect of physical fitness training on intellectual performance in adults. Williams, Collingwood, and Vitalo (1974a), using a factorial design including a no-treatment control group, investigated the impact of parallel physical fitness training on student learning in a social- and problem-solving-skills training course. Although both the experimental and control groups showed significant learning gains, the group receiving the parallel physical fitness training showed significantly greater learning gains over the control group in each of the teaching areas. Studies evaluating the impact of fitness or exercise training on intellectual performance in the elderly have also uncovered a positive relationship (Diesfeldt and Groenendijk, 1977; Powell, 1974; Powell and Pohnorf, 1971) notwithstanding the negative finding of Barry et al. (1966), who attempted to evaluate the impact of fitness training on intellectual performance but failed to achieve significant improvement in the fitness levels of the subjects and hence no change in intellectual performance could be expected.

Correlational studies of the relationship between fitness and grades for younger populations (high school, grade school) report similar significant findings although generally of somewhat less magnitude. Thus, McMillan (1961) found a correlation of .360 between fitness and high school performance, while Kratochvil, Carkhuff, and Berenson (1969) report significant correlations of .27 between fitness and academic performance in grade school and .50 between fitness and students' level of creativity/productivity. Similarly, Ismail, Kane, and Kirkendall (1969) report significant loadings for students' scores on balance and coordination test items on an intellectual development factor, and Verduczo (1969) developed five regression equations predicting intellectual achievement by motor skills performance ranging from .75 to .85 for educationally subnormal children.

Although the research relating physical fitness of students to indices of actual learning achievement overwhelmingly support the significance of fitness for success in learning endeavors, studies attempting to link physical fitness to intelligence test scores have produced mixed findings. Howe (1959), Francis and Rarick (1959), and Sengestock (1966) each found that children of normal intelligence significantly outperform children of sub-normal intelligence on a broad range of physical fitness tests despite matching of groups for chronological age and the exclusion of brain damaged and physically handicapped subjects. Biddulph (1954), however, found no difference in I-Q test performance between his high-fitness and low-fitness student groups. Further, Burley and Anderson (1955) found no relationship between fitness and scores on the Henmon-Nelson Intelligence Test. In contrast, both Smart and Smart (1963) and Rabin (1957) report significant but low magnitude relationships between I-Q's measured by the Stanford-Binet and WISC Intelligence Test and physical fitness. Liese and Lerch (1974) also report a significant relationship between fitness as measured by the AAHPER Youth Fitness Test and scores on the Stanford Binet Intelligence Test for a trainable mentally retarded population. Working with an elementary school population of emotionally disturbed children, Gruber and Noland (1977) found moderate but non-significant canonical correlations ranging from .39 to .60 between measures of fitness and intellectual ability as measured by the Wide Range Achievement Test.

In contrast, research exploring the relationship of improvement in physical fitness to change in performance on intelligence tests has produced more consistent findings. Oliver (1958) found that retarded boys exposed to a ten-week physical fitness program out-performed a matched control group of boys receiving no physical training on three of five tests of mental intelligence. Corder (1966) successfully replicated Oliver's (1958) findings in a study using an additional control group of boys receiving added attention but no physical training. Still, a third study using random assignment of trainable mentally retarded children to an experimental condition of physical fitness training and a control condition of added attention but no physical training also reports significant increment in intelligence test performance as measured by the Stanford-Binet Intelligence Test for experimental subjects over control subjects (Brown, 1977). Finally, Guten (1966) found significant correlations of .355 and .342 between fitness improvement and gain scores on mental tests for two groups of college students. The only negative finding reported is that of Barry et al. (1966). As indicated above, however, the physical training program used in this research study failed to produce significant improvement in the subjects' fitness levels.

Physical Fitness and Performance in the Work Area

Although one might expect to find a large number of studies relating physical fitness and indices of work performance, survey of the literature uncovered only five studies reported in journals indexed in *Psychological Abstracts*. Although each of the five studies supports a significant relationship between fitness and role performance, the roles investigated were in the human service area and therefore may be contaminated by the already established relationship between physical fitness and social effectiveness. Nonetheless, the research merits attention especially since several of the roles investigated are intimately related to the work of a professional helper. Carkhuff et al. (1971)

reports the highly significant correlation of .81 between fitness levels for adults and effectiveness in the helping role, as measured by the levels of communication skills offered by corrections officers in a counseling interview. Collingwood and Stockwell (1973) found a small yet significant (r = .35) relationship between candidate physical fitness levels and their scores on a selection index for choosing state police trainees. In an effort to relate physical fitness levels to teaching-role outcome, Collingwood, Williams, and Holder (1974) factor analyzed the relationship between teachers' scores on physical fitness measures and their scores on ten variables which previous research had identified as significantly predictive of student achievement (Aspy, 1976). Fitness was found to be a first-order factor for six of the ten variables and a second-order factor for one additional variable. Despite this noteworthy trend, however, none of the regression correlations utilizing fitness to predict performance on each of the ten variables was significant.

Conclusions on the Relevance of Physical Fitness for Effective Living

Fifty out of the sixty research findings reviewed evaluating the relationship between physical fitness and evidences of successful implementation of functions associated with the living area report positive relationships between fitness and indices of personal adjustment and social achievement. The physically fit person tends to evidence a healthier personality, greater social confidence and success. A rough estimate of the variance in successful everyday living which is accounted for by fitness is 25% to 30%, based upon correlational studies reported in an earlier research review (Vitalo, 1973). Furthermore, fitness appears to be a significant variable for emotional health for both normal and deviant groups. Additionally, the relationship between fitness and emotional adjustment appears constant across the variety of assessment instruments investigated, including objective and self-report evaluations of social effectiveness, social acceptance, social initiative, and emotional well-being. There was, however, a tendency for more mixed results when written assessments of overall adjustment were used. Finally, there appears to be some increasing significance of the impact of fitness on emotional adjustment as age increases. Since data for assessing this hypothesis is limited, this finding must be considered tentative. Confirmation of the correlational studies reporting a relationship between fitness and success in the living areas is provided by the factor analyses studies which investigated the impact of changes in levels of fitness upon levels of functioning on dimensions associated with successful living outcomes. Eight out of twelve training studies reported that enhanced personal and social effectiveness resulted from systematic fitness development. The impact of fitness training and improving emotional interpersonal functioning appears stronger in groups evidencing initial psychological distress. Finally, research depicting the personality profile of the physically fit person appears congruent to the description of the healthy personality.

Of the twenty-three findings reviewed relating physical fitness to success in learning achievement, only two studies failed to support a meaningful relationship between these dimensions. Furthermore, four out of five factorial studies investigating the impact of physical fitness on intellectual achievement found improved performance in learning associated with improved fitness. These joint sets of findings support the conclusion that physical fitness significantly relates to successful role functioning in the learning area. Research suggests that the functionally fit person tends to be more intellectually achieving. Relatedly, the higher functioning person on a physical dimension tends to be the higher functioning person on intellectual dimensions. Based on the correlational studies reviewed, a rough estimate of the overall amount of learning-outcome variance accounted for by physical fitness across age levels is 20% to 25% (Vitalo, 1973). When the research studies investigating the relationship between fitness and academic achievement are analyzed in terms of age level of the sample being investigated, there appears to be a significant increasing relationship between fitness and intellectual achievement over age (Williams & Vitalo, 1974). At the earlier age levels, including pre-nursery, grade school, and junior high school, fitness appears to account for between 6% to 10% of the intellectual achievement (Vitalo, 1973). In later age groups fitness appears to account for between 16% and 48% of the variance in learning achievement. A Kendall Rank correlation was completed between the age group sampled in studies investigating the relationship between physical fitness and academic performance and the size of the correlation found. The Kendall Rank correlation coefficient was .91 ($p < .05$) (Williams and Vitalo, 1974). This finding suggests that fitness is more critically related to intellectual achievement as the person grows older. This hypothesis takes on an added significance in light of the research reported above concerning the impact of exercise on the retention of intellectual performance in the elderly (Diesfeldt & Groenendijk, 1977).

Only four studies were found which related physical fitness to performance in the career area. Unfortunately, these studies related performance to careers that were all in the human service area and therefore involved effectiveness in social functioning. Hence, the relationship of fitness to career-role performance is somewhat confounded by the already established relationship of fitness directly to social effectiveness. Nonetheless, three of these studies supported the importance of fitness for human service delivery roles.

Clearly, the overwhelming finding of both correlation and factor-analysis studies supports the relationship of physical fitness to effective functioning in the living and learning areas and tentatively supports the relationship of physical fitness to effectiveness in performance in the working area. The postulate (Carkhuff, 1969) that the person who is fully functioning is also the physically fit individual appears supported. The impact of fitness on success in living, learning, and working roles may be both direct and mediated. In a direct impact, fitness does provide the energy resources, strength, and movement capacity to sustain both a wider area of activities and the intense involvement in activities. Indirectly, research suggests a relationship which may be mediated in part by the increase oxygen flow to the brain (Cooper, 1972; Dill, 1960) and the enhancement of this increased oxygen supply to mental activities (Diamond, 1973). Additionally, research has suggested a relationship between blood levels of cholesterol and poor retention of problem-solving ability, concept formation, and other measures of mental ability and alertness in adults over forty years of age (Reitan and Shipley, 1963). Relatedly, Golding (1961) has reported significant reduction in cholesterol levels following a twenty-five week endurance type exercise program suggesting a mediated link between fitness and intellectual performance. One might hypothesize that, especially in persons over forty years of age, the relationship between fitness and intellectual performance may be partly mediated by the control of the development of cholesterol levels in their bodies.

Research also suggests other factors which might act to mediate the impact of fitness on success in the living area. Fitness appears to have a clear impact on self-attitudes. In turn, the concept we have of ourselves appears to relate directly to motivation and to achievement (Leacock, 1968; Rosenthal & Jacobson, 1968). An individual who sees himself or herself as successful is more likely to try to succeed than an individual who sees himself or herself as a failure (Carkhuff, 1971). Thus, the studies by Collingwood (1972) and Collingwood and Willett (1970), which suggest that constructive changes in self-image, heightened sense of self-confidence and well-being are quickly facilitated through fitness training, also suggest a possible mediating link to other areas of life achievement. The research of Oliver (1960) and Layman (1972) suggests that the process of fitness training teaches behavior which is effective in eliciting successful experiences in other areas of living. Specifically, the learning of body control facilitated by fitness training may be helpful in learning control in other areas of personal functioning. The reinforcement of initiative behavior emanating from physical exercise may generalize to initiative behavior in other areas, especially social. Jones (1946) completed a longitudinal study of boys at different levels of fitness over the period of early adolescence. The findings of his study suggest that the life experiences of the less fit individual become progressively restricted and deteriorative. Hence, the living situations that a less fit person enters may in fact retard the person's opportunity for success in the roles he or she assumes.

Clearly, strong implications are suggested for educational and child rearing practices as well as for therapeutic processes. Indeed, Carkhuff's (1969) conclusion that the physical fitness component represents a necessary inclusion in any program geared toward facilitating constructive change appears well supported by the research. The studies suggest that the presence of fitness in the growing child is associated with good adjustment and more positive life experiences, and that fitness training can elicit constructive personality changes. Incorporation of systematic fitness training in child rearing practices, whether family or institutionally based, appears well supported. Similarly, it appears that physical fitness training which is systematic and progressively more difficult effects a meaningful and significant contribution to learning achievement and should be seriously incorporated within academic programs and objectives. The apparent heightened importance of fitness in late adolescence and adulthood as a contributor to learning achievement suggests that fitness training should be incorporated within universities and especially in graduate-level education as a mandatory adjunct to cognitive development. Such training programs should focus upon cardiovascular fitness in addition to muscular endurance because the former dimension has the clearest physiological link to facilitating higher mental processes (Barry, Steinmetz, Page & Rodahl, 1966; Cureton,

1963; Dill, 1960; Golding, 1961). It should be noted, however, that research suggests that a program that fails to achieve significant fitness improvement cannot be expected to effectively support learning and growth in any other areas of functioning.

THE RELEVANCE OF PHYSICAL FITNESS TO PSYCHIATRIC REHABILITATION

The review of research investigating the relationship of physical fitness to various indices of real life performance supports several important understandings. First, physical fitness appears as a significant contributor to the achievement of personally valued life outcomes, especially in living and learning areas of functioning. The conclusions concerning the relationship of physical fitness to success in the working area are limited by the research found to date. However, this research supports the significant relationship of fitness to success in human service roles. Second, physical fitness appears to have a special importance in learning achievement. A student's level of fitness appears to predict his or her acquisition of the content knowledge and skills being studied. The presence of effective fitness training within educational programs appears to augment the learning achievement. Third, physical fitness appears to relate to the presence of personal characteristics deemed significant to mental health and the therapeutic processes. These characteristics include positive self-concept, self confidence, positive body image, calmness, dependability, appropriate assertiveness, resourcefulness, and independence. Finally, successful fitness training has been connected to significant reduction in the excessive presence of client symptoms, especially anxiety and depression.

Essentially, the research supports the tentatively hypothesized relevance of fitness for rehabilitation processes. The absence of adequate fitness can be a source of breakdown in role performance and a cause of problems in living (Jones, 1932; Diesseldt and Groenendijk, 1977; Clark, Wade, Massey, and VanDyke, 1975). However, a more detailed understanding of the relevance of fitness to rehabilitation requires a detailed analysis of the function of rehabilitation.

Rehabilitation as a function of mental-health-care delivery may be viewed from two perspectives — specifically, from a pre-service perspective and from an in-service perspective. The term *pre-service* is commonly used to designate the preparation of professionals prior to their assumption of service roles. The use of this term in the context of this chapter will be broadened somewhat to include student selection, choice of content areas for study, teaching process and evaluation of student competency, all components of the pre-service endeavor. The term *in-service* commonly designates programs of ongoing support to professionals already in service-provision roles. In the context of this chapter the in-service perspective will be broadened to incorporate issues of client populations, client problem areas, the rehabilitation process, and evaluation of service provision, in addition to the more customary component of in-service training to care providers. More detailed review of the relevance of physical fitness to these pre-service and in-service components should facilitate awareness of areas for application of the findings from the literature on physical fitness. Such applications should lead to enhanced efficacy of both pre-service and in-service functions.

RELEVANCE OF PHYSICAL FITNESS FOR THE PRE-SERVICE AREA

Clearly, the implication one may draw from the literature on physical fitness for the pre-service area will be experienced as the most radical and controversial. Readers may gird themselves in an effort to avoid being distracted by the controversy by simply reviewing some basic principles of pre-service education. First, pre-service education functions ultimately to ensure that the community's needs for care are effectively and efficiently met. Unlike non-professional educational programs which may entertain non-specific relations with societal needs, professional training programs are generated out of such needs and exist to serve and thus meet those needs. Therefore, it becomes clear that such pre-service programs should be fully shaped by what will in fact ensure the achievement of their mission and the implementation of their mandate. Second in a more immediate sense, graduate and other pre-service educational programs should deliver what they promise to the students. What they promise is to train their students to be effective in those roles for which the programs were developed. Thus both the outcome objectives and the process objectives of pre-service education shape themselves in whatever form proves functional to the mission, which is ensuring the relief of human need.

With this perspective on pre-service programs the reader may review the following research-based conclusions concerning the relationship of physical fitness to intellectual and emotional-interpersonal functioning and from this base jointly generate implications for pre-service programming. These conclusions are:

1. An individual's level of physical fitness relates positively and significantly to his or her level of intellectual achievement.

2. The relationship of an individual's level of physical fitness to his or her level of intellectual achievement increases significantly as age increases.

3. Training which results in significant improvement in an individual's level of physical fitness tends to result in significant improvement in that individual's level of intellectual achievement.

4. An individual's level of physical fitness relates positively and significantly to his or her level of emotional-interpersonal effectiveness.

5. The relationship between an individual's level of physical fitness and his or her level of emotional interpersonal effectiveness increases significantly with age.

6. Training which results in significant improvement in physical fitness also results in significant improvement in an individual's level of emotional interpersonal functioning.

7. Systematic programs progressively demanding physical exertion of sufficient intensity, duration, and frequency are required to sustain fitness past the period of early adulthood and to maximize fitness during the period before adulthood.

These seven conclusions are wholly supported by the research reported previously. They focus on three dimensions: intellectual achievement, emotional and interpersonal effectiveness, and age. It is apparent that pre-service programs are generally graduate programs directed towards the preparation of individuals for helping roles, and working with candidates who are generally in their early to mid-twenties.

With these last three observations concerning pre-service programming, and with the maintenance of the overall perspective defining the mission and mandate of pre-service programming, and with the seven conclusions based upon research which relates physical fitness to intellectual and emotional interpersonal functioning — it is now possible to generate implications of the research on physical fitness for the pre-service program components of: students, teaching content areas, teaching process, and evaluation of competency.

The research evidence supports the use of physical fitness as a selection criteria in choosing among applicants for entry into pre-service programs. For the age group in question, research suggests that fitness alone is a better predictor than a number of traditional indices and as a component in multiple regression equation should significantly enhance the power of any selection formula. From a substantive point of view, the most fit students will be the most able to learn and benefit from pre-service programs.

An obvious implication in relation to content areas for study is that physical fitness must be introduced to the course work contained within the pre-service curriculum. An awareness and understanding must be developed as to the meaning of physical fitness and its relatedness to positive mental health. Related to the introduction of physical fitness to the content of pre-service curricula is the introduction of training in physical fitness to the teaching programs contained in pre-service education. This introduction, it would appear, should have a dual focus.

The first focus would be on skill modules teaching students to diagnose their own levels of fitness. These modules should teach them skills with which to develop systematic programs for the improvement and sustainment of physical fitness levels for use in their own lives and in their roles as professionals and effective practitioners. Such a learning would serve to augment the students achievement within the pre-service program as well as to facilitate his or her continued intellectual achievement and emotional-interpersonal effectiveness during the course of their professional lives.

The second focus would be on skills modules teaching students how to diagnose levels of fitness in clients they will be serving, and how to develop systematic programs which are responsive to their clients and effective in improving their clients' fitness levels. Further, modules should be included to teach students the skills for instructing their clients in physical fitness self-diagnosis and generation of programs for enhancing fitness. Research suggests that both these inclusions would function to immediately enhance the client's ability to participate and benefit from the rehabilitation process and to enhance and sustain continued benefits and success beyond the treatment process.

Finally, with reference to pre-service evaluation, assessments of physical fitness should be incorporated within the final determination of successful completion of pre-service preparation. These assessments should be in terms of the adequacy of the fitness levels of the candidate, the adequacy of his or her ongoing fitness program, and the competency of the candidate in implementing diagnosis and fitness programming in the rehabilitative process.

Since these conclusions may be controversial, it may be more palatable to entertain the incorporation of fitness into the pre-service system as a research paradigm. Indeed, such incorporation within a re-search design will allow for empirical verification of the implied efficacy based upon existing research findings relating physical fitness to educational achievement.

THE RELEVANCE OF PHYSICAL FITNESS FOR REHABILITATION SERVICE PROVISION

Although the implications that may be drawn from the research on physical fitness in the area of pre-service preparation of mental-health-care providers may indeed be the most controversial, the implications of the research for the actual provision of service are not without their potential for controversy as well. To a large measure the controversy emerges as the result of the directions given for such issues as staff selection and evaluation. The seven conclusions listed above with one addition can serve as a base for generating directions for incorporation of physical fitness into actual service delivery. The additional conclusion is that:

8. Training which results in significant improvement of physical fitness also results in significant reduction of problematic behaviors across a variety of client populations.

Table 6-1 presents data drawn from studies investigating physical fitness training on cognitive, affective, and behavioral functioning. The table facilitates forming conclusions about the relevance of fitness to the in-service components of client population and problem areas. In general, the research supports the relevance of fitness across age levels and the increasing relevance of fitness for the adult and senior populations. This especially holds for the elderly, the mentally retarded, and for persons in exiting chronic care facilities (aftercare clients). With regard to these populations, staff should maintain a heightened awareness of the possible involvement of physical fitness in the client's program.

Table 6-1 also presents a summary of target symptoms or problem areas corresponding to the successful outcomes observed in research applications of fitness training to resolving experiences of human

TABLE 6-1

CLIENT POPULATIONS AND TARGET SYMPTOMS CORRESPONDING TO RESEARCHED APPLICATION OF FITNESS TRAINING TO MENTAL HEALTH CARE DELIVERY

AUTHOR	AGE LEVEL				TARGET SYMPTOM
	0-12	13-17	18-59	60 +	
Brown, 1977		TMR[1]			inadequate social maturity; deficient intellectual functioning
Clarke, Wade Massey & Van Dyke, 1975				X	restricted level of daily activities
Collingwood, 1972			X		negative self-concept; negative body image
Collingwood & Willet, 1971		X			negative self-concept; negative body image
Corden, 1966		TMR			deficient intellectual functioning
Diesfeldt & Groenendijk, 1977				X	deficient recall; visual motor coordinator and task recognition
Dodson & Mullens, 1969			X		internalization of affects; somatization of anxiety (high scores on scales Hy and Ps of MMPI); disturbance of focus on here and now
Duke, Johnson & Norwicki, 1971	6-14				inadequate sense of control of one's experience
Folkens, 1976			X		high anxiety and high depression due to cardiac "at risk" status
Hellerstein et al., 1967			X		depression consequent to identification of heart disease
Knudson & Davis, 1949			X		over-aggressive behavior; use of psychotropic drugs for control behavior
Kramer, 1951			X		over-aggressive behavior; hyperactivity
Lindsey, 1970	X				improved school adjustment in nondiagnosed school children
Marusak, 1952			X		restricted communication; restricted interest in activities
Meyer, 1955			X		psychotic behavior
Oliver, 1958		TMR			deficient intellectual functioning
Smith & Sigitakos, 1970			X		psychotic symptoms; distorted body image
Van Fleet			X		psychotic behavior; inadequate participation in therapy; impaired cognitive performance
Wood, 1977			X		high anxiety

grief. It is clear that a wide variety of symptoms can be impacted through systematic physical fitness training. It is also clear that, for example, among the elderly, fitness training may have a special value in ameliorating cognitive deterioration and restricted activity level. It also appears that physical fitness has a special relevance for improving cognitive functioning among the mentally retarded. Relative to aftercare populations or populations still in long-term-care facilities, fitness training appears to have a positive impact on such problematic behaviors as manifestation of psychotic symptoms, inadequate participation in therapy, impaired cognitive performance, over-aggressive behavior, use of psychotropic drugs to control behavior, restricted communication, and restricted interest in activities. It should be noted that the use of psychotropic drugs is considered problematic because while it may control the manifestation of psychotic behavior it is costly and presents a risk to the physical health of the person involved.

For the general adult client population

lack of fitness appears to have relevance for a wide variety of problem areas. These include: negative self-concept, negative body image, excessive internalization of affect and somatization of anxiety, depression especially where it is consequent to the identification of heart disease, high anxiety, excessive tension due to frustration, over aggressiveness, and inability to focus on the here and now. With younger age groups, fitness appears to have relevance for problem areas around inadequate sense of control, and a possible preventive application in the area of improving school adjustment.

In general, the application of physical fitness to these above-described problem areas incorporates several additional benefits. A fitness program may be designed which is of minimum cost to a client. A properly designed and implemented fitness program is health enhancing — that is, it benefits the physical well being of the client independent of the problem area being addressed. The elimination of problems through the application of a fitness program places the locus of control for relief with the client, thus facilitating a heightened experience of potency and competence. Finally, the fitness approach to problem resolution provides the client with a constructive new competency which he or she may in turn share with others. In essence, the approach not only resolves problems experienced by clients but enhances their effectiveness in roles involving them with responsibility for others.

With reference to the overall delivery process, conclusions drawn from the research on physical fitness clearly suggest implications for *intake*, *assessment*, and *rehabilitation delivery*. The process of intake must include input from clients concerning their experience of their own physical fitness for the roles they are attempting to maintain. It must also include input concerning their activities to sustain fitness. The assessment process must look at the adequacy of a client's physical resources to meet the life areas he or she is attempting to impact, as well as his or her competency in diagnosing and facilitating maintenance of the program.

With reference to the rehabilitation or treatment delivery itself, fitness must be understood in two contexts; first, as indicated above it may be a vehicle for facilitating alterations in a client's problematic experiences. Furthermore, the delivery of the skills of self diagnosis, fitness development, and maintenance may be the singular substantive need of a client especially if the individual is experiencing difficulty as a result of inadequate resources to meet assumed roles. It is interesting to note that in this instance service providers must reopen their understanding and move from a response of recommending the reduction of roles to a response of facilitating the mastery of the skills needed to fulfill roles which have been assumed.

The second area for rehabilitation is augmentation of client participation and learning from the treatment process itself. Treatment is understood as provision of skills and competencies to the client and the facilitation of his or her successful application of these skills to produce beneficial life outcomes. It is in itself a *learning process*. The research suggests that the client must have some requisite level of fitness in order to efficiently benefit from this learning process. The research also suggests that systematic programs geared toward enhancing the fitness of clients and paralleling their learning of skills in other areas would have an augmenting effect on such learning. Thus, if the client's skill deficiency was really in quite another area — for example, an inability to respond to a spouse's needs — fitness may still be incorporated within the rehabilitation process to facilitate the client's ability to learn the skills of communication he or she needs in order to achieve the positive life outcome of a successful marriage.

The conclusions drawn from the research on fitness also have important implications for staff selection and, naturally, for staff in-service training. Clearly, fitness appears as a significant contributor to social effectiveness and, more specifically, to success in helping roles. Thus, the selection process for hiring staff in helping roles should incorporate measures of the candidate's level of physical fitness. Job role requirements for persons assuming helping roles should include responsibilities for maintaining physical fitness in the same way that they are expected to maintain professional skills. Since most professionals find themselves without the knowledge or skills to incorporate the physical fitness component into their delivery of service, in-service training programs will be needed to close this gap.

In summary, the relevance of physical fitness for pre-service functions emerges at each stage of exploration, understanding, and action in relation to the individual whose needs are being served. Within the pre-service realm, that individual is the student. As the pre-service program explores its student candidates, it should obtain input on students' levels of physical fitness. As a pre-service program attempts to understand which candidates should in fact become students, it should use their level of fitness as part of the determination formula. The pre-service program needs to deliver the knowledge and skills concerning fitness to its students both for incorporation in their own lives as well as for use in the service of their future clients. Research on physical fitness would support the fact that the incorporation of fitness into the pre-service preparation programs would have the benefits of: maximizing the quality of students obtained; maximizing the quantity of learning achieved by students; maximizing the quality of preparedness of students to function in their professional helping roles and, ultimately, maximizing the likelihood of benefits to those clients who will finally be provided care by these professionals.

RELEVANCE OF PHYSICAL FITNESS FOR IN-SERVICE PROGRAMS

In relation to in-service programs, the service deliverer must ensure that during the exploration phase the client's input is obtained on his or her experienced level of fitness in relation to assumed life responsibilities. In ensuring the development of adequate client input on the issue of

physical fitness, the care provider should draw from his or her base of understanding concerning the special relevance of fitness to certain client populations, especially the elderly, the mentally retarded, aftercare and the cardiac involved client. The care provider should also draw on his or her prior knowledge of the established impact of fitness on the wide array of problem areas which have already been researched (See Table 6-1). The care provider must understand the client's needs for enhanced fitness or skill acquisition in order to enhance or sustain their own levels of fitness. Service deliverers must incorporate within their range of offerings, special programs for the teaching of the skills of fitness development, not only for their direct impact on the problematic experiences reported by clients, but also for their facilitating impact on the client's ability to learn through treatment. Finally, service delivery managers must incorporate physical fitness criteria in their staff selection process, in their expectation for ongoing staff performance, and in their in-service training programs for existing staff. In this way the staff already on-board can be upgraded in the knowledge and skills necessary for integrating physical fitness into their deliveries to clients.

Existing research would support that the incorporation of physical fitness to the in-service sector of rehabilitative service delivery would have the overall benefit of maximizing the capability of the service delivery system to effectively provide the benefits it promises to those in need. Specifically, such incorporation would: maximize the quality of staff available to serve clients; ensure attention to a critical dimension of effective functioning; provide a skill important to sustaining successful life outcomes; maximize the efficiency of implementing the rehabilitation process by maximizing the client's ability to learn via such processes; reinforce a systems emphasis through building on the client's skills and strengths; enhance the quality of client participation in the rehabilitation process; and support the continued functioning of the client after the conclusion of rehabilitative care.

GUIDELINES FOR IMPLEMENTING PHYSICAL FITNESS AS A REHABILITATION DELIVERY

Irrespective of the breadth of appropriate points for the introduction of physical fitness into pre-service and in-service components in a mental health care system, the most immediate area of application is the introduction of physical fitness as a treatment delivery or vehicle for treatment delivery.

The following guidelines are offered as an appropriate introduction of physical fitness into mental health care. The first set of guidelines address themselves specifically to the care provider and are guided by the principle that the first step in effective delivery to clients is the development by the care provider of functionality in his or her role. Specifically, it behooves the care provider to master the area of physical fitness and its application to his or her own functioning prior to its introduction as a delivery to clients. A variety of materials including training programs are readily available in the area of physical fitness. Programs of fitness training are accessible through the local YMCA's and YWCA's, Jewish Community Centers, schools and neighborhood centers. Two especially good printed resources have been offered by Collingwood and Carkhuff (1976, 1976a). These authors have produced a manual for developing increased physical fitness and a companion volume for training fitness development as a skill. Irrespective of the resource, however, the first task for professionals interested in implementing fitness within treatment is to master the knowledge and skills associated with the area and to develop functionality in terms of his or her own fitness.

Additional guidelines deserve adherence as one approaches the introduction of physical fitness into rehabilitation delivery. First, the primary directive of any treatment delivery is that treatment must begin with the frame of reference of the client. No technique, no new concept, no new teaching delivery supplants the client as a point of initiation for all helping. If physical fitness is to be introduced, it must be introduced in a manner that is responsive to the client's needs. Furthermore, its responsiveness to the client's needs must be understood by the client and not simply by the care provider. In addition to being responsive to the client's understood needs it must also be responsive to his or her values. By values it is meant other concerns which the client may have about the care he or she receives. In traditional psychotherapy such concerns are generally interpreted as evidences of resistance or as derivatives of other personal dynamics. Although with specific clients this conceptualization may be valid, unfortunately, as a universally applied perspective, it eradicates any face validity to client preferences, undermines the client's rights as a consumer, and generally dissuades the care provider from even inquiring about such preferences. If physical fitness is to be implemented effectively within the context of treatment, the client's values must be elicited, respected, and incorporated within the treatment selection and implementation process. Such values often include expressions of concern for cost, the desire that the treatment approach be effective, that the treatment approach provide the client with the capacity to function independently at some point, and that risks of harm be minimized. Whatever the unique composition of a particular client's values may be, the introduction of physical fitness will have to be compatible with them.

The introduction of fitness must also be responsive to the environment in which the client lives. Although the social or physical environment is rarely a negating factor for the introduction of fitness, it is very commonly a limiting factor on the approach to be used in terms of physical fitness development. That is, the particular exercise one selects and exercise regimen one develops must be compatible with the social and physical environment of the client. A jogging routine which takes the client away from home for significant periods of time may be experienced by a spouse as additional evidence of indifference and may lead to the exacerbation of marital discord rather than the first step toward alleviating such discord. Similarly, a walking exercise in a high crime area might have added risks with little compensating value.

The introduction of fitness must also be responsive to the client's physical means and preferences. Physical means include financial resources, basic physique, health, physical strength, and preferences for types of exercise and activity. In regard to physical health, a medical exam prior to fitness training should be mandatory.

Essentially, these four principles of responsiveness serve to ensure the relevance of fitness to the particular client and to maximize his or her engagement in the process of physical fitness development.

Other guidelines tend to ensure the effectiveness of a particular application of physical fitness to the treatment process. First, as a general observation, effective programs are goal oriented. Thus, any physical fitness program should have an operationally defined and behaviorally measurable goal. Additionally, fitness programs that prove effective must be systematic in the design, must include exercises of sufficient duration and intensity, and a regimen of sufficient frequency to ensure the achievement of the desired body change. Fitness programs that succeed begin at a level of exercise which is immediately doable by the client. Programs that prove effective are paralleled in their implementation by a systematic monitoring process that assesses whether the expected changes in body capacity are occurring. Finally, each element of the goal setting, program development, program implementation, and program monitoring must be personalized in order that it continues to be experienced as immediately relevant and valued by the client.

The last set of guidelines are directed towards insuring the maximization of benefit to the client through the introduction of physical fitness development. First, the client is most benefited when he or she is taught the skills with which to solve his or her own problems. When this is achieved, the client becomes the master in his or her own rehabilitation process, and incorporates into his or her repertoire of competencies a skill which will have ongoing relevance for themselves as well as to others.

A second and final guideline is that the benefits to the client are maximized when an opportunity is provided on an ongoing basis for the client to draw learnings from his or her experience with the direction of improving the ongoing effort to develop physical fitness, as well as with the direction for generating learnings which are generalizable to other areas of life. In this regard clients should be encouraged to maintain a journal (Carkhuff, 1976) in which significant experiences are recorded, explored, understood, and directions for action generated. The sharing of these journal entries and the context of the treatment sessions should be encouraged, and the development of significant learnings facilitated by the therapist.

ENDNOTES

[1] Written by Dr. Raphael Vitalo, Director, Consultation and Education, Community Care MHC, Springfield, Massachusetts, and Marianne Farkas, Boston University.

REFERENCES

Allport, G. **Pattern and growth in personality.** New York: Holt Rinehart and Winston, 1961.

Alexander, M. The relationship between the muscular fitness of the well adjusted child and the non-well adjusted child. (Unpublished dissertation, University of Michigan) Ann Arbor, Michigan: University Microfilms, 1956. No. 19672

Anthony, W., Cohen, M. and Vitalo, R. The measurement of rehabilitation outcome. **Schizophrenia Bulletin**, 1978, in press.

Aspy, D. **Kids don't learn from teachers they don't like.** Amherst, Mass.: Human Resource Development Press, 1977.

Arnett, C. Interrelationship between selected physical variables and academic achievement of college women. **Research Quarterly**, 1968, *39*: 227-330.

Barry, A., Seinmetz, J., Page, H. and Rodahl, K. Effects of physical conditioning on older individuals II: Motor performance and cognitive function. **Journal of Gerontology**, 1966, *21*: 192-199.

Biddulph, L. Athletic ability and the personal and social adjustment of high school boys. **Research Quarterly**, 1954, *25*: 1-7.

Bolton, B. and Milligan, T. The effects of a systematic physical fitness program on clients in a comprehensive rehabilitation center. **American Corrective Therapy Journal**, 1976, *30*: 41-46.

Breen, J. Anxiety factors related to some physical fitness variables. (Unpublished dissertation, University of Illinois) Ann Arbor, Michigan: University Microfilms, 1959, No. 59-44495.

Brown, B. The effects of an isometric strength program on the intellectual and social development of trainable retarded males. **American Corrective Therapy Journal**, 1977, *31*: 44-47.

Burley, L. and Anderson, R. Relationship of jump and research measures of power to intelligence scores and arithmetic performance. **Research Quarterly**, 1955, *26*: 28-35.

Carkhuff, R. **Helping & human relations** (2 vols.) New York: Holt, Rinehart & Winston, 1969.

Carkhuff, R. **The development of human resources.** New York: Holt, Rinehart & Winston, 1971.

Carkhuff, R. **Teaching as treatment.** Amherst, Mass.: Human Resource Development Press, 1976.

Carkhuff, R. **The art of helping.** Amherst, Mass.: Human Resource Development Press, 1972 (a).

Carkhuff, R. **The art of problem solving.** Amherst, Mass.: Human Resource Development Press, 1972 (b).

Carkhuff, R. What's it all about anyway? **The Counseling Psychologist,** 1972, *3*: 79-87 (c).

Carkhuff, R., Banks, G., Berenson, B., Griffin, A. and Hall, R. The selection and training of correctional counselors on physical, emotional and intellectual indexes. **Journal of Counseling Psychology,** 1971, *18*.

Carron, A. and Witzel, H. Comparisons of personalities for selected groups of fifteen year old males. **Perceptual and Motor Skills,** 1975, *40*: 727-734.

Cattell, R. **Personality and motivation structure and measurement.** New York: World Book, 1957.

Clarke, H. and Clarke, D. Social status and mental health of boys as related to their maturity, structural and strength characteristics. **Research Quarterly**, 1960, *32*: 326-334.

Clarke, H. and Green, W. Relationship between personal-social measures applied to 10 year old boys. **Research Quarterly**, 1964, *34*: 288-298.

Clarke, H. and Jarmon, B. Scholastic achievement of boys 9, 12 and 15 years of age as related to various strength and growth measures. **Research Quarterly**, 1960, *32*: 155-161.

Clarke, B., Wade, M., Massey, B. and Van Dyke, R. Response of institutionalized geriatric mental patients to a twelve-week program of regular physical activity. **Journal of Gerontology**, 1975, *30*: 565-573.

Collingwood, T. Physical functionality. Paper presented at the Second Human Relations Institute, Amherst, Mass., November, 1972.

Collingwood, T. Effects of physical training upon behavior and self attitudes. **Journal of Clinical Psychology**, 1972, *28*: 583-585 (a).

Collingwood, T. HRD model and fitness. In D. Kratochvil ed. **Human Resource Development Model In Education**. Baton Rouge, La.: Southern University Press, 1973.

Collingwood, T. and Stockwell, D. The importance of physical fitness for the selection and training of state police. Consortium Monograph series on Fitness, Vol. 1, No. 1, Monroe, La: Northern Louisiana University, National Consortium for Education, 1973.

Collingwood, T., Williams, H. and Holder, T. Physical fitness relationship for effective teacher behaviors. Consortium Monograph Series on Fitness. Monroe, La.: Northern Louisiana University, National Consortium for Education, 1974.

Collingwood, T. and Willett, L. Effects of physical training upon self-concept and body attitudes. **Journal of Clinical Psychology**, 1971, *27*: 411-412.

Consumer Reports. Exercise and your heart. **Consumer Reports**, 1977, *42*: 254-258.

Cooper, K. **The new aerobics**: New York: Bantam Books, 1972.

Cooper, K. **Aerobics for women**. New York: Bantam Books, 1972 (a).

Corder, W. O. Effects of physical education on the intellectual, physical and social development of educable mentally retarded boys. **Exceptional Children**, 1966, *32*: 357-364.

Cowell, C. & Ismail, A. Relationship between selected social and physical factors. **Research Quarterly**, 1962, *33*: 40-43.

Cureton, T. Improvement of psychological states by means of exercise fitness programs. **Journal of the Association of Physical and Mental Rehabilitation**, 1963, *17*: 14-25.

Currie, D. and Harris, J. Energy level and personality: Some speculations. **Canadian Counselor**, 1971, *5*: 199-208.

Diamond, E. Can exercise improve your brain? **Readers Digest**, May, 1973, 101-104.

Diesfeldt, H. and Groenendijk, H. Improving cognitive performance in psychogeriatric patients: The influence of physical exercise. **Age and aging**, 1977, *6*: 58-64.

Dill, D. B. Fatigue and physical fitness. In Johnson, A. ed., **Science and medicine of exercise and sports**. New York: Harper and Row, 1960.

Dodson, L. and Mullens, W. Some effects of jogging on psychiatric hospital patients. **American Corrective Therapy Journal**, 1969, *23*: 130-134.

Drowatszky, J. Evaluation of physical fitness and motor fitness of boys and girls in Coos Bay, Oregon, schools. **Research Quarterly**, 1966, *37*: 32-40.

Duke, M., Johnson, T. and Nowicki, S. Effects of sports fitness camp experience on locus of control orientation in children ages 6 to 14. **Research Quarterly**, 1977, *48*: 281-283.

Fenechel, O. **The psychoanalytic theory of the neurosis**. New York: Norton, 1945.

Flieshman, E. A. **The structure and measurement of physical fitness**. Englewood Cliffs, New Jersey: Prentice Hall, 1964.

Folkins, C. Effects of physical training on mood. **Journal of Clinical Psychology**, 1976, *32*: 385-388.

Frances, R. J. and Rarick, G. Motor characteristics of the mentally retarded. **American Journal of Mental Deficiency**, 1959, *63*: 792-811.

Golding, L. Effects of physical training upon total serum cholesterol levels. **Research Quarterly**, 1961, *32*: 499-508.

Graber, J. and Noland, M. Perceptual-motor and scholastic achievement relationships in emotionally disturbed elementary school children. **Research Quarterly**, 1977, *48*: 68-73.

Gustin, B. Effects of increase in physical fitness on mental ability following physical and mental stress. **Research Quarterly**, 1966, *37*: 211-212.

Hall, C. and Lindsey, G. **Theories of personality**. New York: John Wiley, 1957.

Hardy, M. Social recognition at the elementary school age. **Journal of Social Psychology**, 1937, *8*: 365-384.

Harris, D. Comparison of physical performance and psychological traits of college women with high and low fitness. **Perceptual & Motor Skills**, 1963, *17*: 293-294.

Hart, M. and Shay, C. Relationship between physical fitness and academic success. **Research Quarterly**, 1964, *35*: 443-445.

Kratochvil, D., Carkhuff, R. and Berenson, B. The cumulative effects of parent and teacher offered levels of facilitative conditions upon indices of student physical, emotional and intellectual functioning. **Journal of Educational Research**, 1969, *63*: 161-164.

Layman, E. The contribution of play and sports to emotional health. In Kane, J. ed. **Psychological Aspects of Physical Education & Sports.** Routledge & Kegan, Paul: London, 1972.

Leacock, E. B. **Teaching and learning in city schools.** New York: Basic Books, 1968.

Leonardson, G. Relationship between self-concept and perceived fitness. **Perceptual & Motor Skills,** 1977, *44*: 62.

Lilse, J. and Lerch. Physical fitness and intelligence in TMRs. **Mental Retardation,** 1974, *12*: 50-51.

Lindsey, C. H. Effects of health and physical education instruction on East Baton Rouge Parish elementary school children. Doctoral dissertation, LSU, 1970. (Unpublished dissertation, Louisiana State University) Ann Arbor, Michigan: University Microfilms, 1970. No. 70-18, 543.

Linton, J., Hamelink, M. and Hoskins, R. Cardiovascular system in schizophrenia studied by the Schneider Method. **Archives of Neurology and Psychiatry,** 1934, *32*: 712-722.

Maslow, A. **Motivation and personality,** New York: Harper and Row, 1954.

McCloy, E. Factor analysis method on the measurement of physical abilities. **Research Quarterly,** 1938, *6*: 114-121.

McFarland, R. and Huddleson, J. Neurocirculatory reactions in the psychoneuroses studied by the Schneider Methods. **American Journal of Psychiatry,** 1936, *93*: 567-599.

McKinney, F. Case history norms of unselected students and students with emotional problems. **Journal of Consulting Psychology,** 1947, *11*: 258-269.

McGraw, L. and Tolbert, J. Sociometric status and athletic ability of high school boys. **Research Quarterly,** 1953, *24*: 72-80.

McMillan, B. A study to determine the relationship between physical fitness as measured by the NYSPF test to academic index of high school girls. Unpublished master's thesis, Springfield College, 1961.

Meyer, M. The influence of recreation participation upon the behavior of schizophrenic patients, (Unpublished dissertation, New York Univeristy) Ann Arbor, Michigan: University Microfilms, 1955. No. 15, 550.

Morgan, W. Physiological and psychological correlates of depression in psychiatric patients. **Research Quarterly,** 1968, *39*: 1037-1043.

Morgan, W. Physical work capacity in depressed and non-depressed psychiatric females. **American Corrective Therapy Journal,** 1970, *24*: 14-16.

Morgan, W. Physical fitness correlates of psychiatric hospitalization. **Contemporary psychology of sport,** G. S. Kenyon, ed., Chicago: Athletic Institute, 1970 (a).

Morgan, W., Roberts, J., Brand, F. and Feinermain, A. Psychological effects of chronic physical activity. **Medicine and Science in Sports,** 1970, *2*: 213-217.

Nadel, G. and Horvath, S. Fitness evaluation of psychiatric patients. International Journal of Neuropsychiatry, 1967, 3: 191.

Nauthton, J., Brahn, J. and Lategola, M. Effects of physical training in psychologic and behavioral characteristics of cardiac patients. Archives of Physical Medicine, 1968, 49: 131-137.

Oliver, J. N. The effects of physical conditioning exercises and activities on the mental characteristics of educationally subnormal boys. British Journal of Educational Psychology, 1958, 28: 155-65.

Oliver, J. N. The effects of physical conditioning on the sociometric status of educationally subnormal boys. Physical Education, 1960, 156: 38-46.

Olree, H. Relationship between skill in sports, participation in sports and physical fitness on college men. (Unpublished dissertation, George Peabody University) Ann Arbor, Michigan: University Microfilms, 1961. No. 61-5821.

Powell, R. Psychological effects of exercise therapy upon institutionalized patients. Journal of Gerontology, 1974, 29: 157-161.

Powell, R. R. and Pohndorf, R. G. Comparison of adult exercisers and non-exercisers on fluid intelligence and selected psychological variables. Research Quarterly, 1971, 42: 70-77.

Rabin, H. The relationship of age, intelligence and sex to motor proficiency. American Journal of Mental Deficiency, 1957, 62: 507-511.

Rarick, G. and McKee, R. A study of twenty third-grade children exhibiting extreme levels of achievement on tests of motor proficiency. Research Quarterly, 1949, 20: 143-151.

Raven, L. Comparative study of sociometric status and athletic ability of Anglo-American and Latin-American 6th grade boys. Masters thesis, 1951. Dept. of Educ., University of Texas.

Reid, A. The contribution of the freshman year of physical education in a liberal arts college for women for certain personality variables. Dissertation Abstract, 1955, 15: 2091-2092.

Reitan, R. and Shipley, R. The relationship of serum cholesterol change and psychological abilities. Journal of Gerontology, 1963, 18: 350-357.

Rice, D., Rosenberg, D. and Radzyminski, D. Physical fitness of the mentally ill: The effect of hospitalization. Journal of Association of Physical & Mental Rehabilitation, 1961, 15: 73-81.

Rogers, C. A theory of therapy, personality and interpersonal relationships. In Kock, S. ed. Psychology: a study of a science, Volume 3. New York: McGraw Hill, 1959.

Rosenberg, D. and Rice, D. Physical fitness & psychiatric diagnosis. Journal of Association of Physical and Mental Rehabilitation, 1964, 18: 73-81.

Rosenthal, R. and Jacobson, L. Pygmalion in the classroom. New York: Holt, Rinehart & Winston, 1968.

Sengstock, W. Physical fitness of mentally retarded boys. Research Quarterly, 1966, 37: 113-120.

Shaw, B. Sociometric status and athletic ability of Anglo-American and Latin-American boys in a San Antonio Junior High School. Masters thesis, 1960, Dept. of Educ., University of Texas.

Smart, R. & Smart, M. Draus-Weber scores and personality adjustment of nursery school children. **Research Quarterly**, 1963, *34*: 199-205.

Smith, J. and Hurst, J. The relationship of motor abilities and poor acceptance of mentally retarded children. **American Journal of Mental Deficiencies**, 1961, *66*: 81-85.

Tillman, K. Relationship between physical fitness and selected personality traits. **Research Quarterly**, 1965, *36*: 483-487.

VanFleet, P. Some effects of physical education therapy on the personality characteristics of schizophrenic patients. Unpublished doctoral dissertation, University of California, 1950.

Verduzco, R. The relationship between motor and intellectual performance among educationally subnormal children. Cited in Kane, J. ed, **Psychological aspects of physical education and sport**. London: Routledge & Kegan, Paul, 1972.

Vitalo, R. Physical fitness and the fully functioning person I. Fitness and intellectual functioning. Unpublished manuscript. Thunder Bay Family Counseling Agency, Thunder Bay, Ontario, Canada, 1973.

Vitalo, R. Physical fitness and the fully functioning person II. Fitness and emotional-interpersonal functioning. Unpublished manuscript. Thunder Bay Family Counseling Agency, Thunder Bay, Ontario, Canada, 1973 (a).

Vitalo, R. Physical fitness and the fully functioning person. Unpublished manuscript. Family Counseling Agency, Thunder Bay, Ontario, Canada, 1973 (b).

Vitalo, R., Cohen, B and Walker, R. Short-term, crisis-oriented training as treatment. Unpublished manuscript. Child/Adult Mental Health Center, Youngstown, Ohio, 1974.

Weber, J. Relationship of physical fitness to success in college and to personality. **Research Quarterly**, 1954, *24*: 471-474.

Wells, H. Relationship between physical fitness and psychological variables. (Unpublished dissertation, University of Illinois at Urbana) Ann Arbor, Michigan: University Microfilms, 1959. No. 59-599.

Werner, A. and Gottheil, G. Personality development and participation in college athletics. **Research Quarterly**, 1966, *37*: 1-6.

Williams, H. and Collingwood, T. Differential fitness levels and interpersonal skill acquisition. Consortium Monograph Series on Fitness, National Consortium for Education, Monroe, La., 1974.

Williams, H., Collingwood, T. and Vitalo, R. The relationship of physical fitness to intellectual functioning within a specialty area. Consortium Monograph Series on Fitness. Monroe, La.: Northern Louisiana University, National Consortium for Education, 1974.

Williams, H., Collingwood, T. and Vitalo, R. Participation in physical fitness training and its augmenting effects in human achievement skill acquisition of helper-trainees. Consortium Monograph Series in Fitness. Monroe, La.: Northern Louisiana University, National Consortium for Education, 1974 (a).

Williams, H. and Vitalo, R. The relationship of aging to correlations of physical and intellectual functioning. Consortium Monograph Series in Fitness. Monroe, La.: Northern Louisiana University, National Consortium for Education, 1974.

Wood, D. The relationship between state anxiety and acute physical activity. American Corrective Therapy Journal, 1977, *31*: 67-69.

CHAPTER VII

Vocational Rehabilitation Strategies[1]

The problems and complications involved in rehabilitating the psychiatrically disabled client into a work environment are immense. For example, consider these facts:

1. Successful adjustment to a work environment does not correlate significantly with adjustment to living or learning environments.

2. Clients often lose their jobs, not because of an inability to perform job tasks, but because of skill deficits in the emotional-interpersonal area of functioning.

3. Clients who do lose their jobs often do not possess the skills necesary to obtain a new job, and either do not try to find employment or return for further help from the rehabilitation practitioner.

4. There is no relationship between hospital-based work therapy and competitive employment. The work behavior of the psychiatrically disabled helpee is situationally specific.

5. Previous studies of employment success rates show that approximately 30%-50% of discharged patients obtain employment, but that less than 25% maintain full-time employment. With an increasing number of long-term patients being discharged from the hospital, the current full-time employment percentages may be considerably less (Anthony, Cohen & Vitalo, 1978).

If the problems are complex, then the solutions will probably not be simple. Unfortunately, the field of mental health has approached the vocational rehabilitation of the psychiatrically disabled client as if it were very simple. In particular, mental health practitioners often wait until the treatment process is almost complete before they refer their clients for vocational rehabilitation. Or, mental health practitioners consider the vocational rehabilitation process to be simply a matter of placing a person on the job — a process that seemingly can be accomplished within several weeks.

In reality, the process of rehabilitating the psychiatrically disabled client is much more involved. However, one method of understanding the entire process is to envision the vocational rehabilitation process as composed of three basic intervention components: (1) work adjustment training, (2) career counseling, and (3) career placement. Psychiatrically disabled clients may become involved in some or all of these intervention components, depending upon their diagnosed strengths and deficits. A client who needs *work adjustment training* commonly has deficits in the various physical, emotional, and intellectual skills needed to retain any job that she or he gets. A client who needs *career counseling* lacks a career objective and career plans based on her or his interests, values, and the requirements of the world of work. A client who needs *career placement* services lacks the ability to seek out possible jobs and become hired.

A psychiatric rehabilitation practitioner, skilled in each of these three career intervention strategies, as well as rehabilitation diagnostic skills, can identify the specific vocational areas in which the client is deficient. Once the diagnosis has been made, the practitioner can, depending on her or his own role, either write a detailed, comprehensive referral that requests the needed vocational services or begin the career intervention process her/himself.

Table 7-1 illustrates some typical work environment deficits categorized by the more appropriate career intervention strategies. This classification scheme is proposed to give the rehabilitation practitioner a better conceptual understanding of career deficits and the typical modes of career interventions. The categories are not perfectly compartmentalized, nor is there an intent to achieve a perfect classification. Many agencies and practitioners provide all three services, while others might provide only one. For example, some vocational counseling centers might help clients develop a career objective and a career plan (i.e., a career counseling intervention), but ignore the client's career placement and work adjustment deficits. Other agencies may provide training in career placement skills for those helpees who already have a career plan and the necessary work adjust-

TABLE 7-1

TYPICAL WORK ENVIRONMENT DEFICITS CATEGORIZED BY APPROPRIATE CAREER INTERVENTION STRATEGIES

WORK ADJUSTMENT TRAINING	CAREER COUNSELING	CAREER PLACEMENT
Cannot dress appropriately for work	Cannot identify own interests	Cannot identify job-related assets
Cannot use public transportation	Cannot identify own abilities	Cannot identify employment sources
Cannot be punctual	Does not know what occupations relate to interests	Does not use sources of employment information
Cannot control temper at work	Does not know what occupations relate to abilities	Does not look for work frequently enough
Cannot make friends at work		Cannot write a resume
Cannot accept criticism	Cannot evaluate occupational alternatives based on own values (decision-making skills)	Cannot fill out an application
Cannot follow direction		Cannot explain job skills
Cannot give directions		Cannot use stigma reduction skills with interviewer
Cannot work for extended periods	Lacks a career objective	
Cannot evaluate own work performance	Inappropriate career objective	Cannot attend and respond to interviewer
	Lacks career plan to achieve career objective	Cannot dress appropriately for interview
		Cannot ask questions of interviewer
	Cannot identify deficits which are hindering career plan	Cannot explain career plans to an interviewer

ment skills. Some less scrupulous facilities might go so far as to provide career placement independent of whether the client has an adequate career plan or work adjustment skills.

The intervention strategies also differ in terms of their orientation to the rehabilitation model. A career intervention which maximizes a rehabilitation emphasis attempts to teach the client as many as possible of the needed skills. A non-rehabilitation career intervention merely walks the client through the process, with little or no client skills development. For example, a client may obtain a career objective, a career plan, or an actual job placement primarily through the activities of her or his practitioner, without actually learning from the practitioner how to do the process her/himself. In these situations the facility or helper is acting in a *supportive role* rather than a *skills-teaching role*. Other facilities, although still providing support, will much more actively attempt to teach the client the skills needed to overcome the deficits, rather than trying to merely provide compensatory support for the client's lack of skilled functioning.

WHEN SUPPORT IS NOT ENOUGH

Case Illustration 7-1

It wasn't that Henry didn't have a clear-cut goal — he did. His goal was quite simple, to be offered the Zipco Manufacturing job for which he was applying.

And it wasn't that Henry didn't have a program to enable him to achieve his goal — he did. Marsha, the practitioner who had done most to lift him out of the severe state of anxiety and mental depression into which he had fallen, had worked with him to develop a comprehensive series of specific steps leading from where he was — unemployed — to where he wanted to be — employed full-time by Zipco Manufacturing.

The problem was that Henry himself couldn't quite believe all this was happening.

Only a few short months before, Henry had felt about as low as a guy could feel: worried sick, always depressed, sometimes even suicidal. A Vietnam vet, he had just about run through his whole string of benefits and a possessor of a bum leg which had developed the bad habit of giving way under him at the worst possible times — like on an escalator in the middle of a crowded department store. He was forced to live off his parents who could not afford this extra expense, but he had nowhere else to go because no one seemed interested in employing him.

Now things were beginning to look like they might change. Marsha had helped him get his act together — at least to the extent that it *was* together. Having a chance to work with her had made a big difference, all right. And one of the biggest differences was that in a very few minutes Henry would be having his first honest-to-God job interview in a very long time. It was a good job with a chance to move up, not just some sleazy job with little pay and less opportunity!

"Mr. Jameson will be with you in a moment."

Henry nodded and mumbled his thanks to the receptionist before taking a seat. The nervousness that had been threatening all morning now seemed like a giant wave about to sweep over him. He picked up a magazine but his eyes couldn't keep their focus on the page. Giving up the effort, he tried instead to go over the different steps that Marsha had outlined for him.

"Look this Mr. Jameson right in the eye when you meet him," Marsha had said. "Greet him by name and make sure you give him a firm handshake."

"Make sure you answer every one of his questions with a positive fact about yourself," she had told Henry. And she had gotten him to write out a list of such facts which could be used in responding to many different questions.

"Make sure that you ask some intelligent questions of your own," she had said. And once again Henry had written out some appropriate questions.

No doubt about it — Marsha had given him a program. Yet for some reason the whole preparatory stage they had gone through now began to seem blurred and unreal to Henry. What were those facts he had written out? What were the questions? In desperation, Henry realized that he was drawing almost a total blank.

"Good morning!" The hearty voice took him by surprise. An older man was coming toward him, hand outstretched. Mr. Jameson?

"Uh — hi." Getting up, Henry reverted to an old habit and shoved his hands deep in his pockets. His eyes wavered across the other man's face, then dropped until they found the tips of his own highly polished shoes.

A bad beginning, certainly. But rather than improving, things got worse. Henry answered Mr. Jameson's questions in monosyllables, his face usually averted. He couldn't think of a single question of his own. Finally, when Mr. Jameson asked, "Henry, why do you really want to come work for us?" Henry could think of no more effective response than, "I dunno — I just need a job."

Marsha had told Henry what he had to do. She had certainly been supportive. Henry's goal was fine. His program was excellent. But when it came to putting this program to the test of practical action, Henry just wasn't ready. He had never really been taught the necessary skills with respect to job interviewing skills. Henry clearly had not been rehabilitated.

Obviously, an accurate rehabilitation diagnosis is the key to the amount of skills training and support and the type of career intervention which is implemented. Rehabilitation practitioners must be aware that the vocational rehabilitation needs of these clients vary tremendously, and that the amount and type of intervention must vary accordingly. The remainder of the chapter describes each of the three types of vocational intervention strategies. A more detailed description of career counseling skills has been provided by Pierce, Anthony and Cohen (1977) while a more detailed description of career placement skills has been provided by Pierce, Cohen, Cohen and Anthony (1977).

Work Adjustment Training

Even though employment rates are rather gross measures of professional effectiveness (Erickson, 1975; Bachrach, 1976), employment data do indicate that only a minority of clients are employed one year after hospital discharge. These figures lend weight to Olshansky's (1968) belief that professionals are only beginning to find out what patients have known for some time — that is, employers are disinclined to risk hiring emotionally disabled clients. Although practitioners may decry the attitudes displayed by the business community, rehabilitation efforts must clearly do more to dispel the community's concerns and stereotypes. Work adjustment training, in its attempt to specifically improve the client's work-related behaviors, is certainly one potential method of changing the potential biases of the employer. Community rehabilitation programming, specifically designed to change employer attitudes and behavior, is a more direct method of reducing employer prejudices (See Chapter VIII for a further discussion of community rehabilitation programming).

WORK ADJUSTMENT TRAINING DEFINED

Work adjustment training programs are designed for those clients who lack the basic work and social skills needed to maintain a job (Neff, 1968). Many chronically disabled clients have either never acquired work habits or lost many of the work habits they once possessed, for example, attending skills, punctuality skills, production skills, and so on. In addition, many clients lack the social skills needed to relate effectively with peers, supervisors, and supervisees. In effect, these clients need a whole new vocational structure (Lamb et al. 1969). It is important to note that although work is the main focus of work adjustment training, social skills training is an essential aspect of the program, because there are many social norms that are demanded by work settings. Unfortunately, some work adjustment programs focus on work to the exclusion of social skills training, often with deleterious effects.

Thus, work adjustment training attempts to re-shape a client's working and social attitudes and behavior so that he or she can function adequately in a work environment. It is essentially an in vivo training setting which imposes gradually increasing demands and tasks on the client as the client learns new skills. Neff (1970) has stated that the primary features of work adjustment training are the non-verbal features of the total work situation. A comprehensive program, however, must integrate work as a therapeutic mode with other interventions to achieve its greatest impact. Work adjustment settings include hospital wards (Fairweather et al. 1969), hospital workshops, community based workshops, and groups or individual placements in industrial settings (Brown, 1977; Lamb et al. 1970). More innovative programs consist of client-owned businesses (Fairweather et al. 1969). In essence, the settings for work adjustment training are limited only by the practitioner's creativity, program development skills, and community resource development skills. So long as the focus of training is on the acquisition and application of work and social skills, work adjustment training can occur anywhere.

It is important for the practitioner to remember that *work adjustment training is only part of a total career intervention program.* All too often what starts out as a training program gradually becomes a sheltered work placement. Both the practitioner and the client should have some idea of where the individual's program is ultimately going, and how the client is supposed to get there. The client and practitioner are therefore involved in a collaborative diagnostic effort in which the goals and the means of reaching these goals are explored and agreed upon by both practitioner and client. Such a process may mean that the client may opt for a program other than what the practitioner deems appropriate. In the end, however, it is the client's treatment program, and if he or she is to understand it and be invested in it, then with the practitioner's

help, the client must ultimately choose.

In essence, work adjustment training involves a goal-directed program which begins to integrate psychiatrically disabled clients into the vocational development process in order to teach them job maintenance skills. Comprehensive work adjustment programs not only work on basic work habits; they also seek to orient the client to the world of work and to prepare the client for the next phase of vocational rehabilitation — career counseling and placement. Work adjustment training is *not* occupational training. That consists of specialized job-skills training based on the client's interest and aptitudes and usually will occur after the work adjustment training and the career counseling phases, although theoretically it could parallel work adjustment training.

THE MEANING AND IMPORTANCE OF WORK ADJUSTMENT TRAINING

Although the importance of work has been observed by a number of theoreticians and practitioners (Olshansky, 1968; Super, 1957; Super & Bohn, 1970; Zook et al. 1976), its importance is not reflected in current therapeutic practice. Typically, work programs occur in segregated sheltered environments after the client has been "treated" or "cured" by the use of various combinations of chemotherapy and psychotherapy (Olshansky, 1975). Historically, vocational rehabilitation in the mental health system has not been perceived as a high-status activity; this status is reflected in the pay scales and administrative hierarchy in state and federal mental health systems.

In contrast to its perceived importance within the mental health field, Olshansky (1969) notes that work does serve several very important purposes for clients: First, it provides structured and meaningful activity for individuals who have difficulty using their time well; second, it provides a means of "shedding one's patienthood" and acquiring some semblance of normalcy; and third, by functioning in an approved adult role and by becoming more self-supporting, clients improve their self-concept.

Work becomes even more important when deviance is viewed from a sociological perspective, which deems that deviance is largely measured by an individual's inability to work and to be self-supporting (Levine & Levine, 1969). It is sufficient to say that despite predictions that work will play a less important role in people's lives in the future, currently it is a primary criterion of normalcy.

It is important, therefore, that vocational training or counseling and placement services occur early in the client's rehabilitation program; for if the client is ever to shed the role of patient, he or she must learn the skills to function as independently as possible in the community. It is clear, then, that work adjustment training for the severely disabled becomes even more important when the low percentages of successes as measured by employment rates are considered.

Moreover, when one considers that skills training is possible in spite of severe psychiatric delusions and hallucinations (Anthony & Margules, 1974), the value of initiating work adjustment training early in a client's program is even more apparent. In addition, Olshansky (1968) has observed that an individual's ability to work is not determined by the degree of his or her disability. So it is neither necessary nor wise to wait until a client's symptoms have subsided before initiating vocational training, since that only exacerbates the problem of no structure and encourages secondary deviance (Goffman, 1961; Rosenhan, 1973; Scheff, 1966).

In addition, work adjustment training is a meaningful vehicle in which to teach more easily defined behaviors and to provide a base from which to teach more complex interpersonal skills. For example, it is relatively more difficult to describe and teach the behaviors needed to make friends. In contrast, work behaviors are more observable and the contingencies for rewarding productive behaviors and extinguishing distracting behaviors are clearer and more immediate (Olshansky, 1969). Moreover, within the structure of work adjustment training, incidental socialization and the acquisition of interpersonal skills

is possible (Schwartz, 1976). The work training program can reinforce these interpersonal skills by building a social skills training component into the program. Additionally, other skills such as hygiene, money management, decision-making and transportation skills can be included in a work adjustment training program, because these skill areas may have an impact on the client's ability to succeed in independent living (Foote et al. 1976).

It should be noted that work adjustment training is a time consuming, difficult task that seeks to teach a number of different skills other than just work behavior. Work adjustment training demands a high degree of technical knowledge and expertise, and a commitment on the part of the practitioner to facilitate a client's development in the working environment. The following principles are presented as guidelines for the practitioner so that he or she might develop the skills to either develop or reorganize a work adjustment training environment that is capable of enhancing a client's potential for growth.

PRINCIPLES OF WORK ADJUSTMENT TRAINING

1. **Work adjustment training must be designed so as to achieve a more prominent role in the rehabilitation process.**

   Although work has been a model of treatment for more than a century (and probably longer), there is very little data available with which to evaluate these programs. Moreover, descriptions of various programs which discuss various techniques, assumptions, goals, and problems are scarce. Only in the past five to ten years has such material become available (Lamb et al. 1970; Fairweather et al. 1969; Schwartz, 1976).

   This is especially disturbing because the problems facing work adjustment programs and their clients are imposing, and they reflect some of the basic inadequacies of psychiatric rehabilitation practice today. That is, the fact that work adjustment is usually saved for the latter stages of treatment indicates a misplaced priority on the resolution of "more important" matters such as intro-psychic conflicts, to the detriment of everyday matters such as work, earning a living, and supporting oneself.

The fact that work adjustment training maintains a low treatment priority is manifested by such problems as unappealing work settings and jobs, intermittent work, and low pay for clients (Olshansky, 1975). In addition to these conditions clients must overcome other obstacles, such as staff who make decisions for them while expecting that clients will show more initiative and independence (Fairweather et al. 1969). The fact that clients survive these conditions at all is a statement of the clients' strengths, a fact that is not commonly acknowledged by helpers. Nevertheless, their cumulative effect is to sustain a client's dependence on others and to negate any efforts to enhance a client's self-esteem. It also conveys the message that work is not important and encourages a client's preoccupation with his or her emotional problems.

It is important therefore that several steps be taken by practitioners to protect themselves and clients from some of the problems listed above. First, program evaluation efforts, formal or informal, should be an integral part of any program. Statements regarding the purpose of a work adjustment program, the assumptions underlying why the service exists, and how it hopes to achieve its goals should be visible and subject to criticism from within and outside the program (Spaniol, 1977). Second, mechanisms must be built into the program in order that staff and clients can give and receive feedback regarding their performance and their relationships with one another. Third, staff should assume an expectation of success for their clients. That is, they should assume that, given the proper conditions, their clients can do better (Lamb et al. 1970; Wolfensberger, 1975). Fourth, the practitioner should attempt to phase himself/herself out of a job. This means that the client should assume increasing responsibility for making decisions. Therefore, clients should not be passed on or retained in programs. Rather, the client

should move according to decisions made with the practitioner's help. Fifth, efforts should be made to stimulate and facilitate staff members' growth and development (Goldenberg, 1970). Sixth, staff must advocate more strongly for work adjustment programs for their clients. And lastly, more information regarding the content of work adjustment programs, the problems they encounter, and their successes and their failures must be shared with others.

2. **The work adjustment environment must be designed to exert a therapeutic effect on the client.**

One of the greatest challenges facing work adjustment training programs is the blending of a therapeutic environment with a competitive working environment. That is, if the goal is to help the client function as independently as possible, and at the same time to teach appropriate work habits, a sensitive balance between treatment and work must be attained. This balance may be achieved by maintaining competitive employment expectations while at the same time providing opportunities for clients to explore with each other their deficits, strengths, difficulties, and how to function more effectively in the work environment. Although work adjustment programs attempt to approximate a working environment, practitioners must not lose sight of the fact that such settings are created in order to rehabilitate. In order to achieve that goal, some programs may have to sacrifice profit and productivity as an overriding objective (Lamb et al. 1970).

Within a work environment, a wide variety of knowledge and techniques should be utilized by practitioners. They are as follows:

a) **Utilization of Organizational Knowledge and Techniques:** Effective management can serve as a useful rehabilitation tool in creating an environment which involves clients in the decision-making process, and which encourages productive behavior on the client's part. Techniques such as participative management, providing change within the environment, nominal group brainstorming, and performance evaluation are proposed as a means to develop a stimulating environment. Such techniques also help clients learn to problem solve — a factor which appears to have a significant impact on a client's ability to adjust to new situations outside protected environments (Meichenbaum & Camerson, 1973; Fairweather et al. 1969). They also increase a client's investment in the work he or she is doing and, at the same time, encourages group cohesion among clients and staff through structured, task-oriented interaction (hersen & Blanchard, 1972).

b) **Skills Training Groups.** The use of a skills training approach within a group setting is often an effective means for teaching appropriate job-seeking and job maintenance behavior. A good deal of research indicates that primary and secondary groups may have a considerable impact in mediating behavior (McGuinnes, 1970). Structured skills training groups are therefore suggested in order to help clients learn specific skills and information and to discuss common areas of concern. Groups provide the opportunity for peer feedback, so that clients may begin to develop a more realistic picture of their strengths and deficits. In addition, structured groups are only one step removed from more unstructured group settings such as work. By participating in structured skills training groups, the client can learn skills that he or she may generalize to other group settings.

c) **Ongoing Rehabilitation Planning.** Practitioners must be available to work adjustment training clients in order to help them explore problems and successes encountered in their work settings. Clients need individualized programs, and practitioners may need to further develop programs and evaluate progress with the client as the client advances through the work adjustment training process.

3. **Work must be meaningful and clients should be paid according to their levels of competence.**

As mentioned earlier, many work adjustment training settings and tasks reflect the low priority ascribed to vocational rehabilitation. Typically, the work is tedious (Olshansky, 1969) and intermittant (Schwartz, 1976). In addition, pay scales tend to be low and homogenous regardless of the kind of work involved and the productivity of the trainee. Work adjustment training environments also tend to be deficient in that they are drab and uninviting (Olshansky, 1975). At the same time, it is not clear that the job skills taught in these settings are readily generalized to other work settings — especially if the settings and tasks do not approximate the natural environment.

There is anecdotal material available that indicates that work adjustment training may occur in a variety of settings, and may consist of a multitude of interesting and meaningful tasks (Schwartz, 1976; Fairweather et al. 1969; Lamb et al. 1970). If the goal for a trainee is to leave a relatively protected environment for a more natural one, then work settings should be as "normal" as possible, with reasonable demands placed on the client. The work should be "real" and relevant and should vary in kind and complexity to avoid boredom (Olshansky, 1975). Wages should match the complexity of the tasks so as to provide a career ladder incentive system that rewards performance (Fairweather et al. 1969). Moreover, importance should be placed on the performance of work tasks rather than an obsessive introspection as to why someone is having difficulty. This is especially important because employers are loathe to act as quasi-therapists for their workers and care little about why a person is not performing a job.

Evidence indicates that we have not been very successful at teaching clients skills that will make them workers, citizens, friends, and so on. In contrast, we have been very successful at teaching them to be clients. If we want a client to be a worker, then we must treat him or her like one, and provide the trainee with opportunities that reflect the world of work in the way it really is. We must also provide the client with the means to learn those skills necessary to function in the natural environment. Practitioners must therefore philosophically adopt "normalization"

(Wolfensberger, 1975) and "high expectation" (Lamb et al. 1970) points of view for their clients.

4. **Work adjustment training is but one component of a total vocational rehabilitation process.**

As has been pointed out earlier, work training programs have been sold as an over-simplified process. Specific techniques and approaches have been viewed as the answer in rehabilitation, when in fact they are only part of the answer. Comprehensive work adjustment training needs to take into account the social context in which services are developed, the direction of an individual's program and how it will fit into the client's community, the impact that the treatment environment has on the client, and the optimal practitioner techniques and skills that will facilitate and maintain behavior change.

In addition, the goals of work adjustment training must be kept in mind because all too often training programs inadvertently evolve into permanent placement programs, either because no opportunities exist for the client or because the client has not been able to progress beyond the work training setting. If a client is to remain in that setting, he or she should be involved in that decision, because that permanent placement then becomes part of the client's career plans.

CAREER COUNSELING

It is not uncommon to hear at an admissions staffing for a psychiatrically disabled individual that one of the overall rehabilitation goals is the helpee's pursuit of an occupational goal. Indeed, this is not an uncommon goal for the bulk of American society as well. Occupational concerns begin early in life; children in their preschool years often quiz others as to what they want to be when they grow up. The importance of the role of "worker," "provider," "breadwinner," to name a few, cannot be stressed too lightly as it has meaning for the individual, for the individual's family, and it fulfills a portion of the American ideal. Certainly the reverse is true. To be unemployed or on welfare evokes strong negative reactions in others, a poor self-image, and it creates an uncertain role function to replace the lost, highly cherished role, which comprised a third to a half of one's daily life. Unfortunately, however, the field of mental health has historically not valued the practice of career counseling in a fashion that reflects the major importance of work.

CAREER COUNSELING DEFINED

"Career development" is the process by which a person efficiently and effectively develops and pursues occupational goals (Pierce, Anthony & Cohen, 1977). Career counseling is that part of the career development process which identifies the client's career objective and develops the plans to achieve that career objective.

THE PURPOSE OF CAREER COUNSELING

The purpose of career counseling is to assist a psychiatrically disabled individual in the exploration of his or her unique value and interest systems; to reach an understanding about the interplay between the helpee's unique set of values and interest and those realistically expected or demanded by employers in the field; and to develop an action plan to assist a helpee in the selection of possible career choices. Stated more simply, its purpose is to equip the psychiatrically disabled individual with the skills and knowledge which are needed to choose a career goal and develop a career plan. It is also the purpose of career counseling to teach clients the process of career counseling to the extent to which it is possible given the client's level of functioning. As a result of this teaching procedure the client is able to replicate the process by him/herself and thus becomes less dependent upon agents of the helping profession.

There are many ways of choosing or, more correctly, not choosing a career. Research reported by Friel suggests that something less than a quarter of the population make decisions by weighing the facts and planning carefully (Friel & Carkhuff, 1974); and even these few do not approach the decision-making and planning process in a systematic fashion.

In terms of the psychiatrically disabled population, many clients simply comply in a passive manner with the wishes of others. If their friends, family or other relatives find them a job, they will take it. If the rehabilitation or mental health practitioner recommends an occupation, they will pursue it. These clients make no real choice of their own. They accept no responsibility for the decision. It is not they who succeed or fail but the advice which has been given them. And since it is frequently the case that the advice is not derived from a system which will ensure that the client's needs are met, the risk of failure is great.

Other clients impulsively leap before they look. They do not explore themselves or the world of work. They do not try to understand themselves or the world of work. They just act. For many, the consequences of these hit-or-miss decisions are quite negative.

There are many other ways in which clients make career decisions. Some are fatalistically resigned to whatever happens, others rely on intuition, and the remainder just agonize or are paralyzed in the face of the decision. Career counseling meets an overwhelming need for many psychiatrically disabled clients.

WHEN AND WHERE CAREER COUNSELING IS CARRIED OUT

Career counseling is appropriate for any client who has been diagnosed as having deficits related to identifying a career goal or career plan. The career counseling process may begin at any point in the treatment process or as soon as deficits are diagnosed. There is no prior need for the client to gain therapeutic insights or to first have all his or her symptoms reduced. The process of therapy and the development of new skills to replace deficits can be complementary processes. While the therapist is working to make the person less "sick," the rehabilitation practitioner is working to make the client more "well." Beginning career counseling in the hospital setting can provide an opportunity for the psychiatrically disabled clients to attain career planning skills in a protected environment. Here an individual will have the opportunity to learn and practice new career counseling skills as well as to receive feedback from staff and other psychiatrically disabled individuals. Depending upon the level of functioning of the individual, he or she may not have the time or the ability necessary to learn all of the skills required to efficiently and effectively develop and pursue occupational goals. If the practitioner and client agree that more skills training is required, then the practitioner will need to facilitate a referral to another rehabilitation practitioner who possesses the needed skills, or to an agency which has the reputation of training the client in career counseling skills.

For many psychiatrically disabled individuals, referral is made to the local state office of vocational rehabilitation. At this agency, the initial focus of the process is upon determining eligibility for services. If the client is determined eligible, then the focus is on either providing evaluation and training, or job placement. Career counseling, in the context of the state agency, may mean the administration of a battery of aptitude and interest tests, and the sharing of the results with psychiatrically disabled individuals for placement purposes. It has often been termed a "magical" approach since this process from eligibility determination to career choice selection has often been largely directed by the practitioner without adequate involvement of the client. Reasons for lack of involvement are situationally determined according to the individuals involved, and according to the pressures and requirements of the state agency. But no matter the reason, the end result is that often "it's faster" to determine career choices for psychiatrically disabled individuals that it is to involve the clients in learning some of the skills necessary to determine their own career choices.

THE OVERALL PROCESS OF CAREER COUNSELING

The career counseling process flows from the goal of career counseling. To reiterate, the ultimate goal of career counseling is for the client to develop a career objective and a specific and effective plan for reaching that objective. Clients may only need to engage in various aspects of the career counseling process, depending upon the client's unique pattern of strengths and deficits. In essence, the complete career counseling process is composed of three basic and developmental phases. In the initial *exploration* phase, the practitioner helps the client explore both the world of work and her or himself. In particular, the client first explores her or his interests and the values which she or he feels are important in selecting an occupation. The client then explores how the world of work is organized in terms of interest patterns. Finally, the client explores how the world of work is organized in terms of occupational requirements. The outcome of the exploration phase is the identification of a number of realistic job alternatives.

The exploration phase eventually gives way to the *understanding* phase. During this phase, the practitioner seeks to help the client understand exactly what his or her values mean. The practitioner then works with the client to evaluate various occupational alternatives in terms of these values. The outcome of the understanding phase is the selection by the client of the realistic occupational goals with which he or she would be most satisfied.

Finally, the client is ready for the *action* phase of career development. During this phase, the practitioner first works with the client to develop a specific plan which will lead to achieving the occupational objective developed in the second phase. During the implementation step of the action phase, the practitioner must work with the clients to develop an implementation schedule. But even more importantly, the practitioner must work with the client to teach her or him to modify the career route if necessary. This is necessary because for a variety of reasons (e.g., new opportunities open up, new things are learned), the client's plans often change. The client must learn to modify his or her career route so that she or he can continue along the path to the career objective or modify the objective. This will enable the client to continue to have a plan. The outcome of the action phase is the client's possession of a step-by-step plan of action to achieve specific career goals. The major steps involved in an effective career counseling process are portrayed graphically in Table 7-2.

TABLE 7-2
MAJOR STEPS INVOLVED IN CAREER COUNSELING

ACTING

Implementing a career plan to achieve objective

Developing a career plan to achieve objective

UNDERSTANDING

Understanding world of work in relation to client's career value system (deciding on an objective based on client's values)

Understanding client's unique career value system (those things the client wants from work)

EXPLORING

Exploring information about world of work in relation to client's world. (work requirements and occupational-interest categories)

Exploring information about client's world (previous experiences, interests, values, and abilities)

139

Clearly, clients may not have deficiencies in all these phases, although they frequently do. Some of the more common client deficits in the career area are as follows:

I. Exploration Deficits

A. Client lacks information about self.

(1) Client does not know what general things are important for him or her to consider in choosing an occupation.

(2) Client does not know what abilities she or he has in relation to the world of work.

B. Client lacks information about the world of work.

(1) Client does not know what occupations are related to his or her interests.

(2) Client does not know what occupations relate to her or his abilities.

II. Understanding Deficits

A. Client lacks ability to make a systematic decision about which occupation she or he should enter.

(1) The client does not know how to use the things that are important (his or her values) in order to evaluate occupational alternatives.

(2) The client does not have the detailed occupational information she or he needs to thoroughly evaluate potential occupations.

(3) The client does not have a systematic method for making a career decision.

III. Action Deficits

A. The client does not have a step-by-step plan to reach his or her occupational objectives.

(1) The client cannot identify in concrete and specific terms the deficits which are interfering with reaching his or her occupational goals.

(2) The client cannot identify in concrete, specific, and achievable terms the steps she or he can take to overcome these deficits.

Where there is a deficiency in only one of two areas, then obviously the practitioner needs only to use the skills necessary to facilitate the client's career development in those specific career areas where the client is deficient. For example, the client may only need to develop an action plan for reaching his or her occupational objective or the client may only want to evaluate a decision which she or he has already reached. While any particular client may not need all the skills contained in the career counseling process, the rehabilitation practitioner must master all the skills so that she or he can mix and match the skills to suit any one client's pattern of career deficits.

EXAMPLES OF THE UNDERSTANDING PHASE OF CAREER COUNSELING: AN UNSKILLED AND SKILLED APPROACH

Case Illustration 7-2

Understanding Career Alternatives:
An Unskilled Approach

It wasn't that Marion was totally without skills. She was fully aware of how important it was for a client to explore her or his career options. The problem was that she felt exploration alone was sufficient.

There was no doubt that she had helped Ernie Dominguez. At the start of their session he had been totally adrift, totally without direction. Helping him to explore his background and interests, Marion had found that Ernie loved to work outdoors. Further exploration revealed a good deal of information about his other interests as well as about his educational and work background. Finally Marion had been able to play her trump cards — showing Ernie how the information he had come up with fit into a specific area of interest and a specific level of education.

"Hey . . ." Fascinated, Ernie had gazed down at the scratch pad on which Marion had been writing. "Hey, that's me, huh? I'm a 'People/Thing' guy! And a — what is it? — a Level 2, huh? Wow, I never knew any of that before."

Marion always enjoyed the way clients reacted to her introduction of systematic interest and educational categories. It often seemed to them like magic of some sort.

Which was silly, of course. The real magic involved getting clients to really act on the results of their exploration!

Which had been, as it turned out, exactly the sort of magic that was missing in Ernie's case. She had helped him list four different career possibilities which fit into his interest and educational categories. One of these, a job with a landscaping firm, seemed perfect to Marion and she had told Ernie so. In so doing, Marion skipped the understanding phase of the career counseling process.

"Landscaping, huh?" He had looked at Marion, then down at the scratch pad again. "Huh. I never thought about that." For a moment he looked puzzled. Then he seemed to shrug this mood off. "Well, what do I know; I guess I can't argue with the facts."

Encouraged, Marion had listed some contacts he could make in order to find out about jobs with landscapers. Ernie had accepted all of this passively, almost as though he were willing his own doubts away. Leaving, he had thanked Marion profusely. For her own part, she had spent a silent moment hoping that the magic of effective action would strike Ernie and bring him success.

Alas, it didn't turn out that way. Less than a month later, Marion had run into Ernie at a downtown gas station. He was pumping gas, his face an expressionless mask. At first she wasn't even sure he recognized her.

"Oh, yeah, Ms. Martin," he'd said at last. "How's it goin'?"

"Fine, Ernie, fine. But what about you? What about   ?"

"That landscaping thing?" Ernie had shrugged. "Ah, no one wanted to hear from me. Maybe it wasn't my thing anyway. This job's O.K. for a month or two anyway."

"And — and then?"

"I dunno — I was thinking maybe of going out to the Coast. Getting out of here, anyway. There's nothing around here for me."

And the thing that hurt, the thing that Marion thought of now, as she sat in her office alone, was the way in which Ernie's expression had included her in the "nothing" that made up his life!

As the preceding example indicates, it is often not enough to just explore him or herself and the world of work. The client may also lack the ability to make a systematic decision about which specific occupation she or he should enter. As was the case in Ernie's situation, this problem can arise for several reasons. First, the client may not *understand enough about him or herself*. That is, the client may not know enough about what she or he wants from a career in order to really use this information to evaluate occupational alternatives. Second, the client may not *understand enough about his or her* occupational alternatives to come to a definite decision. Third, although the client may have all the information she or he needs, the client may have no *systematic decision-making method* for using this information to make the choice. The result of any or all of these client deficits is the client's inability to choose one occupation with which he or she feels satisfied. In direct contrast to the preceding example of Ernie is the case illustration which follows. Fortunately for this client his practitioner checked into whether or not the client had deficits in the understanding phase. Once identified, the practitioner taught the client a skilled method of overcoming these deficits.

Understanding Career Alternatives: A Skilled Approach

Sara had helped Jim develop a number of personal values related to his career options: a local area, independence, specialized training and specialized work.

"Great," she said. "Now we've got to pin these values down a bit more carefully." She overviewed the process of operationalizing values with Jim and then took him through the actual process. His value of a "local area" turned out to involve any area which could be reached by the local bus system. "Independence" really meant the amount of time Jim could actually spend working alone. "Specialized training" meant the number of courses he could take in a training program that would be directly applicable to his intended job. And "specialized work," of course, meant the number of specific technical tasks he would have to perform.

Next, Sara took Jim through the procedures involved in developing a favorability scale. He caught on quickly and had soon developed a specific rating for each value. For his value of "local area," for example, Level 5 (Most Favorable) turned out to be a job within a thirty-minute bus ride of his apartment, while Level 1 (Most Unfavorable) was a job more than one hour away by bus.

Once Jim had worked out a favorability scale for each of his occupational values, Sara helped him to assign numerical weights to each value. On a one-ten scale where ten was "most important," Jim gave a full ten to "independence" and lower relative weights to all his other values.

They were ready for the next phase of activity. Sara knew that, although it was certainly important for him to understand himself and his own values, it was equally important for him to gain an understanding of the specific nature of his career alternatives themselves. After all, how else could he see how his values fit with a particular job?

Sara and Jim had already developed a list of seven possible occupations that fit into the general categories of Jim's interests and educational background. Now they narrowed the original list of seven down to three: electrician, computer programmer, and x-ray technician. Each could be approached through a specialized training program. But before Jim could make an intelligent decision between the three, he had to gain additional information about all of them. Sara worked with him to develop a list of specific 'people' and 'thing' sources of information. Calling the local technical school, for example, she was able to get Jim an appointment with several different teachers, each with a background in one of Jim's three possible career fields.

It was almost a week before Sara saw Jim again. But when he reappeared, he was carrying a notebook crammed with information. Now she was able to sit down with him and develop a matrix which would allow him to quantify the relationships between each job and each of his occupational values. Working with numbers and precise definitions, Jim was in his element. He confided to Sara his suspicion that the job as an electrician was going to come out on top. But it didn't. Given the primary importance which he placed upon independence and the data he had unearthed about the inevitable subservience of apprentice electricians to their supervisors or foremen, this job finished second. His best option turned out to be the career in computer programming.

"Huh!" Jim exclaimed, looking at the results as his face broke into a huge grin. "How about that? I guess what made the difference was finding out how much freedom a good programmer has once he gets started — especially one who works for a relatively small company."

Sara answered his grin with one of her own. "It feels good to know just where you want to get to," she told him. "Now the only thing we have to do is figure out just how to get you there!"

SOME PRESENT PROBLEMS IN CAREER COUNSELING

As mentioned previously, the treatment of the psychiatrically disabled client typically does not include attention to vocational rehabilitation until the last phase of the treatment process. The presumption appears to be that when psychiatric problems have been eliminated, or at least reduced enough for a return to the community and a work environment, the client automatically will be prepared for the expectations of work. Since the problems and complexities involved in rehabilitating the psychiatrically disabled client into a work environment are numerous, career counseling should be integrated as part of the treatment process from the early stages of treatment. The highly pressured executive, for example, after experiencing emotional stress requiring treatment may never wish to withstand such pressure again, and may need to redirect his or her vocational goals. For many, this is a difficult step capable of directly influencing the psychiatric disability, since frequently a career change to a less pressured (and therefore often less prestigious) job can affect pride, ego, and cause a major shift in economic status. If these problems are addressed early in treatment, the shock of career change and the corresponding implications of that change might be anticipated and reduced.

Currently, too many clients at the point of termination of treatment are: 1) left with no career plan at all, 2) have plans made for them without exploration and understanding by staff, or 3) have plans made for them by significant others. Many clients who have spent many years at one job are virtually unaware of the types of alternative jobs available or are not informed of the skills needed for other work. In the highly specialized work world of today, many people do not have transferable skills and therefore will require training programs in addition to an understanding of what might be an appropriate career goal.

Another difficulty in career counseling is the almost total avoidance of a career counseling approach for low level functioning clients. Competitive employment for these clients is a very long term goal, and perhaps more of a hope than a goal. Yet even these helpees can go through parts of the career development process. For example, parts of the career counseling skills can be used to decide what sheltered workshop experience would be best for the client, or, the client might begin to learn career decision-making skills by deciding which job he or she will perform in a particular sheltered workshop. The determining criterion is the point at which it becomes functional for the client to begin planning his or her occupational life in a more systematic way.

Another problem for practitioners of career counseling is that in many mental health facilities the hierarchy of disciplines reflects the attitude toward career counseling services. There is often no position specifically geared toward dealing with this area. Thus, not only does no vocational rehabilitation occur, but there is no effective referral for rehabilitation services either. If the referral for rehabilitation is not detailed and a follow-up of the referral made, chances are increased that the referral will never be acted upon. Practically speaking, if the mental health system is preparing clients for functioning in all areas of life, it is essential that the system remember that most clients could spend eight hours per day, five days per week — that is one half of their waking hours in a work environment.

SUGGESTED DIRECTIONS

Although it is easy to point out deficits in the present system of career counseling, it is also necessary to suggest ways in which the present system might improve. One suggestion is a re-education process for rehabilitation practitioners and therapy staff with respect to the need for a comprehensive career counseling approach. In the re-education effort, rehabilitation practitioners must learn to become skilled in all the skills necessary to assist psychiatrically disabled individuals in career goal attainment. Besides engaging in career counseling with clients, rehabilitation practitioners must also be able to articulate the comprehensiveness of their approach to other professionals. This articulation of the scope of a rehabilitation practitioner's skills will communicate expectations to psychiatrically disabled helpees and therapy staff personnel as to what they might expect to gain from career counseling services. A side benefit of a more comprehensive articulation of unique career skills is the likelihood of more accurate referrals for these services.

The re-education effort has implications for rehabilitation practitioner training. In most cases, the major focus in rehabilitation practitioner training has often been on "counseling theory and various theories of personality." Although useful in itself, theory only teaches the practitioner to be more understanding of the client's emotional living area of functioning. Also typically necessary for rehabilitation success is that the psychiatrically disabled helpees have achievable goals in the working environment. To accomplish this end, rehabilitation training programs must incorporate detailed information concerning the composition of the world of work as a whole and ways to ensure that the psychiatrically disabled individual reaches desired or realistic work objectives. Universities providing training (and agencies providing re-training programs) must develop a core curriculum consisting of diagnostic interviewing, rehabilitation programming, and career counseling skills as the basic skills necessary to conduct effective career counseling. Technical information regarding the knowledge of occupations, and their entry requirements are also essential to the process.

Lastly, rehabilitation practitioners must increasingly focus their attention on the development and implementation of a career plan throughout the treatment process. The purpose of this would be to increase the expectations of the psychiat-rically disabled individual to achieve and accomplish more, as well as to emphasize "normal" role functioning. In the treatment setting itself, whether for inpatients or outpatients, a job board could be placed which would provide listings (for example, newspaper ads) regarding available jobs in many categories).

Inpatient therapy or counseling groups, whose focus may be on the psychiatrically disabled individuals' "feelings," must be supplemented by career skills training groups which focus on "what happens when you get out of the hospital?" A focus on projected work goals might also serve as a chance for the psychiatrically disabled to explore their interests and values in the context of a supportive setting.

If a particular rehabilitation setting emphasizes career counseling, it is also incumbent upon that setting to act as an advocate for the employment of psychiatrically disabled persons. By using their community marketing skills (See Chapter VIII), practitioners must also see their role as attempting to increase the number of employers willing to train or hire the formerly psychiatrically disabled.

CAREER PLACEMENT

Career placement intervention is presently undergoing a renewed evaluation by some rehabilitation practitioners. For the last several decades, placement activities have often been perceived by the professional practitioners as secondary to the more desirable activities of career counseling. More recently, however, has come the realization that many clients may be failing in the working area because of poor or nonexistent career placement interventions.

CAREER PLACEMENT DEFINED

Career placement is a process in which a rehabilitation practitioner assists a client to obtain the best possible job available to him or her. In order to accomplish this end, the client must first come to recognize and then to understand his or her job-related assets which an employer would consider beneficial. Secondly, the client must understand how to find available jobs for which he or she is qualified. Lastly, the client must be able to present his or her job-related assets to the employer in both oral and written formats. Simply stated, the practitioner helps the client learn *what* she or he has to offer, *where* to offer it, and *how* to go about offering it. It is the responsibility of the rehabilitation practitioner to operationalize the process for the client by making each aspect of the process a clearly defined skill which can be learned. By actively involving the client in the process, it is hoped that the client will be more fully motivated to gain the skills and knowledge required to obtain his or her desired vocational objective.

SOME CURRENT PROBLEMS IN CAREER PLACEMENT

Placement presents many problems for psychiatric clients. Job placement often requires skills that clients have never developed or which have atrophied. Even for the most skillful job seeker, a career change imposes some amount of stress because each new job demands different skills, relationships, and situations. Miller and Form (1957) note that in any decision to change jobs, the individual must resolve the process of job exploration, establishment in that job, maintaining the job, and possibly leaving the job for another. For many clients — especially those who have purposefully or inadvertantly made a career of being a patient — the task of actually seeking a legitimate job imposes demands that create even more severe stress in their lives. They must develop strategies to explain uncomfortable issues, for example, hospitalization, periods of unemployment, sporadic employment, etc. Also, they may often not possess some rudimentary job-seeking skills such as knowing where to look for a job, developing a resume, contacing an employer by phone or mail, or interviewing for a job.

In essence, placement requires a continued period of adjustment. Clients may not be able to handle full-time employment or full responsibility initially (Lamb et al. 1970). The fact is that the quality of care provided during the placement process is one of the most crucial but neglected aspects of a career intervention program. Inadequate preparation and support may destroy months of hard work and career planning on the part of the client and the practitioner.

Another problem is that even for the most qualified worker, jobs are very difficult to find, and for the client who has few skills, little experience, and a psychiatric history, it is extremely difficult. As long as social programs do not reflect a commitment to the vocational development of its disadvantaged and chronically unemployed populations, the psychiatrically impaired will face a formidable task in securing employment.

Although it is true that ex-mental patients run a higher risk of being discriminated against when seeking employment, some studies suggest that a client who is skilled in interviewing techniques and work behaviors is less susceptible to employer prejudice (Farina et al. 1973; Farina & Felner, 1973). The psychiatric label is most harmful when certain behaviors of the client him/herself reinforce a popularly held stereotype of the psychiatrically disabled. The mastery by the client of certain career placement skills can help the client increase the chances for employment.

THE PURPOSE OF CAREER PLACEMENT

The overall purpose of career placement is to equip the client with the skills and knowledge she or he needs to compete more effectively for a position. There are two major reasons that this skill is critical.

First, the more skilled the client is in placement skills, the better the chances are that he or she will be able to obtain his or her preferred placement. The reasons are both qualitative and quantitative. On the quantitative side, clients should be able to generate more application options. On the qualitative side, they can present themselves in a better light to interviewers or other placement decision-makers.

Second, psychiatrically disabled clients frequently have trouble in the area of job retention. The more skilled the client is in placement activities, the better the chances are that the client can obtain the type of position which she or he will be motivated to retain. This is partially due to the fact that with the development of placement skills, the client should have more and better opportunities for placement. In addition, the client is less likely to just "up and leave" because she or he develops an investment in the placement objectives by actively participating in the process. Finally, if the client wants or needs to change jobs he or she has a better chance of obtaining new employment without the renewed services of the rehabilitation practitioner.

In short, placement skills are important because they can contribute to both the acquisition and retention of positions by the psychiatrically disabled client.

WHEN AND WHERE CAREER PLACEMENT CAN BE USED

Career placement is appropriate for any psychiatrically disabled client who is diagnosed as having deficiencies in the career placement areas. Common client deficits in the placement area may include the following:

1. Inability to Identify Assets

The client is unable to articulate factually based assets which would make him or her attractive for a potential position.

(a) The client cannot articulate factual evidence indicative of his or her *ability to perform the tasks* required by the position.

(b) The client cannot articulate factual evidence indicative of his or her *dependability* (e.g., attendance, punctuality).

(c) The client cannot articulate factual evidence indicative of his or her *ability to relate to other people* (e.g., get along with peers and supervisors or to supervise others).

2. Inability to Develop Potential Job Position

The client is unable to identify a sufficient number of sources where she or he could obtain the type of position desired.

(a) The client cannot list *general types of places* where she or he might secure the desired position.

(b) The client cannot list *specific places* where she or he might secure the desired position.

3. Inability to Present Self in Writing

The client is unable to present him/herself in a written format in a manner which would facilitate his or her obtaining the desired position.

(a) The client cannot fill out necessary *application forms*.

(b) The client cannot write a *cover letter or a résumé* which effectively presents assets.

4. Inability to Present Self in Person

The client is unable to present her/himself in an interview in a manner which would facilitate acquisition of the desired position.

(a) The client lacks *interpersonal skills* needed to relate in an interview situation.

(b) The client lacks the *knowledge* and skills needed to answer interviewer's questions and ask own questions.

A client may or may not have all of the placement deficits outlined above. For example, one client may be able to fill out an application form but still may not have the interpersonal skills to get through an interview. In another situation, the client may not need all the placement skills because his or her unique situation simply does not require them. For example, the client may not be able to identify any potential employers, but knows that the state employment service has a record of all job openings in the area. Or the client may not need to be able to write a cover letter because the rehabilitation practitioner may have already made the contact for the client.

In the cases cited above, the practitioner would only need to work with the client on overcoming those particular deficits that the client possessed and that were relevant to reaching the desired position. Thus, although any particular client may not need all the placement skills, the practitioner her/himself must have all the skills. Such a highly skilled practitioner has a response repertoire that will enable her or him to meet the placement needs of any individual case.

Placement strategies are seen as appropriate skills to master for anyone who is working or planning to work with older adolescent or adult psychiatrically disabled clients in order to assist them in living, learning, and working more independently. The clients may be inpatients or outpatients; they may be preparing for placement in competitive or sheltered environments. In the latter case, the client's mastery of the placement skills will usually be viewed as preparation for later competitive placements. It should be noted that the process of career placement, with its emphasis on identifying client assets, can make many psychiatrically disabled clients feel more positive about themselves.

Case Illustration 7-3

There wasn't anything special about Brad — or so he felt, at least. Since his release from the hospital he had been receiving therapy from Clara on an outpatient basis. She had been quite pleased with the way he had regained a real degree of self-confidence. Faced with the prospect of looking for work, however, Brad now seemed in danger of losing everything he had gained.

"Ah, they're not even going to talk to a jerk like me," he told Clara, gesturing to the advertisement on her desk which she had clipped from that morning's paper.

"I know you feel really helpless because you don't have any experience in this area." Clara responded. "But after all, 'vending machine salesman' was right at the top of that list of possible jobs that we drew up together. And this ad says that Samson, Inc., is looking for exactly that kind of salesman."

"Yeah, I know," Brad said glumly. "But let's face it — I never sold supplies for vending machines in my life. There's bound to be a whole lot of guys applying who are real pros. I wouldn't have a chance!"

But Clara felt sure that Brad would have a chance. And she was determined to see that he made the most of it. After talking with him for a few minutes, she introduced the idea of exploring his occupational assets.

"What do you mean, my assets?" The idea confused Brad at first. But Clara was able to clear up this confusion quickly.

"Sure, previous experience is one important thing that most employers look for right away," she said. "But it's not the only thing. In many cases, an employer is even more concerned with what kind of worker you are in general. What we need to do is explore some ways of showing your strengths — and doing it in such a way that Samson ends up being willing to overlook your lack of specific experience."

"Yeah?" Brad may have been unconvinced but he was clearly interested. "It sounds good. How do we do it?"

"We give them *proof* of how well you've done in the past," Clara said. "We take a good long look at your past jobs, your outside activities — everything we can. And we come up with as many hard-and-fast facts as we can to show that you're the best person for this particular job.

And this is precisely what they did, beginning with Brad's earlier jobs. He had already mentioned that he had worked as a door-to-door salesman some time before. With Clara's help, he remembered that his own sales during the first four months of the job had been nearly double that of the two other salesmen who had started work at the same time.

"I never thought about that before," he said. "Hey, that makes me sound pretty good, huh?" Moving on, there was a real degree of enthusiasm in his new exploration.

"Listen, I got something," he exclaimed after a few more minutes. "For a job like this you got to do a lot of driving, right? Well, you're looking at a guy with an A-number-one perfect driving record! Not one accident in fourteen years of driving — not even a ticket!"

"That's beautiful," Clara said, grinning and taking notes furiously. "And listen, didn't you say you never used to get sick on the jobs like a lot of the other men?"

"Right, right!" Brad nodded vigorously. "Sure — that's how I did so good on my door-to-door job! I only missed one day the whole time I worked there. Those other guys, they must have been out three or four times a month!"

"Missed only one day on job," Clara murmured as she wrote, "Lowest absentee rate of all employees . . ."

In the end it was a cheerful, confident Brad who walked out of Clara's office and headed for Samson, Inc. And if Clara's strong streak of practical realism kept her from feeling totally confident, she still felt far more pleasure than surprise when Brad called the next day, his voice high and excited. "Hey, guess what!" he exclaimed. "I got the job! I did!" And Clara thought, "sure you did. There's something special about all of us if we just know how to look for it . . ."

TABLE 7-3
STEPS TO CAREER PLACEMENT

ACTING TO GET A JOB

    Present self in person
    Present self in writing

**UNDERSTAND
THE CLIENT'S WORK
OPPORTUNITIES**

    Identify unlisted job openings
    Identify listed job openings

**EXPLORE
THE CLIENT'S
ASSETS**

    Identify assets from work and educational experience.
    Explore work and educational experience

The practitioner can work with clients to develop opportunities for placement in either individual or group contexts. The number of clients will depend upon the amount of individual attention the individuals require in order to be able to complete the needed tasks. It should also be noted that career placement skills can be introduced at any point in the psychiatric treatment process. More specifically, placement opportunities may be developed with clients prior to therapy being initiated, concurrent with the therapeutic process, or after this process has been completed.

THE PROCESS OF CAREER PLACEMENT

There are three major steps involved in a total career placement intervention. These steps are presented in Table 7-3. As suggested by Table 7-3, the steps are of a developmental nature. That is, one must first identify *what* it is she or he has to offer before one begins to look for a place to offer it. In like manner, one must know *where* one can offer something be-

fore she or he can learn *how* to apply for the job itself.

Thus in most cases, the client must proceed by initially *exploring* his or her past work and educational experiences in order to specify what she or he has accomplished. Once this exploratory process has been completed, the client must work to understand the specific businesses, agencies, or institutions where she or he can use her or his assets to obtain the desired position. Finally, the client must *act* to offer his or her assets both orally and in writing.

The client can achieve the maximal amount of independence if she or he not only completes each of the major steps, but also learns how to do each of the steps her/himself. Obviously the amount of client learning will vary depending upon the client's level of functioning. Whenever appropriate, the practitioner must work with the client to help him or her actually learn the career placement process. In this manner, the client will be able to replicate the placement process independent of the practitioner at some future point.

FUTURE DIRECTIONS

Placement is the final stage that in fact determines whether the practitioner's and client's vocational rehabilitation efforts have been relevant. It is a criterion against which all other career intervention efforts can be judged. In order to maximize the chances for success, the following guidelines are offered.

1. Because placement is a critical life event for the client, intensive planning and support are needed by the client. Such support may include on-site visits with the client and his or her employer. Both parties may benefit from anticipatory guidance in terms of predicting what problems to expect, what kinds of stresses a new career brings, and how to cope with them. Possible techniques might include "walking the client through" the process of taking the correct route to work, meeting his or her supervisor, becoming acquainted with the work site, and understanding the routine and regular work tasks. On-going visits with the client and the employer should be an integral part of a placement program in order to deal with issues before they become overwhelming problems. In addition, the use of groups is a useful, supportive, and problem-solving mechanism for clients. Also, enlisting the help of a co-worker on the job is another option to help a client acclimate to the working environment. A placement program gradually increasing attendance and responsibility is another way to help the client adjust to a new job and career.

2. As mentioned before, clients often lack the skills or responses to deal with new work or interpersonal situations. The use of skill training with respect to job seeking, job interviewing, and anticipated work problems is an effective tool in developing a response repertoire for a variety of circumstances.

3. Typically, practitioners have focused on limited avenues of job opportunities for clients. Outside of those usual opportunities described in government publications, there are many jobs that exist that are not mentioned. It is important that practitioners not bias their options based upon their own values, background, and training. Experience has shown that clients can develop their own jobs either individually or as groups (Fairweather et al. 1969; Lamb et al. 1970). Practitioners may have to focus on more creative options outside the usual avenues of employment, especially when unemployment is high and even non-disabled groups experience difficulty finding jobs.

CAREER INTERVENTION STRATEGIES – A CONCLUDING COMMENT

Levine and Levine (1969) have observed that deviance is largely defined by a person's inability to live independently by earning a living. Until the time that our social value system accepts a life of dependence and welfare existence, work will continue to be a highly visible criterion of mental health. For that reason alone, vocational rehabilitation will continue to play a significant role in psychiatric rehabilitation. More than that, however, work provides a structure in which social contact and purposeful activity is facilitated for a population which has limited resources in order to develop and structure activities. Work will therefore also be a significant therapeutic activity for many clients.

Unfortunately, however, many mental health professionals do not seem to attach much importance to career intervention strategies. An obvious reflection of this situation is the low status, low pay, and low profile of career intervention specialists within the mental health system. Much of the fault for this situation appears to lie with vocational rehabilitation practitioners. Often they have allowed their function to become that of a "job person," that is, the person responsible for "getting the client a job." They have not been articulate in describing the importance of what they do and the complexities involved in doing it. They have acted as if the employment outcome for psychiatrically disabled clients was much better than it actually is. They have not served as effective spokespersons for what they have to offer the mental health system.

The present chapter categorized the career intervention process into three distinct categories for the purpose of highlighting the complexities involved in vocational rehabilitation. Each of these strategies (work adjustment training, career counseling, career placement) takes time and tremendous skill on the part of the practitioner. The practitioner must not only learn the skills involved in these career intervention areas, but must also articulate the career intervention process to other mental health practitioners. In this way, mental health practitioners will be able to make more useful referrals to vocational rehabilitation practitioners. This will also allow those professionals who specialize in vocational rehabilitation more time to effectively achieve a vocational outcome for their clients.

ENDNOTES

[1]This chapter was written with the assistance of Roger Davies and Linda Boucher.

REFERENCES

Anthony, W. A., Cohen, M. R. and Vitalo, R. The measurement of rehabilitation outcome. **Schizophrenia Bulletin**, 1978, in press.

Anthony, W. A. and Margules, A. Toward improving the efficacy of psychiatric rehabilitation: A skills training approach. **Rehabilitation Psychology**, 1974, *21*: 101-105.

Bachrach, L. A note on some recent studies of released mental hospital patients in the community. **American Journal of Psychiatry**, 1976, *133*: 73-75.

Brown, B. S. Responsible community care of former mental hospital patients. **New Dimensions in Mental Health**. NIMH, Rockville, Md, 1977.

Erickson R. Outcome studies in mental hospitals: A review. **Psychological Bulletin**, 1975, *62*: 519-540.

Farina, A., Felner, R. and Boudreau, L. Reactions of workers to male and female mental patient job applicants. **Journal of Consulting and Clinical Psychology**, 1973, *41*: 363-372.

Farina, A. and Felner, R. Employment interviewer reactions to former mental patients. **Journal of Abnormal Psychology**, 1973, *82*: 268-272.

Fairweather, G. W., Sanders, D. H., Maynard, H., Cressler, D. L. and Black, D. S. **Community life for the mentally ill: An alternative to institutional care**. Chicago: Aldine, 1969.

Foote, J. R., Wilson, R., Ollerich, D. W., Latimer, J. L., Ruppert, R. J., Fisher, F. W. and Waxler, R. Programs for patient-workers: Approaches and problems in four institutions. **Hospital and Community Psychiatry**, 1976, 93-97.

Friel, T. W. and Carkhuff, R. R. **The art of developing a career: Helper's guide**. Amherst, Mass.: Human Resource Development Press, 1974.

Gergen, K. J. **The concept of self**. New York: Holt, Rinehart & Winston, 1971.

Goffman, E. **Asylums: Essays on the social situation of mental patients and other inmates**. Garden City, N. Y.: Anchor Books, 1961.

Goldenberg, I. I. **Build me a mountain: Youth, poverty, and the creations of new settings**, Cambridge, Mass.: MIT Press, 1971.

Hersen, M. and Bellack, A. Social skills for chronic psychiatric patients — rationale, research, findings and future directions. **Comprehensive Psychiatry**, 1976, *17*: 559-580.

Hersen, P. and Blanchard, K. H. **Management of Organizational behavior: Utilizing human resources. 2nd Edition.** Englewood Cliffs, N. Y.: Prentice-Hall, Inc., 1972.

Lamb, H. R., Heath, D. and Downing, J. F. **Handbook of community mental health practice.** San Francisco: Jossey-Bass, 1969.

Lamb, H. R. **Rehabilitation in community mental health.** San Francisco: Jossey-Bass, 1971.

Levine, M. and Levine, A. **A social history of helping services: Clinic, court, school, and community.** New York: Appleton-Century-Crofts, 1970.

McGuinnes, E. **Social behavior: A functional analysis.** Boston: Houghton-Mifflin, 1970.

Meichenbaum, D. and Cameron, R. Training schizophrenics to talk to themselves: A means of developing attentional controls. **Behavior Therapy**, 1973, *4*: 515-534.

Miller, D. C. and Form, W. H. **Industrial sociology.** New York: Harper and Row, 1957.

Neff, W. **Work and human behavior.** New York: Atherton Press, 1968.

Neff, W. Rehabilitation and work. In **Rehabilitation Psychology: Proceedings of the National Conference on the Psychological Aspects of Disability.** October, 1970, American Psychological Association.

Olshansky, S. Changing vocational behavior through normalization. In W. Wolfensberger, ed. **Normalization: The principle of normalization in human services.** Toronto, Canada: National Institute on Mental Retardation, 1975.

Pierce, R. M., Anthony, W. A. and Cohen, M. **Psychiatric rehabilitation practice: The skills of career counseling.** Amherst, Mass.: Carkhuff Institute of Human Technology, 1977.

Pierce, R. M., Cohen, M. R., Cohen, B. and Anthony, W. A. **Psychiatric rehabilitation practice: The skills of career placement.** Amherst, Mass.: Carkhuff Institute of Human Technology, 1977.

Salomone, P. R. A client-centered approach to job placement. **Vocational Guidance Quarterly**, 1971, *19*: 266-270.

Schwartz, D. A. Expanding a sheltered workshop to replace non-paying patient jobs. **Hospital and Community Psychiatry**, 1976, *27*: 98-101.

Shrey, D. Post-employment services for the severely disabled. **Rehabilitation Counseling Bulletin**, 1976, *19*: 564-570.

Spaniol, L. A program evaluation model of rehabilitation agencies and facilities. **Journal of Rehabilitation Administration**, 1977, *1*: 4-15.

Super, D. E. The psychology of careers: An introduction to vocational development. New York: Harper and Row, 1957.

Super, D. E. and Bohn, M. J. Occupational psychology. Belmont, Calif.: Wadsworth Publishing Co., 1970.

Test, M. and Stein, L. Practical guidelines for the community treatment for markedly impaired patients. Community Mental Health Journal, 1976, 12: 72-82.

Wolfensberger, W. Normalization: The principle of normalization in human services. Toronto, Canada: National Institute on Mental Retardation, 1975.

Zooke, J., Bell, M., Pakstis, J. and Struck, W. A group employment program for rehabilitating clients with severe emotional disabilities. Hospital and Community Psychiatry, 1976, 27: 81-87.

CHAPTER VIII
Community Rehabilitation Programming

Within the last twenty years, large numbers of previously hospitalized psychiatrically disabled helpees have been discharged (Ozarin, 1976). During that period the implicit policy of most public mental hospitals has been one of de-institutionalization, resulting in the presence of many more psychiatrically disabled helpees in the community. Unfortunately, the policy of de-institutionalization was prompted more by economic and political considerations than by any understanding of the treatment and rehabilitation implications (Jones, 1975). Thus, one of the greatest determinants of a particular patient's chances of being discharged became the discharge policy of the hospital in which she or he was a patient, rather than the actual clinical functioning of the patient (Cumming & Markson, 1975).

In retrospect, it appears that *the practice of discharging large numbers of psychiatrically disabled helpees into the community was an idea whose time had come but whose method had not.* Within recent years, professional journals and the public media have recounted numerous horrors regarding the plight of many discharged helpees. These studies ring familiar, as it was only a few years earlier that alarming accounts of the institutionalized patient appeared regularly in these same media. *Only the time and place seems to have changed; the descriptions and faces of the patients are strikingly familiar.*

This dismal picture does not suggest that there were no patient benefits from the former policy of de-institutionalization. Some patients are in fact functioning at higher levels, with more freedom and responsibility, and in more humane environments. Yet much more in the way of community rehabilitation programming needs to be done, a fact that was not generally appreciated when the policy of de-institutionalization was initiated. For example, it was about twelve years after the initial 1963 legislation creating the community mental health center concept, before legislation was enacted which recognized rehabilitation services as essential treatment components. The Community Mental Health Center Amendments of 1975 (Public Law 94-63) mandated that federally funded mental health centers provide specific services to patients discharged from mental health facilities, including follow-up care and transitional halfway houses (Ozarin, 1976).

History has taught us, however, that simply legislating a service does not produce an effective service. In order for community-based rehabilitation efforts to reflect positive patient outcomes, the rehabilitation intervention must be carried out by skilled rehabilitation practitioners equipped with relevant rehabilitation programs. The remainder of this chapter outlines some of the current problems in community rehabilitation programming and discusses some of the rehabilitation practitioner skills necessary to make a successful rehabilitation intervention in the community.

COMMUNITY NON-COORDINATION: AN ACTUAL TRANSCRIPT

(Case Illustration 8-1)

Family and Juvenile Court: Case of "C": Age 14

> The Court: Good morning "C," how are you? Mr. and Mrs. B. how are you? This is a review today, so let me hear how your plans have progressed.
>
> C: Probably OK.
>
> The Court: Probably?
>
> C: Yes.
>
> The Court: How is "C" doing, Mr. and Mrs. B?
>
> Mrs. B: He is learning to accept things more, but Mr. J. will tell you that we have tried to get help for "C."

Mr. J:	Well, we had an appointment with T. Hospital and
(the practitioner)	they are in the process of assessing "C;" we also applied to Q. Hospital and they referred us to L. Hospital. L. Hospital suggested P. Family Services, since the family was involved.
The Court:	So, in three months, this is all that has occurred. I hear that you are frustrated, "C" is frustrated and the family is frustrated. What exactly were you looking for?
Mr. J:	Our assessment showed that "C" needed a lot of inpatient treatment, but that "C's" relationships at home were his only thing, so we didn't want to take that away. So we have been looking for an outpatient facility. A lot of people have said that it is not within their boundary, or that it is not desperate enough.
The Court:	Well, it seems to me that part of all this circular activity is a result of community problems. The point is that it is a frustrating experience for you and that isn't getting anything solved. I don't have a very good idea of what is happening to "C" other than the fact that an outpatient facility is thought good. I wonder if being more clear wouldn't be helpful. . . . "C," how do you feel about school? Are you enjoying it more, or is it difficult or what is it like?"
C:	I'm doing better.
The Court:	Oh. What does it mean when *you* say you are doing better. Can you tell me what that means to you?
C:	It means that I am getting along better at school. Except that the guy in front of me is always turning around and belting me, or something.
The Court:	And what do you do then?
C:	I just ignore him and do my work. That's what doing better means. . . .
The Court:	So all told, it seems that the family needs counseling in order to understand their own feelings and how they deal with them. "C" needs help to understand what other things he can do besides punch people out when he is furious; he needs help in being able to catch up to his grade level in school. It looks like being specific about what particular problems we need a service for would help them to decide if they can help and would help us all to know who should be held responsible. . . .
After Comment:	As the Family Court judge noticed, the lack of a clear understanding and the goals set for the child led the service agency involved to have a great deal of difficulty in deciding which facility would be the appropriate one to press for assistance. Second, given the ambiguity, the practitioner could not convincingly present his client to the requested agencies. The facility, therefore, ended up designating the client as low priority and did not provide the service.

Some Current Problems in Community Rehabilitation Programming

1. **Patients who are discharged to the community are generally not functioning at a "normal" or adequate level.**

This fact is perhaps most clearly evidenced by the recidivism and employment data reported in Chapter II. Many psychiatrically disabled helpees who have been discharged into the community or treated in the community are not functioning very productively.

2. **Many rehabilitation settings in the community lack rehabilitation programs.**

The types of community rehabilitation settings are multitudinous; e.g., community residential facilities may be categorized as boarding homes, apartments, family care, foster care, home care, foster communities, group homes, halfway houses, lodge programs and nursing homes (Mannino, Ott & Shore, 1977). Unfortunately, the practitioners of many of these facilities often lack rehabilitation diagnostic skills and rehabilitation programming skills. As a result, the program emphasis is too often placed on symptom removal or custodial care rather than prescriptive skill building. Typically, group discussions, rather than group skill training are the modus operandi.

3. **Many psychiatrically disabled helpees refuse aftercare or terminate services prematurely.**

As indicated in Chapter V, the research suggests a rather horrendous no-show and premature termination rate for psychiatrically disabled helpees. Obviously, aftercare facilities cannot expect to demonstrate a significant effect on such indices as recidivism unless the helpee uses the aftercare service. One study attempted to judge the effects of recidivism on the initiation of formal aftercare programs in three Tennessee counties (McNees, Hannah, Schnelle & Bratton, 1977). Results indicated no overall reductions in recidivism rate as a result of the initiation of aftercare programs. However, recidivism rates were lower for those individuals who contacted the aftercare program than for those who did not. Clearly, not enough helpees chose to use the aftercare programs.

4. **Interventions with the patient's significant others is not a strong enough emphasis of most community rehabilitation programs.**

Too often the focus of the rehabilitation intervention is only on the patient. Yet what is becoming increasingly clear is that one of the factors associated with hospital admission is the perceptions of the patient's functioning by significant others (Carpenter & Bourestom, 1976; Cumming & Markson, 1975; Franklin, Kittredge & Thrasher, 1975). At the present state of our knowledge it would be inconceivable to conduct a rehabilitation intervention without involving the significant others in the patient's living, learning, and working environment.

5. **The community rehabilitation intervention often places too little emphasis on teaching the helpee various emotional-interpersonal or social skills.**

In the past the primary skill teaching focus in many rehabilitation programs has often been on ADL activities in daily living skill development or various sheltered or transitional work activities. An additional focus must be placed on the emotional-interpersonal skills which the helpee must have in order to function in his or her living, learning, and working environment. Recent research suggests that the patient's interpersonal or social functioning is a significant source of variance in recidivism outcome (Franklin et al. 1975; Miller & Willer, 1976).

6. **Not enough utilization has been made of community volunteers.**

Too often the community support system is only conceived of as either professional persons, facilities, or agencies. Yet one of the most effective deterrents to recidivism is the presence of a person in the community responsible for the patient's well-being (Katkin, Zimmerman, Rosenthal & Ginsburg, 1975). This person does not need to be a professional working out of an agency; rather, excellent outcomes can be achieved by volunteers working out of their homes. These volunteers can assist the patient in a number of ways, by stimulating the patient to perform his or her skills, reinforcing this skill behavior, serving as a model or teacher, and collecting evaluative information needed for program modification.

7. **The community rehabilitation settings often lack an evaluative component.**

If community rehabilitation programming is going to improve, then the community settings must evaluate their on-going rehabilitation efforts. Otherwise, ten years from now we will know little more about psychiatric rehabilitation than our present minimal level of understanding. In order for this evaluation effort to occur, each rehabilitation practitioner must be equipped with rehabilitation evaluation skills (Chapter IX provides a further discussion of rehabilitation program evaluation skills).

8. **Strong community resistance often exists against development of community rehabilitation facilities.**

Newspaper accounts routinely report on community antipathy toward the development of rehabilitation facilities within certain community boundaries. Neighborhood opposition has often been vocal and effective in preventing new facilities from opening. Rehabilitation practitioners must be extremely skillful in developing programs capable of changing the community's opposition.

Relevant to attempts at overcoming community antagonism toward such settings is the research on changing attitudes toward disabled persons. Anthony (1972) reviewed this research and found that in order to run an effective attitude change program, the target of the program must be exposed to positive information about the disability and have contact with the disabled person(s). Neither contact nor information alone is generally successful in developing more positive attitudes. Thus, programs designed to overcome community opposition toward rehabilitation facilities should probably contain both information about and contact with psychiatrically disabled persons. Smiley (1972) has pro-

vided a good example of an attitude change program designed to recruit community volunteers for a halfway house for the mentally retarded. The information component included several speeches on mental retardation, normalization, and community care. The contact component of the attitude change program consisted of entertainment by a rock-and-roll band comprised of mentally retarded musicians.

9. **Many employers possess negative attitudes toward the psychiatrically disabled.**

However, this problem may to some extent be mitigated by rehabilitation programming. The research seems to suggest that these negative attitudes can to a great extent be overcome if the helpee makes an effective in-person presentation to the potential employer (Brand & Claiborn, 1976; Farina & Felner, 1973). It may not be the stigma associated with psychiatric disability that most prevents the former psychiatrically disabled person from finding employment; a greater deterrent to employment may be the helpee's failure to present him/herself adequately in the employment interview.

Thus, one very effective way of combating negative employer attitudes is through the helpee's own behavior. This skill has been referred to in previous chapters as stigma reduction. In these instances the helpee is providing both the contact and information experience. An experimental study by Evans (1976) is an excellent example of a stigma reduction program carried out by a person with a disability and which produced positive attitude change in non-disabled persons.

10. **Low expectations of community behavior by the helpee and significant others can reduce the helpee's ability to function effectively.**

If individuals and agencies within the community do not expect and demand more skillful and less pathological functioning, the chances of the helpee performing more competently are reduced. A rather large body of research exists which suggests that psychiatrically disabled helpees have a significant amount of control over their behavior and that they can, in fact, demonstrate more healthy behavior if that is what is expected (Braginsky & Braginsky, 1967; Chesno & Kelman, 1975; Krieger & Levin, 1976; Kroger, 1967; Kroger & Turnbull, 1970; Price, 1972). In one study, for example, inpatients who were labeled and treated more normally than in the traditional psychiatric labeling and treatment process were discharged to the community much more quickly than the control group of inpatients who were treated as if they were "sick" (Chesno & Kelman, 1975).

11. **Many clients are not sufficiently prepared to effectively use community resources.**

The figures alluded to earlier with respect to the rates of no show and premature termination are a direct reflection of the client's inability to use mental health resources. Clients are often equally unskilled in using resources such as the social security office, employers, vocational rehabilitation resources, banks, recreational facilities, and others. Many psychiatrically disabled helpees often accept institutional life because they lack the skills to cope as an outpatient (Townsend, 1976). The rehabilitation practitioner must do much more than suggest or refer the helpee to various resources in the community. The practitioner must also teach the client how to use and benefit from the resource.

12. **Many resources are not sufficiently prepared to service psychiatrically disabled clients.**

Just as the client must be prepared to use the resource, the resource must often be prepared to receive and service the client. Even if the resource is a mental health facility, a need may still exist for education in the type of program each particular helpee needs. The alarming rate of premature terminations suggests that more resource preparation is needed.

13. **Many communities still lack the community resources they need.**

Even though a multiplicity of rehabilitation settings have been developed, there are many times when the specific community resource needed by a particular client is lacking. In these instances, the rehabilitation practitioner must have the skills to either modify existing resources or develop new resources.

14. **Many rehabilitation practitioners do not possess a sufficient repertoire of community rehabilitation programming skills so that they can most effectively use the helpee's community to achieve rehabilitation goals.**

This problem should come as no surprise, as these community rehabilitation programming skills are still being developed and evaluated. The next section of this chapter outlines the ingredients of some of these community rehabilitation programming skills.

THE SKILLS OF COMMUNITY REHABILITATION

The practitioner skills used to facilitate community rehabilitation programming are called *community coordinating skills* (Cohen, Pierce, Anthony & Cohen, 1977). These practitioner skills are needed by rehabilitation practitioners in addition to the rehabilitation diagnostic and programming skills outlined in Chapters IV and V.

A more detailed explanation of these community coordinating skills has been provided by Cohen, Pierce, Anthony and Cohen (1977). The present section serves as an introduction to familiarize the reader with some of the essential skill components of community coordinating.

In essence, community coordination involves making effective decisions concerning the resource which will best serve a particular client, and then developing and implementing a plan to actually use the resource. Effective practitioner functioning in this area will minimize inappropriate use of resources and maximize the client's ability to take advantage of the resources which are used. More specifically, community coordination involves three basic steps: 1) *evaluating and deciding* upon the environment or resource which will best allow the client to overcome deficits (or build assets) or will best accommodate his or her existing strengths and deficits; 2) *obtaining the commitment* of the environment or resource to provide specific services needed by the client; and 3) *devel-*

oping and implementing a program to overcome potential client or environmental problems in using the environment or resource. Practitioners capable of performing each of these steps are said to possess: 1) community decision-making skills, 2) community marketing skills, and 3) community programming skills.

It is important for practitioners to possess these skills because many times the use of a community resource is a critical step in the rehabilitation process. If a client fails a training program, or returns to a setting with which she or he cannot cope, or is not hospitalized when she or he needs to be, the results can be disastrous. Even if the results are not disastrous, another failure becomes one more problem with which an already harrassed client must deal. Thus the practitioner must do all that she or he can in order to evaluate the community resources available, make the best decision possible about which particular resource will have to be used, and plan what has to be done to make that resource most effective for the client.

I. DECISION-MAKING SKILLS

Any time there is more than one potential community resource (i.e., a person, agency, or program) that can be used to help achieve the client's rehabilitation goals, the practitioner can employ decision-making skills in order to make the decision more knowledgeably and systematically. The advantages of using a systematic decision-making process are: a) the decision process is made more comprehensible to the helpee, significant others, and the practitioner, b) the reasons for preferring one resource alternative over another are articulated clearly and observably, and c) it is possible to evaluate the various alternative resources from a number of frames of reference, that is, based on the helpee, the helpee's significant others, or the practitioner's value system. The decision-making skill component of community coordinating is composed of several steps (Cohen, Pierce, Anthony & Cohen, 1977). In brief, some of these major steps include: 1) brainstorming resource alternatives, 2) identifying the

values relevant to this specific decision, 3) operationalizing the values, 4) researching the potential alternatives, and 5) choosing the preferred alternative based on how well it will satisfy the previously identified values.

1. Brainstorming Alternatives

In identifying alternative resources, the basic idea is to consider all possible means for achieving the client's rehabilitation goal. Non-goal-related resources can then be eliminated from future consideration. If the client's goal is to live independently, then a group home should not be considered as a potential alternative resource since the client cannot live independently under these circumstances. Thus, each possible resource must be put to the test; can it achieve the goal? All possible alternatives which "pass" this test should be considered. In addition, the brainstorming process should occur within a "reality" context. In other words, the practitioner may need to identify one or two real factors that would limit the possible alternatives. For example, Paul, a client who was looking for a group residential facility limited himself by two reality factors. First, he did not want to relocate. This meant that he would limit his alternatives to the city in which he lived. Second, because he had no transportation of his own, any group home which he selected would need to have access to public transportation. Thus, when the practitioner and this client brainstormed alternatives, they included these two parameters in their search for potential resources.

2. Identifying Values

Once the list of possible resources has been developed, the next decision-making step is to identify the values or criteria that should be used to evaluate which resource will be best for the client. For example, the question facing Paul is: "What values should be considered in deciding whether a particular group-home facility, supervised apartment-living program, or the family-care program would be best."

In developing a comprehensive list of

values, it is helpful to use value categories. Using categories ensures the completeness of the values list. One strategy which is applicable to the development of almost all value lists is to categorize values as physical, emotional-interpersonal, and intellectual.

Physical values are those considerations which have primarily a physical effect on the client (e.g., location, availability). Emotional-interpersonal values refer to those criteria which affect the way the client feels about him/herself or others (e.g., supervision, opportunity for making friends). Finally, intellectual values refer to those things which cognitively impact the client (e.g., opportunity to make own decisions, go to adult education classes).

3. Operationalizing Values

As values are identified, they should also be operationalized. Operationalizing something means defining it in an observable and measurable way. The basic strategy for doing this involves using *time* and *amount* to define behavior. Formats that can be used to do this are: 1) amount of _____ and 2) amount or percent of time doing _____. For example, "expense" may be defined as "the amount of money it costs." "Independence" might be defined as "the amount of time I can do what I want to do."

In the process of operationalizing values, it may become clear that what initially appeared to be a single value is, in fact, two or more values. For example, a client may indicate that she or he wants to live in a place which is "convenient." When the practitioner explores what the client means by this value, she or he discovers that "convenience" refers both to being close to work and to being close to follow-up treatment. Each of these values may then be defined:

Convenience to work — amount of time it takes to get to work.

Convenience to treatment — amount of time it takes to get to treatment.

The check step for knowing when a value has been operationalized involves making sure that it contains only one major element. The process of operationalizing values will make clear to all concerned exactly what is meant by the value. All the relevant persons who are capable of participating in the decision-making process should help identify and operationalize the values. This will usually mean the practitioner, the client, experts, and significant others who are affected by the decision. For example, the practitioner could ask a halfway house director what values should be considered in making a decision about whether or not to use a halfway house as a resource. If a client was considering whether or not to live with relatives, the relatives' values concerning this situation would also have to be introduced into a decision-making process. Clearly, significant others will often be affected by the decision.

4. Researching Potential Alternatives

The research process involves gathering any information which is necessary to assess the value characteristics of each alternative resource. For example, in investigating the value of "expense," the client or practitioner might investigate the rental fee for the supervised apartment program, the family-care program, and transitional facilities (halfway houses). In some cases, it may be most appropriate to use general sources of information. For example, one might go to the central office of a family-care program for information rather than to individual family homes.

Either the practitioner, the client, or significant others may be doing the research. This will depend on the client's and significant other's capabilities as well as the accessibility of needed information. In general, the more the client or significant others can do, the better. Their active participation will lead to more investment in the ultimate decision.

5. Choosing the Preferred Alternative

The actual decision-making process involves evaluating each alternative in terms of how well each resource satisfies the values which have been developed. The informational base for doing this is the research completed in step number 4. There may be times when no alternative is capable of satisfying a significant portion of the client's values. In such a situation the practitioner may work to develop other alternative resources. At this point, there are three possible approaches the practitioners may take to develop additional alternatives for the client: 1) evaluate other alternative resources not originally considered 2) modify the alternative resources already evaluated to make these alternatives more favorable, and/or 3) develop new resource alternatives.

CHOOSING THE COMMUNITY RESOURCE CAREFULLY: AN APPLICATION OF DECISION-MAKING SKILLS

(Case Illustration 8-2)

Wes was determined to stay off drugs. But Shari knew full well that determination alone would not be enough. She had seen too many young people make what they felt was a total, absolute commitment, only to weaken in a matter of a few short weeks when things got tougher than they had anticipated.

"You don't need to be in the hospital," she told Wes. "What would probably be best is a group-living facility where you can get the kind of support you need to stay drug free."

Wes agreed with this. As it turned out, he was also familiar in a very limited way with one particular facility near his family's home. "A place called — Westward House, something like that," he said. "I remember a buddy of mine had an older brother who spent time there."

"Yes, I've heard of that one," Shari told him. "I think the name is Westwood House. It might be a good place, too. But I think it's probably too early to pick a facility right now. There are a lot of things we need to know in order to choose just the right house for you."

"What kind of things?" Wes wanted to know.

"Oh — like how many people are there, for example. Remember, you said you didn't like being crowded wherever you lived, so we wouldn't want to pick a place where everyone lived dormitory-style."

"Yeah, that makes good sense," Wes admitted. "Huh, I never would have thought to check that out."

"There are other considerations, too," Shari told him. "Like whether the people are your age or older or younger. Whether the types of drug problems being treated are like yours or of a different kind entirely. What kinds of activities go on. What the supervision is like. All sorts of things. The important thing is to pick the place that is best for you as an individual!"

Before her next meeting with Wes, Shari did a good deal of research into the residential facilities in the area. In the end, she was able to develop a list of some nine different facilities, each described in terms of its population, programs, client problems, supervision, and other significant features. When Wes arrived, she and he began to explore the alternatives reflected on this list. They did this in terms of a specific set of personal values which Shari helped Wes to develop; values like living in an uncrowded situation, living with people his own age, and so on.

Given Wes's clearly stated values and the information which Shari had gathered, the two were able to make considerable progress. Westwood House and several other facilities were eliminated because their client-populations were largely heroin addicts undergoing a methodone maintenance treatment; since Wes's drugs-of-choice had been marijuana and "speed," such facilities really didn't seem appropriate. Other facilities were eliminated because of one or another of Wes's own personal values. In the end, one facility — a group home called The Downey House — emerged as the clear favorite.

But then the powers-that-be threw a monkey wrench into Wes's and Shari's careful plans: Downey House, they learned, had just lost part of its funding and was thus unable to accept any more new residents!

This was a setback. Fortunately, Shari knew how to deal with it. None of

Wes's other alternatives were really favorable. But one — a place called Exodus House — had only posed one significant problem. Wes placed a lot of value on "privacy" and Exodus House generally placed new residents in four-bed dormitory rooms.

Would it be possible, Shari wondered, to modify this particular alternative — to get Wes a private room at Exodus House?

It was certainly worth a try. So Shari contacted the director of Exodus House and outlined Wes's situation and the crucial need for privacy.

"Well. . ." The director considered the matter. "We usually can't handle requests for private rooms. As it happens, however, we're not very full at this particular time. We've been moving some of our present residents into singles and I don't see any reason why we couldn't give Wes a single as well."

Full of fresh excitement, Shari and Wes recycled the decision-making process to include this new information. Sure enough — the possibility of "privacy" at Exodus House transformed this setting into the preferred and clearly favorable alternative for Wes!

"That's it, then," Wes said, real pleasure in his voice. "Man, I'm glad you thought to check out the chances for a single at Exodus! I really would have been crawling up the walls at some place like Westwood."

"It feels good to know you've chosen the best spot for your own particular situation," Shari responded. "And that positive feeling makes a lot of difference to your chances!"

Shari wasn't kidding. She knew that the confidence which Wes felt about his stay at Exodus House was a crucial ingredient in his overall program of treatment. Finding himself in a totally inappropriate facility, he might well have used this as an excuse to get back into drugs — "Man, this just isn't where my head is at!" But like Shari, Wes himself knew that Exodus House represented his best possible option. And knowing this, he would also know that if he didn't make it there, he probably couldn't make it anywhere.

II. MARKETING SKILLS

The second major set of community coordinating skills are marketing skills. The term marketing is not used in the sense of selling a product but in the professional sense of providing a service to both the helpee and the community resource. The purpose of marketing skills is to obtain the agreement of the resource to help the client. In many instances, this is a simple task. The resource exists and is designed to provide psychiatric rehabilitation services. It has openings available, and is familiar with clients with deficits similar to those of the client being referred. In cases where the preferred resource is a designated psychiatric rehabilitation program with services available to clients with needs similar to the referred client's, a request for service may be all that is needed. After obtaining the resource's agreement to provide the service to the client, the practitioner would begin working to ensure the client's successful use of the preferred resource.

In some cases, however, the referral will require more effort by the practitioner. When the preferred resource has been chosen as a result of the modification of a resource alternative, the practitioner must work to get the agreement of the resource to provide the modified service to the client. For example, consider the case of John, a client whose preferred alternative was a modified educational program at the local university. To obtain the desired program, the practitioner might need to persuade the admissions director and the dean of curriculum to change the eligibility and course requirements and to offer more internship experiences. The practitioner would then need to negotiate a contract or agreement about the changes the university is willing to make in order to meet John's rehabilitation goals. In other words, the practitioner would need to use his or her marketing skills to get the firm commitment of the university personnel to help this client.

Another common situation is one in

which the practitioner is limited in the rehabilitation options available to meet a client's needs. Here it becomes necessary for the practitioner to select as the preferred resource, a resource that is not designated for psychiatric rehabilitation purposes. For example, when the practitioner needs an educational tutor to help a client learn to read English, he or she may have a local community action program as the only alternative. The practitioner will need to persuade the community action program to designate a reading tutor to work with the psychiatric rehabilitation client. It may require special skills to negotiate an agreement with this program to provide services to this "different" type of client.

Lastly, the preferred resource may be unavailable. It may be either temporarily unavailable (e.g., has a waiting list because of large demand for service) or permanently unavailable. The preferred resource will frequently be temporarily unavailable and the practitioner will need to work hard to get the resource's immediate commitment to help the client. Less often, the practitioner will have chosen to develop an entirely new resource as the preferred resource. When the practitioner has chosen to develop a potentially new resource for the client, he or she will clearly need to make the resource *aware* of the problem, *persuade* the resource to agree to help, and *negotiate* an agreement about what services the resource will provide to the client.

1. Awareness Skills

Before the practitioner can begin working to implement the overall program goal, he or she must first obtain the agreement of the resource to provide services to the client. In John's case, the practitioner must get the commitment of the university to provide a modified program to John. The first step in getting their commitment is to make them aware of the client's problem and goal. To prepare for the initial contact with the preferred resource, the practitioner must have the answers to five questions.

First, the practitioner must have a clear statement of *what* service he or she is requesting from the resource. Second, the practitioner must know *who* to contact at the resource. Third and fourth, the practitioner will need to be prepared with a clear introductory statement of *who* he or she is and *who* the client is. For the practitioner, presenting him/herself will usually be a simple task. To present the client, however, may require planning to discriminate what facts are initially important and appropriate to share with the new resource. Minimally, a brief statement of the client's situation will need to be shared.

Lastly, the practitioner must indicate *why* he or she is contacting the specific resource. The reasons for contacting the resource will include a statement of how it was selected to meet the needs of the client. A description of the decision-making values in which the preferred resource alternative scored relatively high, would provide these reasons.

John's practitioner developed the following answers to the five questions:

What Is Requested?	A modified university program (lower eligibility requirements to include a previous grade-point average of 2.5, flexible on course requirements and capable of providing internship opportunities).
Who to Contact?	The admissions director will need to be contacted concerning John's acceptance; the dean of curriculum will need to be contacted regarding course requirements and internships.
Who Am I?	My name is Nancy Cosgrove. I am a counselor at the North Valley Mental Health Center.
Who Is the Client?	John is a young man who is very interested in continuing his education at your university.

Why Resource Was Chosen? The university was chosen because it offers John the opportunity to earn a degree, to participate in courses in which he has an interest and to interact closely with his instructor.

After completing the answers to these five questions, the practitioner is prepared to present the relevant facts necessary to make the resource aware of the client's problems and goals. In some instances, this will be all that is needed to get the resource's agreement to provide services to the client. In other cases, this will be just the beginning of the practitioner's efforts to gain the resource's commitment to help the client. Before actually contacting the resource, therefore, the practitioner should be prepared to persuade the resource to accept his or her client.

2. Persuading Skills

The second step in getting the agreement of the resource to provide services to the client is for the practitioner to persuade the resource of the benefits in helping the client. Typical benefits or advantages that could be presented include: generating new funds, getting positive publicity, increasing good will, reducing work load, realizing the stated objectives of resource, increasing productivity-efficiency, and saving money. The advantages that apply to a particular resource will vary. Therefore, the practitioner must begin by listing the advantages which specifically apply to the preferred resource. In order to list these advantages, it is helpful first to identify from the preceding list any advantages that might result from the preferred resource's agreement to help the client. Second, if there are any other advantages which are not on this list but which apply to this particular resource, they should be added to the list. An approach in generating advantages to the resource is to think about the resource's values — what is important to the resource — and whether helping the client would contribute to the attainment of these values.

After the list of advantages is completed, the practitioner will want to describe how each identified advantage could be attained. For example, if John's practitioner identified "publicity" as an advantage for the university, then a description of how it will be achieved might include the practitioner's submission of an article about the university to the local newspaper.

Another way to persuade the resource to accept the client is to present the assets of the client. The assets of the client, especially those that relate to the possibility of success in achieving the overall program goal, will be important in encouraging the resource to help the client. The practitioner may begin by listing the assets or strengths of the client. Many of these assets are identified during the rehabilitation diagnostic process which operationalized the client's assets in relation to her or his specific living, learning, and working environments. In addition, the practitioner may add assets that have become apparent through continued client exploration during the community coordination process.

Once the list of assets is complete, the practitioner will want to write a description of how the client's assets provide "assurances" that the overall program goal can be achieved. For example, the fact that John is in good physical condition assures that he has the energy to study and attend classes.

Even though the practitioner may present the advantages to the resource and outline the client's own assets, the resource may still object to providing services. The practitioner must therefore be prepared to respond to the objections of the resource. Objections may stem from client deficits or liabilities (e.g., lack of social skills) or from the resource's own situation (e.g., staff resistant to working with psychiatric patients).

To overcome possible objections of the resource, the practitioner has a number of potential strategies available to him or her. *One strategy is to turn a client liability into an asset:* For example, a potential liability for John is that he was a past drug user. One way to turn this into an asset might be to point out the excellent treatment that John received and indicate that the treatment has resulted in a deep commitment to not using drugs. Additionally, if appropriate, the practitioner can point out that because of John's experience and treatment, John is probably less likely than most other students to experiment with drugs. *A second strategy is to compensate for a liability* by showing how other client characteristics help alleviate that particular liability. For example, another potential liability for John is that he was a psychiatric patient. The university might state that his past hospitalizations would scare other students. In response to this objection, the practitioner might point out that John's outgoing and friendly manner has helped him in the past to win many friends. *A third strategy is to deny that the liability is critical.* This means being able to show that what the resource fears will not come true. For example, in John's case the university might be concerned that their instructors are unprepared to meet the needs of a psychiatrically disabled patient. The practitioner might counter this objection by indicating that John will continue to rely on his practitioner and make only appropriate demands of his instructors.

To prepare to handle the potential objections of the resource, the practitioner must anticipate the objections. The practitioner must, therefore, begin by listing the possible objections that the resource may have to helping the client. In order to list the objections, the practitioner may review the client's deficits as identified during the rehabilitation diagnostic process. The practitioner should then select those deficits of which the resource will probably become aware, and put them on the list of potential objections. Also, the practitioner will want to be sensitive to any client deficits that might conflict with the resource's unique situation. For example, if the university has received poor publicity regarding its increase in student drug use, John's practitioner would want to include John's past drug usage on the list of potential objections. To complete the list, the

practitioner will have to include the resource's problems that might make it difficult to comply with the program needs of the client.

But what if the resource either delays making a decision or decides negatively? At this point, it is important for the practitioner to have a response that at least keeps open the possibility of further discussion with the resource. If the resource delays its decision, the following are the types of actions the practitioner may request: another meeting with the resource person to further discuss the referral; a meeting with the resource person's colleague(s) to further discuss the referral; a meeting with the resource person and his or her colleague(s) to further discuss the referral or a telephone call or visit within a short period to further discuss the referral. The purpose of additional opportunities to discuss the referral is to give the practitioner an opportunity to prepare additional persuasive responses (e.g., reasons that will overcome objections, a new list of client assets, etc.).

If the resource decides negatively, the practitioner may either work to open up additional opportunities to discuss the referral or attempt to get the resource to help find another resource to help the client. Some possible responses might include: a request to call back within a short period in case there has been a change in the decision; a request that the resource telephone another resource which might be able to help the client; or a request to see if the resource can give the name of another resource which might be able to help the client. The purpose of these responses is to find another alternative to help the client and to try to end with a positive relationship with the initial resource. In the case where the resource decides negatively and no other resource can provide the service to the client, the practitioner must recycle the decision-making process in order to identify a new preferred resource. If the resource decides positively to help the client, however, the negotiation of the best possible services for the client is the last step in getting the commitment of the resource.

3. Negotiating Skills

Prior to actual agreement-negotiations with the resource, the practitioner will need to know specifically what agreement issues are to be negotiated and the favorability of potential alternative agreements for each issue. The issues and the favorability of alternative agreements provide the practitioner with a clear picture or statement of what he or she would specifically like to get the resource to agree to provide for the client. For example, John's practitioner was pleased that, after his or her persuasive efforts, the university expressed openness to accepting John and modifying the course requirements and internship possibilities. Yet neither the specific changes in course requirements and internships, nor the terms of acceptance had been specified. Before meeting with the university personnel to negotiate the agreement, therefore, John's practitioner defined the three issues to be negotiated; acceptance terms, course requirements, and internships. The next task for John's practitioner was to explore the possible alternative agreements for each issue. For example, acceptance terms might range from John's unconditional acceptance to requiring John to successfully complete prerequisite courses.

When exploring agreement alternatives, the practitioner needs to define the favorability for the client of each alternative. Using a variation of the decision-making skills described in this chapter, the practitioner may assign a favorability scale score ranging from very favorable (level 5) to minimally acceptable (level 1) to potential alternative agreements.

Once the practitioner has developed the client's favorability scales for possible alternatives on the agreement issues, he or she is almost ready to meet with the resource. In negotiating the agreement with the resource, the practitioner will be trying to get the resource to agree to the most favorable terms for the client. However, he or she may not always succeed in getting the most favorable agreement. It is important, therefore, for the practitioner to know when to compromise or to agree to less favorable terms. Where necessary,

the practitioner will need to develop, either with or without the resource, a favorability scale for the alternative agreements from the resource's own perspective. For example, John's practitioner knew it would be difficult for the university to agree to unconditional acceptance of John; some type of trial period would be most favorable to them.

The guideline in developing the resource's favorability scale is that the more consistent the alternative is with the resource's usual way of functioning, the more favorable it will be to the resource. By considering the client's and resource's favorability scales, John's practitioner was prepared to expect a full range of alternatives and to negotiate the best possible program for John.

In essence, the agreement is the point of best possible match between the client's and resource's frames of reference. During the negotiating period the practitioner will also need to use the persuasion skills previously discussed. Once the agreement issues have been resolved and both the resource and practitioner are satisfied with the agreement, a written agreement can be developed and signed. A written agreement, though not binding, ensures that the resource, client, and practitioner all understand the agreement. It also helps to ensure the commitment of the resource and client in completing their part of the agreement. A written agreement should specify *who* is to do *what*. What is to be provided will have to be operationalized. To operationalize the service, a statement of *how* the provision of service is to be measured should be included. The agreement should also include the reasons *why* the service is to be provided. Additionally, the location or *where* services are to be provided, and the time *when* they are to be completed should be spelled out.

III. PROGRAMMING SKILLS

The third major set of community coordinating skills are called programming skills. These skills involve the development and implementation of the plans needed to ensure the success of the client's use of the resource. The plans include developing programs that prepare the client to use the resource *as well as programs that prepare the resource to help the client*. For example, if the resource to be used is the state employment service, client preparation might involve helping him or her to identify the criteria she or he could use to evaluate job possibilities, teaching him or her to fill out applications and rehearsing the employment interview. Just as important, however, the practitioner may also need to develop a plan to prepare the resource for the client. For example, the practitioner might ask the employment service to monitor the client's performance during employment interviews. Lastly, the practitioner may work with both the client and the resource to implement the plans. Implementation of the plans may involve evaluating the progress of the person carrying out the steps of the program and modifying the program as necessary.

The programming skills referred to in this section are the same programming skills presented previously in Chapter V and discussed more extensively in Anthony, Pierce, and Cohen (1977). These practitioner skills include the skills needed to both develop and implement programs.

The discussion of these programming skills will not be repeated here. The practitioner simply uses his or her rehabilitation programming skills to overcome anticipated problems in the client's use of preferred community resources.

However, one aspect of community programming needs to be deliberately emphasized — the development of programs to ensure that the resource is prepared to receive the client. Obviously this is particularly important for resources that have had little experience in dealing with psychiatrically disabled clients. Yet even professionals and agencies with an established track record in dealing with psychiatrically disabled clients may need programs or program steps for certain clients. It may be that community agencies could increase client involvement by modifying their programs to meet unique client needs. Community rehabilitation programs and agencies are often geared for the psychiatrically disabled client *in general*. The client's own rehabilitation practitioner may be able to contribute to the community resource's preparation for *particular* disabled clients.

THE SIGNIFICANT OTHER AS A COMMUNITY RESOURCE

(Case Illustration 8-3)

Felipe knew that the choice confronting Elda was a crucial one. Things had not been going well for her. She had managed to get into far more than her share of trouble. Now everything hung in the balance. She could either remain in the hospital on weekends, a move guaranteed to disrupt not only her own life but also the life of her family even more than it had already been disrupted, or she could start spending weekends at home, a possibility full of risk for Elda, her husband, and her small children.

Felipe moved cautiously. He helped Elda to lay out her alternatives in clear-cut terms. It was critically important that she understand the assets and liabilities of both possible ways of spending weekends. They spent a long time together exploring and evaluating the two possibilities. In the end, both Felipe and his client felt that the best

decision involved Elda going home on weekends and returning to the hospital during the week.

But Felipe knew that his real work was just beginning. If Elda was going to make it, she was going to have to know just what her goals were and just how she could reach them.

"Like I told you before, one of my biggest problems is just finding the time to do all the things I need to do at home," Elda told Felipe. And so he helped her set a specific goal for herself which involved organizing necessary weekend tasks in terms of essential rest, available time, and the priority of each task. And he went on to help her develop a careful step-by-step program with built-in reinforcements which would enable Elda to reach this goal. He then went on to help her set goals and develop appropriate programs in other areas of potential difficulty.

Nor did Felipe stop there. He knew how important significant others could be to any client's progress. One of the people he contacted was Elda's husband, Jess. As the person whose efforts would do most to sustain and promote Elda's achievement of her rehabilitation goals, Jess represented a very real "resource" in his own right.

At first Jess was quite hesitant. While emphasizing how much he wanted Elda to work things out, he just wasn't sure he could handle things well at this point if she started coming home on weekends. Felipe understood this hesitancy. But he took pains to make Jess aware of how important this weekends-at-home step was to Elda. He was persuasive in pointing out that progress for Elda would quickly translate into real benefits for Jess himself — he'd have his wife back again! Finally winning Jess over, Felipe worked out an agreement concerning the ways in which Jess would handle things at home. In effect, this meant helping Jess to set his own goals and develop his own program. All of these goals were simple yet meaningful ones: things like "no raising of voices," "at least three specific compliments given to wife each day," and "at least 30 minutes of quiet conversation each night after the children are in bed."

A straightforward objective was to get Elda's husband to serve as a valuable "supporting" resource. Yet even here Felipe had to use specific skills to promote the other man's awareness, to persuade him to help, to get him to agree to specific terms.

In the end, Felipe felt he had done all he could to prepare both Elda and her husband for Elda's weekends at home. Still, he knew quite well that the proof of his effectiveness could only be given through Elda's success. Her growth and Felipe's own capability were inextricably twined together.

"It's good — it feels really fine!" Elda's high spirits at their next session were testimony to the success of Felipe's careful planning and preparation. Even at this point he knew that there were no guarantees. He would have to do a great deal of follow-up work with Elda — and with her husband, too — before he could relax and let things take their course. But for now, Felipe felt confident. He had helped Elda avoid a longer unbroken period of hospitalization which would have been extremely disruptive for the whole family. He had made it possible for Elda to live at home on weekends, a far more "normal" situation than remaining in the hospital. Most of all, he had helped both Elda and her husband develop the specific goals and programs they needed to make a go of things together during a most difficult time.

COMMUNITY COORDINATING: ADDITIONAL CONSIDERATIONS

Rehabilitation practitioners skilled in community coordination should be able to have a positive impact on many of the problems outlined in the first part of this chapter. By approaching the task of community coordination systematically, the client can take a more active part in the choice of resources. Often the psychiatrically disabled client will comply in a passive manner with the wishes of others. If the rehabilitation practitioner or others make a referral, many psychiatrically disabled clients will accept it. Unfortunately these clients accept no responsibility for the decision. This often leads to only a minimal amount of effort on their part to make the referral work. Frequently, community coordination will involve the *practitioner working with the client* to identify the preferred resource, and to develop a plan to use the resource. But it is also conceivable that the practitioner or client could work alone or with significant others to make and implement many of these same decisions.

In general, the lower the functioning of the client, the more the *practitioner will need to work independently of the client*. For example, in decision-making with a low functioning client, the practitioner might only get input from the client about what values the client considered important and how the values should be operationalized. The practitioner would then carry out the research and evaluation steps on her or his own.

In some cases with a high functioning client, however, the practitioner may choose to teach the client community coordinating skills and then have the client alone use the skills to make and implement decisions regarding the use of resources. Equipping the client with community coordination skills is especially helpful when it is anticipated that the client will need to use many resources. For example, with a high functioning young person who has many living, educational, and career choices to make and who will be relating to many resources (e.g., housing, school, employment, etc.) in his or her lifetime, the practitioner may decide to teach the client to use community coordinating skills.

Systematic community coordination may also serve to involve significant others in the decision-making process. Since the behavior and attitudes of significant others will frequently affect the client's perceptions of the resource, it is often appropriate to give these significant others an active part in the decision. This is, of course, particularly important when the significant other is intimately involved with the decision (e.g., should the client live with them). When the practitioner increases significant others' involvement in the decision, she or he will also be increasing active support for the decision.

Systematic coordination of community resources by the practitioner also allows both the client and significant others to understand exactly why a particular decision was made regarding the use of a resource. This understanding will lead to increased motivation for effective use of the resource on the part of both the client and the significant others. At the most basic level, clients will be more likely to use the resources to which they are referred. Since Wolkon has pointed out that as many as two-thirds of referred psychiatric clients do not make contact with the referral agency, it would seem that increased involvement and motivation for the use of resources is sorely needed (Wolkon, 1970). In short, if the practitioner really

cares if the client uses and benefits from the resource, she or he must be both careful and systematic in the choice. For example, if a client has four alternative resources, in all likelihood one is the best for him or her. It may even be that only one of the alternatives will actually be used and produce benefits for the client. Thus a poor decision about the use of resources may add to rather than resolve problems.

Systematic coordination of community resources by the practitioner also allows resource staff to understand why that resource was selected for the client. The clearer the community resource's understanding of its role in the contribution to the rehabilitation of the client, the greater the possibility of it being able to help the client achieve his or her rehabilitation goal. When the practitioner uses community coordination skills, she or he also helps the resource to understand how it can benefit from working with the client, and how the client's assets will help the client achieve the rehabilitation goal. The understanding of 1) how it can gain from helping the client (resource benefits) and 2) the likelihood of the client's successful rehabilitation (client's assets) will increase the motivation of the resource to participate effectively in the rehabilitation of the client.

In addition, the practitioner might want to make a decision about resource use from his or her own perspective. For example, the practitioner might want to decide whether she or he or some other agency should work with the client to teach job interviewing skills. Although the client's values would be considered, other values such as the practitioner's caseload size and amount of available time would also be used to make the decision from the practitioner's point of view.

Another situation in which the practitioner might emphasize working independently of the client is when the time is very limited. For example, a client might be getting discharged the next day; at the last minute the client's relatives decide that the client cannot live with them. The practitioner is asked to find a living situation for the client. In this situation the practitioner might simply see the client long enough to get the values regarding his or her living situation. The practitioner would probably add any additional values based on his or her experience, use his or her current knowledge about existing resources, and choose a living situation which satisfies as many as possible of the client's values.

Table 8-1 presents some sample problems in which all or parts of the community coordinating skill may be useful. In particular, the marketing skills involved in getting the commitment of the resource to help the client can be used in response to any living, learning, or working problem requiring a systematic approach. For example, marketing skills may be used to handle the living problem of getting the commitment of a volunteer lay helper to visit the client in his or her post-hospital living setting. These marketing skills may also be used to obtain the agreement of a resource to provide money to help pay for the client's education. In addition, these same skills may be used to get a resource to agree to provide inexpensive career testing. The main point is that the marketing skills are appropriate whenever a person (practitioner or client or significant other) needs to systematically get a resource or person to agree to provide help. The need to employ marketing skills stems from: 1) the anticipation of difficulty in obtaining the agreement, and 2) the importance of the agreement.

Additionally, there are many problems for which the development and implementation of programs to facilitate the use of the resource are appropriate (i.e., programming skills). The problems are a result of physical, emotional, or intellectual liabilities of either the client or resource. For example, the client may have a physical problem (e.g., difficulty in staying awake longer than six consecutive hours) that would interfere with her or his ability to remain employed, or the resource may have an intellectual problem (e.g., being unable to develop appropriate reinforcers for the client). Programs to ensure effective use of the resource are necessary whenever client or resource problems are anticipated.

Marketing and programming skills can be used by the practitioner and client, by the practitioner and significant others, or by the practitioner jointly with the client and significant others. For example, the practitioner or significant others might initiate the first contact with the resource and, by so doing, make the resource aware of the client's problem and goals; or after the practitioner has obtained the resource's commitment to help, he or she might develop with the client or significant others the client favorability scales needed for agreement negotiations. In implementing the client programs to use the resource, the practitioner can get the help of the client or significant others in developing the timelines and reinforcers, and in monitoring specific behavioral steps in the program. Again, the level of functioning of the client and of significant others determines their level of participation in the community coordination process.

In addition to the different types of problems and people who use the community coordinating skills, the decision-making skill component may be used for different *purposes*. One way to use the skills is to evaluate decisions which have already been made on at least a tentative basis. For example, suppose that a client had decided that she or he was going to leave the hospital to go home against medical advice. The practitioner could *evaluate the effectiveness of this decision* about going home by obtaining the values that the client considered important to the decision, operationalizing the values and then evaluating the effectiveness of "home" and "hospital" as resources in terms of the client's relevant values. The practitioner and client could then see which resource might be most satisfying. Thus the client could see if she or he was really making a wise decision.

The decision-making process can also be used as an *exploration tool*. This is suggested in the above example. By going through the decision-making process with the client, the practitioner could see exactly what it was about the hospital which was bothering the client so much that she

TABLE 8-1

SAMPLE LIST OF PROBLEMS APPROPRIATE FOR COMMUNITY COORDINATING SKILLS

LIVING	LEARNING	WORKING
1. Where to live	1. What school, college or training program to attend	1. Where to get career counseling
2. Who to live with	2. What specific courses to take	2. Where to go for job placement
3. What to do with free time	3. How can education or training be funded	3. Where is the best place to work
4. Where to go for a substance abuse program.	4. What school would best serve the child	4. Where to go for occupational information
5. Where to spend weekends (e.g., home or hospital?)	5. Where to go for leisure time learning	5. Where to go for career testing
6. What clubs to join	6. What testing services to use	6. Where to get internships
7. What type of treatment to use (e.g., full, partial or no hospitalization)	7. Where to get tutoring	7. Getting commitment of employer to provide job for client
8. Where to get a volunteer lay helper	8. How to get school books	8. Getting commitment of internship experience for client
9. What resources to release client information to	9. Getting school to accept client	9. Getting client accepted into a job-training program
10. Where to get help for a marital or child-rearing problem	10. Getting tutors to agree to tutor client	10. Getting testing service to provide experienced career testing of client
11. Getting the commitment of a volunteer lay helper to help the client	11. Getting loan to help pay for client's education	11. Getting the commitment of a specific career counselor to counsel the client

or he was willing to proceed against medical advice.

Another way in which the decision-making process can be used is as a *tool to evaluate decisions which do not necessarily involve the use of resources*. For example, a client might be trying to decide whether or not to risk getting involved with soft drugs (e.g., marijuana). The decision-making process could be used to evaluate whether using or not using soft drugs was the best decision. A side benefit, of course, would be that the practitioner could come to understand why the client wanted to start using drugs. If appropriate, this would enable the practitioner to begin to expand alternative resources which could be used to meet these same needs.

With clients functioning at higher levels, the practitioner can also help the client learn to make *independent decisions about the use of resources in her or his everyday life* (e.g., deciding what school to attend). But the skills may also be used in non-resource decisions — for example, determining whether spanking is a good method for disciplining a child. In order to teach the client the skill of decision-making, · the practitioner should follow three basic teaching steps. First, she or he should explain how to do each skill step to the client (i.e., how to brainstorm alternatives, develop and operationalize values,

and evaluate alternatives). As each skill is explained, the practitioner should show the client an example of how the skill is done. Finally, the practitioner should have the client do each skill at least once and preferably several times. The more practice the client has in the use of each skill, the better he or she will learn it.

In summary, community coordinating skills can be used with a variety of problems. They can be used by the practitioner alone or in conjunction with a client or with significant others. The skills can be learned by clients to make and implement their own decisions about the use of resources and other life problems.

In essence, community coordinating skills help to ensure that the client does make contact with the most appropriate resource and that she or he is prepared to take advantage of the opportunities offered. For many psychiatrically disabled clients, good intentions about community functioning are not enough. The clients need to be able to do the things which are required for success with the resource. By the same token, good intentions on the part of the resource may not be enough. They must be able to do the things necessary to capitalize on the strengths of the client and accommodate his or her weaknesses.

REFERENCES

Anthony, W. A. Societal rehabilitation: Changing society's attitudes toward the physically and mentally disabled. **Rehabilitation Psychology**, 1972, *19*: 117-126.

Anthony, W. A., Pierce, R. M. and Cohen, M. R. **Psychiatric rehabilitation practice: The skills of rehabilitation programming.** Amherst, Mass.: Carkhuff Institute of Human Technology, 1977.

Braginsky, B. A. and Braginsky, D. Schizophrenic patients in the psychiatric interview: An experimental study of their effectiveness at manipulation. **Journal of Consulting Psychology**, 1967, *31*: 543-547.

Brand, R. C. and Claiborn, W. L. Two studies of comparative stigma. Employer attitudes and practices toward rehabilitated convicts, mental and tuberculosis patients. **Community Mental Health Journal**, 1976, *12*: 168-175.

Carpenter, J. O. and Bourestom, N. C. Performance of psychiatric hospital discharges in strict and tolerant environments. **Community Mental Health Journal**, 1976, *12*: 45-51.

Chesno, F. A. and Kelman, A. Societal labeling and mental illness. **Journal of Community Psychology**, 1975, *3*: 49-52.

Cohen, M. R., Pierce, R. M., Anthony, W. A. and Cohen, B. F. **Psychiatric rehabilitation practice: The skills of community coordinating.** Amherst, Mass.: Carkhuff Institute of Human Technology, 1977.

Cumming, J. and Markson, E. The impact of mass transfer on patient release. **Archives of General Psychiatry**, 1975, *32*: 804-809.

Evans, J. H. Changing attitudes toward disabled persons: An experimental study. **Rehabilitation Counseling Bulletin**, 1976, *19*: 572-579.

Farina, A. and Felner, R. D. Employment interviewer reactions to former mental patients. **Journal of Abnormal Psychology**, 1973, *82*: 268-272.

Franklin, J. L., Kittredge, L. D. and Thrasher, J. H. A survey of factors related to mental hospital readmissions. **Hospital and Community Psychiatry**, 1975, *26*: 749-751.

Jones, M. Community care for chronic mental patients: The need for a reassessment. **Hospital and Community Psychiatry**, 1975, *26*: 94-98.

Katkin, S., Zimmerman, V., Rosenthal, J. and Ginsburg, M. Using volunteer therapists to reduce hospital readmissions. **Hospital and Community Psychiatry**, 1975, *26*: 151-153.

Krieger, M. J. and Levin, S. M. Schizophrenic behavior as a function of role expectation. **Journal of Clinical Psychology**, 1976, *32*: 463-467.

Kroger, R. D. Effects of role demands and test cue properties upon personality test performance. **Journal of Consulting Psychology**, 1967, *31*: 304-312.

Kroger, R. D. and Turnbull, W. Effects of role demands and test cue properties upon personality test performance: Replication and extension. **Journal of Consulting and Clinical Psychology**, 1970, *35*: 381-387.

Mannino, F. V., Ott, S. and Shore, M. F. Community residential facilities for former mental patients: An annotated bibliography. **Psychosocial Rehabilitation Journal**, 1977, *1*: 1-43.

McNees, M. P., Hannah, J. T., Schnelle, J. F. and Bratton, K. M. The effects of aftercare programs on institutional recidivism. **Journal of Community Psychology**, 1977, *5*: 128-133.

Miller, G. H. and Willer, B. Predictors of return to a psychiatric hospital. **Journal of Consulting and Clinical Psychology**, 1976, *44*: 898-900.

Ozarin, L. D. Community alternatives to institutional care. **American Journal of Psychiatry**, 1976, *133*: 69-72.

Price, R. H. Psychological deficit vs. impression management in schizophrenic word association performance. **Journal of Abnormal Psychology**, 1972, *74*: 132-137.

Smiley, C. W. The advocacy program. **Perspectives in Psychiatric Care,** 1972, *10*: 220-225.

Townsend, J. M. Self-concept and the institutionalization of mental patients: An overview and critique. **Journal of Health and Social Behavior,** 1976, *17*: 263-271.

CHAPTER IX
Rehabilitation Program Evaluation

While Chapter II provided us with an overall answer as to the general effectiveness of various psychiatric rehabilitation techniques, the present chapter is primarily concerned with the procedures necessary to evaluate the ongoing effectiveness of specific rehabilitation personnel and programs. It is not enough to know generally what works and what doesn't. Psychiatric rehabilitation practitioners need to know whether their own specific techniques and programs are uniquely affecting their psychiatrically disabled helpee's rehabilitation outcome. By using various evaluative procedures, individual rehabilitation agencies can ascertain the particular benefits that the psychiatrically disabled helpee does or does not receive from their services, and then use this information to further improve their services.

Agencies and practitioners engaged in psychiatric rehabilitation, as well as human service agencies in general, typically do not evaluate the outcome of their specific services. Historically, human service agencies have responded neither directly nor accurately to the question — "How effective is your agency in doing what it purports to be doing?" Some agencies answer such a question by reciting the figures which show how many clients have used their services, for how many hours, with what type of professional, etc. Although these figures are necessary for the administrative operation of the facility, such data are in no way the only indication of agency effectiveness. Unfortunately, many funding agencies which help financially support rehabilitation facilities request only this superficial type of information in order to determine the extent of monetary support which they will provide. Apparently the funding agencies also incorrectly believe that figures such as the number of contact hours between rehabilitation practitioners and their helpees are an index of the effectiveness of that particular rehabilitation facility.

Such a misperception arises out of the inability of the field of psychiatric rehabilitation to define a unique set of rehabilitation goals for each psychiatrically disabled helpee. Rehabilitation program evaluation demands, among other things, the ability to set observable rehabilitation goals. As was discussed in Chapter III, the fields of psychiatric treatment and psychiatric rehabilitation seem to be operating on the assumption that their main goal is "to provide continuous and comprehensive care." When operating from such a goal, an agency's justification for continued operation is the figures which indicate the number and type of helpee contacts. However, these figures must not be misconstrued to be anything more than they really are — an index of process, not outcome.

In general, rehabilitation agencies respond to questions about their effectiveness by describing what they do, rather than the *outcome* of what they do. These answers suggest that the agency is effective because the services provided by the agency are somehow inherently "good services." For example, rehabilitation facilities may attempt to show their effectiveness by stating that psychiatrically disabled helpees who attend their facility can receive psychotherapy, work therapy, industrial therapy, and other forms of therapy from credentialed rehabilitation practitioners. The illogical reasoning upon which this answer is based seems to be that if the facility has properly credentialed professionals providing the proper services, then the rehabilitation facility must be effective.

However, what's proper is not always the same as what's effective, and it behooves rehabilitation practitioners and their respective rehabilitation facilities to specifically ask themselves questions concerning effectiveness. Answers to such questions can only be provided by continual rehabilitation program evaluations. Answers which merely provide a numerical description of the clients served or a description of therapeutic activities provided by the agency are clearly not enough.

Unfortunately, few mental health facilities routinely conduct rehabilitation program evaluations. If rehabilitation agencies were typically engaged in rehabilitation program evaluations, they would be able to respond to questions about their agencies' effectiveness in a manner similar to the following example of an aftercare clinic director:

"We routinely assess how well we are doing what we purport to be doing. Our data from last year indicate that in terms of our main goal of independent living, within six months after hospital release only 15% of our helpees returned to the hospital. Concerning our secondary goal of competitive employment, at six months follow-up our figures indicate that 40% are working full time and 25% part time. These figures compare favorably to both the base-rate figures for psychiatrically disabled helpees as well as the figures for psychiatrically disabled helpees in this community who choose not to use our facilities. In addition, we have found that our helpees reach 68% of the goals which were set for them at ·the beginning of rehabilitation. More specifically, we have found that when we break our helpees' goals down into living, learning, and working goals, we find that we are most successful in meeting our helpees' living goals, followed by working goals, and educational goals, respectively. Our helpees achieve 85% of their living goals, 55% of their working goals, and only 40% of their educational goals. Many more goals are both set and achieved in the living goals area.

In terms of client satisfaction with our services, our helpees rated our service thus: 40% extremely satisfied, 40% satisfied, and 20% unsatisfied. Each helpee's closest relative evaluated our services as follows: 25% extremely satisfied, 50% satisfied, and 25% unsatisfied.

Data from these rehabilitation program evaluations are compiled by each staff member and unit; each staff member is provided with monthly feedback on his or her efforts. The data is specifically used to improve both our rehabilitation programs and staff. Within the past year a number of changes have been made, based in large part on our previous rehabilitation program evaluations. These changes include. . ."

A response of this type to the question of agency effectiveness is exceedingly rare. Yet at the same time it is exceedingly informative, useful and refreshing. It is also a response within the realm of possibility if rehabilitation practitioners act on the unique principles of psychiatric rehabilitation outlined in the previous chapters and conduct rehabilitation program evaluations according to the guidelines to be described in this chapter.

The present chapter addresses itself to the issue of rehabilitation program evaluation by first discussing the several reasons why rehabilitation program evaluation should be a required activity of psychiatric rehabilitation practitioners. However, even though the rationale for rehabilitation program evaluation seems to be compelling, systematic rehabilitation program evaluation rarely takes place. The present chapter identifies some of the typical excuses given by psychiatric rehabilitation agencies for not conducting rehabilitation program evaluations. Following this examination of the rationale for and against rehabilitation program evaluation in general, a rationale is developed for equipping each individual rehabilitation practitioner with evaluation skills. Finally, some of the practitioner skills necessary to conduct a rehabilitation program evaluation are outlined.

REHABILITATION PROGRAM EVALUATION: A RATIONALE

It is certainly not difficult to develop a list of reasons as to why rehabilitation programs should be evaluated. The necessity for program evaluation in social service agencies in general has been well described by Suchman (1967), who has analyzed the rationale for program evaluation into three major types of reasons. It would appear that this general analysis of the usefulness of program evaluations applies equally well to the specific need for program evaluation in psychiatric rehabilitation facilities. Thus, the following rationale for psychiatric rehabilitation program evaluation is based on Suchman's (1967) classification system.

Economic reasons are one of the major factors why psychiatric rehabilitation agencies need to systematically evaluate their rehabilitation efforts. There are indications that the coming years may be characterized as the "age of accountability" (Walker, 1971). The buyer or consumer of services is beginning to demand to get what he or she has paid for or has been promised. It would seem only a matter of time before consumer groups, such as psychiatrically disabled helpees or their relatives, request that psychiatric rehabilitation agencies document their helping effectiveness. It would seem a matter of even less time before the buyer of psychiatric rehabilitation services, who is often the taxpayer, demands that rehabilitation agencies justify their continued financial support.

The recent tendency of both the general public and psychiatrically disabled helpees themselves to inquire more deeply into the effectiveness of psychiatric rehabilitation agencies has direct implications for the necessity of psychiatric rehabilitation program evaluation. It is the results of the rehabilitation program evaluation that can help show society that the rehabilitation facility's services are effective. As public money is needed for an ever increasing array of services, discriminations must be made between those agencies which demonstrate outcome and those which do not. Rehabilitation program evaluation provides a means for making these increasingly necessary discriminations.

Another of the major reasons for the necessity of rehabilitation program evaluation is an *administrative* reason. Administrators of psychiatric rehabilitation facilities need to know what works and what doesn't so that they can modify and improve their services based on the results of their rehabilitation program evaluations. Rehabilitation program evaluation loses its value if the results of the evaluation are not used to attempt to increase the effectiveness of the agency's services. A rehabilitation program evaluation not only assesses the agency's overall effectiveness, but also permits administrators to make within-agency comparisons. For example, a rehabilitation program evaluation can provide knowledge pertaining to what particular program is most effective, what staff members are most effective in achiev-

ing certain goals, what type of helpee is best serviced, what kinds of helpee goals are most often obtained, and so forth. Besides using the feedback from rehabilitation program evaluation to improve the agency's services to its helpees, rehabilitation program evaluation can also lead to improved administrative planning in such areas as public relations, budget preparation, and case assignments.

Ethical reasons comprise the final class of reasons related to the necessity of psychiatric rehabilitation program evaluation. Psychiatric rehabilitation practitioners have a moral obligation to provide their helpees with the most effective services. It is *not* enough to simply believe that an agency is effective. It is *not* enough for psychiatric rehabilitation practitioners to merely have high hopes. The path to effectiveness must include a place for rehabilitation program evaluation.

Most psychiatric rehabilitation practitioners do *hope* that they are offering their helpees the best possible services, within their particular agency's realistic limitations. Yet ethically it would seem that psychiatrically disabled helpees deserve a rehabilitation program which is based on more than good faith. A rehabilitation program evaluation can provide our hopes with a foundation based in reality.

THE CASE AGAINST REHABILITATION PROGRAM EVALUATION

Although the rationale for the necessity of rehabilitation program evaluation is compelling, the reasons used to explain the absence of psychiatric rehabilitation program evaluations are many and varied. The following analysis focuses on the major reasons which are typically used by those psychiatric rehabilitation agencies which do not conduct rehabilitation program evaluations. The list of reasons is by no means exhaustive; the ingenuity of the opponents of psychiatric rehabilitation program evaluation to constantly come up with new reasons for avoiding program evaluation remains a source of constant amazement. The various reasons why psychiatric rehabilitation practitioners do not routinely conduct rehabilitation program evaluations can be loosely classified into the following three categories: 1) rehabilitation program evaluations interfere with the agency's purpose; 2) rehabilitation program evaluations adversely affect the rehabilitation helpee; 3) rehabilitation program evaluations cannot be undertaken because of agency deficiencies. Each of the above reasons which impede rehabilitation program evaluation will be considered along with an analysis of why these obstacles to rehabilitation program evaluation need not be a serious deterrent.

The argument that rehabilitation program evaluation interferes with the purpose of psychiatric rehabilitation practice may be stated in several ways. One familiar line of reasoning holds that rehabilitation program evaluations reduce the amount of money and staff hours spent on the actual practice of rehabilitation. This argument is often advanced with respect to follow-up procedures. However, the exemplary follow-up program described by Lacks and Plax (1972) effectively discounts this argument. Their evaluation included a six-to-nine-month follow-up of a sample of the rehabilitation helpees served by one agency. By hiring an interviewer at an hourly rate and reimbursing her for travel expenses, the cost of follow-up per helpee was only $7.00, a figure which would seem to be a small expense considering the value of the information obtained.

Because the follow-up interviewer was not a regular employee of the agency, the follow-up procedures did not detract from the amount of staff time available to helpees. In addition, the staff time and money which is needed in the initial development of the follow-up procedures and processing of the data could be reduced by using one of the follow-up instruments already available (Lacks & Plax, 1972). Unless the rehabilitation agency is totally unaware of how relatively simple and inexpensive follow-up can be, it is difficult to legitimize the excuse of follow-up costing too much in terms of either staff time or money.

A second way in which rehabilitation program evaluations are accused of interfering with the agency's purpose is perhaps best typified by the following remark of one rehabilitation practitioner when he was queried as to why his agency did not conduct program evaluations. "We are here to provide services for our clients, not to do research on them." This type of statement illustrates not only an antagonism towards research, but a misperception as to the purpose of a rehabilitation program evaluation. A rehabilitation program evaluation, as typically carried out, is not research in its most traditional sense (Campbell & Stanley, 1963).

In contrast to evaluation, research is generally considered ". . . to be more theory-oriented and discipline-bound, exerts greater control over the activity, produces more results that may not be immediately applicable, is more sophisticated in terms of complexity and exactness of design, involves less use of judgment on the part of the researcher and is more concerned with explaining and predicting phenomena. Conversely, evaluation is more mission-oriented, may be less subject to control, is more concerned with providing information for decision makers, tends to be less rigorous or sophisticated, and is concerned primarily with explaining events and their relationship to established goals and objectives. One of the main differences between the two activities is that evaluation is done at the site of the intervention (in the field, usually), which allows much less control over all variables" (Burck & Peterson, 1975, p. 564).

In addition, evaluation need not involve statistics any more difficult than percentages, nor need it involve any secret manipulations of the helpee. As a matter of fact helpees should be told of the evaluation procedures and that after their contact with the agency is concluded they will be asked at a later date to help evaluate the agency's services. A rehabilitation program evaluation is neither an exploitation of the helpee nor a luxury that a rehabilitation agency can do without. It is an integral part of an agency's services and one which can be valuable in planning even more effective services.

The second category of arguments against rehabilitation program evaluation is based on a concern about the adverse effects which the program evaluation might have on the rehabilitation helpee. These concerns typically are based on the mistaken belief that the follow-up procedures used in program evaluations will either infringe on the helpee's privacy or exacerbate the helpee's symptoms. Rarely, if ever, do the directors of program evaluation report that the helpees were adversely affected in any way by the follow-up contacts. The chances of this rare effect occurring might be lessened even more by informing the helpees of the evaluation procedures and follow-up contacts when they apply for help and once again when formal contact is terminated. Many helpees, when they are contacted at follow-up, seem to appreciate the fact that the agency is still interested in their welfare; other helpees seem to enjoy the opportunity to critique the rehabilitation agency; very few if any helpees consider the follow-up an intrusion into their privacy; no evidence exists to suggest that the follow-up aspects of program evaluations exacerbate the helpees' symptoms.

The final type of obstacles to rehabilitation program evaluation seem to be the major stumbling blocks, that is, rehabilitation agency deficiencies which preclude the undertaking of a systematic rehabilitation program evaluation. It may be that if these deficiencies were overcome, the other two types of arguments against evaluation might disappear. No doubt the major agency deficiency is the staff's lack of ability to conduct rehabilitation program evaluation activities. That is, even if the practitioners were motivated to conduct programmatic evaluations, probably few staff members would have the skills necessary to undertake the evaluation. This is no doubt due to the fact the traditional educational programs in counseling, psychiatry, nursing, psychology, occupational therapy, and social work have not routinely trained their respective students in evaluation skills. Thus most rehabilitation facilities have had to rely on outside experts to either conduct the evaluation or provide an inservice training program for agency staff. The long-range solution to this predicament is the teaching of program evaluation skills in the human service professions.

The specific program evaluation skill most often lacked by psychiatric rehabilitation practitioner seems to be goal-setting skills. Both the agencies' overall goals and the goals for individual clients are often written in vague, subjective terms. In such situations meaningful program evaluation is virtually impossible to conduct. Rehabilitation practitioners must not argue that the benefits which their clients receive are too intangible to be seen or measured. It is the responsibility of the providers of the service to identify the observable effects of the service. Goal-setting skills pave the way for rehabilitation practitioners to evaluate the effects of their interventions.

Another rehabilitation agency deficiency which prevents program evaluation from occurring is the significant number of staff who feel threatened by the prospects of an evaluation of their efforts. They may fear exposure or the termination of their job or program. Yet this rarely if ever occurs. The purpose of evaluation is to modify and improve programs and not to throw people out of work!

AN OBSTACLE TO REHABILITATION EVALUATION

Case Illustration 9-1 ▬▬▬▬▬▬▬▬▬▬▬▬▬▬▬▬▬▬▬▬▬▬

Kathy turned her little Volkswagen onto Maple Street and caught the next three lights in a row just as they were turning green.

"I must be doing something right," she congratulated herself. She slowed down to wave at Harvey, a fellow practitioner working at Parkwood whose battered Studebaker she spotted just nosing out of a side street.

Poor old Harv. A heck of a nice guy. It was just a shame that he didn't know where he was going with the kids. Pleased with herself and the world in general on the gorgeous May morning, Kathy had plenty of sympathy to spare for Harvey.

It really was a beautiful morning, too. The daffodils and irises planted along the wide median strip were in full bloom. The sky was that absolutely crystal-clear blue associated with spring mornings. And Kathy was looking forward eagerly to the tasks she had set for herself for the day. Today, for the first time as a psychiatric rehabilitation practitioner, she was going to try evaluating herself on some of her outcome goals.

The simple fact that she actually had some goals probably meant she was ahead of the game. Kathy reminded herself of this as she turned right on Federal Street and then right again into the drive that led to Parkwood School's staff parking lot.

Parkwood was a school for emotionally disturbed adolescents. Kathy was proud of herself for having landed a job there. As the first job following her professional training, the position was quite a good one. Kathy enjoyed the work. She cared about the kids who were her clients. And she felt sure she was accomplishing something very worthwhile.

Although she didn't yet realize it, Kathy was about to lose some of her easily gained confidence in herself.

All of Kathy's conferences that morning seemed to go well. Ted Jorgenson had apparently been having some problems in one of his classes but with Kathy's help was able to get a handle on them. Alfred Hardin had announced he was on a hunger strike but Kathy talked with him and got him to agree to go down to lunch with the others in his group. She herself didn't waste much time eating lunch. She was going to start evaluating her work that afternoon and the prospect excited her.

When the prospect transformed itself into a reality, however, a good deal of Kathy's excitement seemed to degenerate into confusion.

She began by laying out the outcome goals which she had set up — goals which reflected the needs both of her youthful clients and of the institution for which she worked. There was a number of these

goals. Kathy arranged them in the order in which she had prioritized them and began trying to figure out how she was doing. But somehow all of her efforts just seemed to produce more confusion.

She concentrated on one of her highest-priority goals: "to normalize the lives of my clients." She wrestled with her statement of this goal for some time. And it finally dawned upon her that, when all was said and done, she really didn't have a clue as to what this statement meant!

"What it really comes down to is the meaning of 'normalize,' " she told herself. And, of course, she was right. But being right didn't help. Kathy couldn't help feeling, with something very like despair, that she had left something out in all her careful work up to this point.

Here again, of course, Kathy was quite right. She had neglected to operationalize in any meaningful way her perfectly valid definitions of outcome goals. Which mean that she really had no way of telling how either her clients or she herself were doing.

Kathy never operationalized the term "normalcy." As a result, she didn't know whether this meant returning a certain percentage of children to regular school settings or simply reducing by a certain percentage the number of temper flare-ups among her clients — or both. Because she had not operationalized her terms, she had developed no intermediary steps or process goals to help achieve the desired outcome. Moreover, the absence of operationalized definitions of goals meant that she had not been able to plan her own evaluation in any systematic fashion. She had no system for keeping track of the number of temper flare-ups among her clients, for example, because she had never pinpointed such flare-ups as outcome criteria that would require measurement.

In this end, all Kathy could tell herself was "I'm helping to normalize the lives of these kids — I think." Somehow the effect of this statement was not very reassuring.

THE CURRENT POPULARITY OF PROGRAM EVALUATION

At present, journal articles abound with references to program evaluation. An excellent new journal appropriately entitled *Evaluation* first appeared in 1972. Although it may be true that more people are *talking* about evaluation than actually *doing* evaluation, there has certainly been an increase in the number of professionals writing and hopefully reading about program evaluation. Entire books and yearly reviews are now being devoted to the issue of program evaluation in mental health settings.

As might be expected, a number of divergent points of view have developed. The present chapter does not attempt to review the current issues in the field; such a survey may be obtained by reviewing the last several years of *Evaluation*. Rather, the present chapter specifically focuses on those practitioner skills which are needed to evaluate rehabilitation interventions. It is the thesis of this chapter that in order for program evaluation to become a regular component of most rehabilitation facilities, *each rehabilitation practitioner must possess program evaluation skills.*

A RATIONALE FOR PRACTITIONER SELF-EVALUATION

As suggested by Glaser and Backer (1972), the various persons who conduct program evaluations fall into three categories: 1) the practitioners themselves (self-evaluation), 2) inside evaluators, and 3) outside evaluators. The term "self-evaluation" means that the practitioners who are actually conducting the program do the evaluation. Inside and outside evaluators are persons who are not themselves part of the treatment program; they are either employed inside the agency or are outside consultants.

The practitioner self-evaluation model has a number of advantages. First, systematic practitioner self-evaluation should maximize the probability that the practitioner will use the evaluation results. The results of inside or outside evaluators may fail to achieve this purpose because the evaluative feedback is not understandable or useful to the practitioner. In addition, evaluation attempts frequently fail because practitioners feel threatened and therefore resist participating in the evaluation or using the evaluation results. Systematic practitioner self-evaluation is more effective because it increases the likelihood that the practitioner will use the results, since the

results were achieved through their own efforts.

Systematic practitioner self-evaluation is also effective because the practitioner is in a unique position to help design and carry out the evaluation process. He or she understands the rehabilitation process and can help make the evaluation relevant to this process. The practitioner also has more ready access to every aspect of the rehabilitation process for each client. He or she can best assume responsibility for carrying out many of the evaluation procedures.

In addition, systematic practitioner self-evaluation is an effective technique because it requires that the practitioner have the skills to carry out a meaningful evaluation of his or her performance. It provides training for the practitioner to determine not only his or her client outcome goals but also the administrative outcome goals needed to insure the agency's survival. If practitioners are engaged in self-evaluation of their rehabilitation efforts, then they must of necessity be trained in how to set goals for their individual helpees. The mere process of setting goals with individual clients may exert a positive effect on client rehabilitation outcomes and thus be an unintended effect of a practitioner self-evaluation procedure.

Practitioner self-evaluation also includes benefits for the practitioner. In general, the effect of the evaluation will be that the practitioner can do a better job. The resulting improved performance will add satisfaction and pride to his or her job. The ability of the practitioner to describe her or his improved performance will also aid the practitioner in gaining economic security and developing her or his own career. Lastly, systematic practitioner self-evaluation provides the practitioner with an opportunity to monitor and improve his or her own delivery of services.

In summary, if the practitioners conduct the program evaluation themselves: 1) they will be more *motivated* and *capable* of using the results, 2) they will be able to collect much of the needed information in the regular conduct of their jobs, 3) they will be trained in skills (e.g., goal setting) that could positively affect their rehabilitation efforts, 4) they will experience personal satisfaction in knowing how well they are doing and how they might improve, and 5) they will be able to further their own careers by becoming capable of observably describing their professional accomplishments.

THE SKILLS OF PRACTITIONER SELF-EVALUATION

All of the many skills needed by the practitioner to conduct a self-evaluation are included in Cohen, Pierce, Anthony, and Vitalo (1977). The present section will focus on the more major skills which rehabilitation practitioners must possess in order for them to contribute to the evaluation effort. The four major skills which must be possessed by a practitioner who engages in self-evaluation are:

1. The ability to determine delivery and administrative outcome goals.

2. The ability to prioritize these delivery and administrative outcome goals.

3. The ability to operationalize their high-priority outcome goals.

4. The ability to collect, organize, and use the results of the evaluation.

Practitioners who are equipped with these self-evaluation skills will be able to take an active role in the evaluation process, rather than feeling manipulated by persons and techniques beyond their control or understanding.

Skill 1. The ability to determine delivery and administrative outcome goals.

Delivery goals relate to helping clients. Administrative goals relate to meeting supervisory or administrative demands, needs, or wants. In essence, practitioners who wish to conduct an evaluation must first consider their goals in relation to the clients in the delivery system and, next, their goals in relation to their administrations and supervisors. The identification of delivery outcome goals flows from the practitioner's understanding of the rehabilitation process, while the determination of administrative outcome goals may require that the practitioner read various

written materials and talk to administrators. Obviously, there may be an overlap between delivery goals and administrative goals. However, administrators also have goals typically related to budgeting, practitioner supervision, practitioner workload, and others.

One basic concept that applies to both delivery and administrative goals is the distinction between process and outcome goals. Goals may be classified as either *process* or *outcome* goals depending on whether they are the end goals or the intermediary goals which lead to the end goals.

Delivery outcome goals are defined as those goals which, when reached, result in clear change or benefit in the client's everyday life. *Delivery process* goals are defined as all the intermediary goals that take place in the rehabilitation process, leading to the achievement of outcome goals but falling short of "real life" client change or benefit. An example of a delivery outcome goal might be preventing client hospitalizations; an example of a delivery process goal might be client level of problem exploration.

Administrative outcome goals are defined as those goals that directly result in agency funding or client "real life" benefits, while *administrative process* goals are defined as all the intermediary goals that lead to the achievement of administrative outcome goals. An example of an administrative outcome goal might be the number of clients receiving rehabilitation services; an example of an administrative process goal might be the workload of an individual practitioner.

The distinction between delivery process and delivery outcome goals is an important distinction to remain aware of in using evaluation skills. The quintessential evaluation is one that provides information with respect to client *outcome* goals. The prime purpose of the rehabilitation *process* is to bring about real-life client skill change and real-life client benefits. While ideally process and outcome are related, one cannot assume that process changes bring about real-life client skill changes and benefits. The practitioner must directly evaluate delivery outcome goals, and then evaluate process as it affects outcome goals. Too often in the past it has been process goals rather than outcome goals that have been evaluated.

This is not to say that an evaluation of process goals is unimportant. For example, the research reviewed in earlier chapters indicated that the rate of "no shows" and premature terminations is exceedingly high. Thus the process goals of "increasing the number of helpees who show up for their first appointment" would be an important process goal to evaluate. Yet an improvement in this "no show" percentage does not necessarily mean that the increased number of clients who appeared for services actually changed or received any benefits due to their appearance.

A distinction that can be made with respect to delivery or client outcome goals is that of real-life client skill change as opposed to ultimate client benefits. Real-life client skill change implies that the client's observable performance of some skill behavior has changed. Ultimate client benefits are the benefits which the client is now receiving from using the skill.

For example, a student client may have a deficit in attention skills. She or he may not be able to continually face and look directly at the teacher when the teacher is speaking. Since people tend to pay attention to the things which they face and look at, the ability to engage in this behavior becomes critical for this client. A *process* goal for this client might be to attend rehabilitation treatment sessions in order to learn attention skills. A client skill outcome goal for the student might be to use his or her newly learned attention skills with the teacher in the classroom. The "ultimate outcome" or *benefit* of the client's increased attentiveness in class might be earning a satisfactory grade from the teacher, thereby allowing him or her to stay in school. Another example might be that of an employee whose real-life client skill change might be an improvement in her or his self-control skills in the working environment. The ultimate client outcome or benefit would be the client's steady employment throughout the follow-up period.

Skill 2. The ability to prioritize the delivery and administration outcome goals.

Once the outcome goals have been determined, the practitioner has a picture of the areas important in evaluating the rehabilitation services. Most practitioners identify numerous outcome goals. The busy practitioner obviously cannot give equal attention to evaluating and improving his or her performance on all outcome goals. Also, without determining the comparative importance of each goal, the practitioner will have no way to compare his or her performance with that of other practitioners. For example, imagine that Practitioner A has a higher percentage of clients achieving rehabilitation goals than Practitioner B. Yet Practitioner B has a higher client-satisfaction level. Without some method of prioritizing the goals, comparison of the performances of Practitioner A and Practitioner B is arbitrary.

Cooper and Parker (1975) use an analogy from the world of business which aptly illustrates the need for the development and prioritization of a variety of outcome goals: "What would be the consequence if one insurance salesman sold one hundred policies a year and another salesman sold only fifty policies? If the rules of rehabilitation administration are applied, then the man who sold one hundred policies would be considered the better salesman simply based on quantity. More likely, however, rules of business would apply which would necessitate closer scrutiny of additional outcomes such as: buyer satisfaction, annual premiums earned, policy rejection rate by underwriters, refusal rate by policy holders, and first year cancellation rates" (page 18).

The solution to such a problem lies in setting priorities for the delivery and administrative outcome goals that have been determined. Priorities also allow the practitioners to gain a clearer perspective of the conflicting pressures, for example, to both "do a good job" with their clients and "see more clients."

For practitioners to determine which outcome goals are most important, they must consider the clients and the agencies' values. The practitioner will want to take into account the "urgency or need" of the outcome goal to both the client and the rehabilitation agency. "Urgency or need" means that the client or agency will suffer some negative consequence if the goal is not achieved. For example, client "urgency" might mean that the client will lose his or her job; agency "urgency" might mean that the agency will lose its funding. Additionally, client and agency "benefit" can be considered. For example, client "benefit" may mean moving to a more desirable, independent living setting; agency "benefit" may mean achieving the projected annual goals. Practitioners must also consider their "job description" to determine what is legitimately expected of them. A job description should reflect the agreement of services to be provided for the salary to be collected. Ethically, practitioners will be concerned with those goals included in their description of job responsibilities. Although there are other relevant values in prioritizing goals (e.g., time, practitioner skill), practitioners should limit themselves to the most crucial values. Once the practitioner has prioritized the outcome goals, she or he needs to determine how many of the highest priority goals she or he will have the time and energy to devote to evaluation efforts.

Skill 3. The ability to operationalize the high-priority outcome goals.

Before the high-priority outcome goals are operationalized, the practitioner should first determine the process goals needed to achieve the high-priority outcome goals. For each outcome goal there are intermediary steps or subgoals that the practitioners must achieve before they can achieve the outcome goals. Determining the process goals related to the high-priority outcome goals to be evaluated is important. It is important to determine these related process goals because practitioners may not be in the position to evaluate and improve their performance on the outcome goals without first evaluating and improving their performance on the related process goals. For example, practitioners cannot improve their per-

formance on the outcome goal of "helping clients to achieve their rehabilitation goals" if they are not satisfactorily doing the intermediary step or process goal of "setting rehabilitation goals." Practitioners may need to improve their performance on the related process goals before they can improve their performance on their outcome goals. In most cases, practitioners will need to determine the process goals related to their high-priority outcome goals and include in their evaluation an analysis of their performance on the related process goals.

In the operationalization process, the practitioner makes the outcome and related process goals both observable and measurable. The operationalized goal becomes the variable to be evaluated. The key to operationalizing goals into evaluation variables is to specify the observable behavioral components of the goal and how the behaviors can be measured. For example, the outcome goal of "preventing client hospitalization" might become the evaluation variable of "the percentage of clients who are still living outside a hospital one year after termination of the rehabilitation process." In essence, the program evaluation operationalization process sets goals for the individual practitioner, just as the rehabilitation "diagnosis" set goals for the individual client. For example, "practitioner work level" might be defined as "the number of clients seen by the practitioner in a week at the rehabilitation center." When the practitioner is operationalizing the goal, he or she may also find that there is more than one behavioral component to the goal. For example, "practitioner work level" might also be defined as "the number of hours of rehabilitation contact with clients in a week." The practitioner may therefore want to use both "number of clients seen weekly" and "weekly client contact hours" as process variables with which to evaluate his or her performance.

The delivery and administrative outcome goals represent both *quantitative* and *qualitative* goals. The practitioner can read each identified goal and consider whether or not the goals relate to *how well* the job is done. The goals that primarily relate to being more *effective* are labeled *"quality"* goals. For example a practitioner's administrative outcome goal of "client satisfaction" relates to the client's rating of *how well* or *how effectively* the rehabilitation services were delivered by the practitioner. Therefore, it could be labeled a "quality" goal. Other goals will relate to *how many* or *how much* of the service or job is done. The goals that primarily relate to being more *efficient* are *"quantity"* goals. For example, a practitioner's administrative outcome goal of "increasing the number of clients served" relates to *how many* clients are served. Therefore it could be labeled a "quantity" goal.

Skill 4. The ability to collect, organize and use the evaluation results.

There are usually many people and devices to help collect the data for evaluating the performance on each of the high-priority outcome and related process goals. In the majority of cases, it will be either the client's or the practitioner's behavior that will be measured. The decision about who is to do the measurement is more complicated. The practitioner, his or her supervisor, clerical staff, or even the client may be appropriate choices. In some cases, significant others or community resources' staff will be in the best position to measure the behavior. The deciding factor about who is the best person to do the measuring should be that person's ability to provide accurate measurement, including the necessary time and accessibility to the behavior being measured. At times, the practitioner and others can equally provide the measurement. The decision then may be based on practical (e.g., time, cost) or political (e.g., believability) factors. For example, both Practitioner A and the center receptionist are capable of measuring the number of clients the practitioner sees weekly at the rehabilitation center. Practitioner A chose the receptionist as the person taking the measurement for this variable. Her decision was based on political (e.g., easier for others to believe receptionist results) and time considerations. The persons doing the measure-

ment may vary as evaluation variables vary; but all results should be reported to the practitioner.

The most difficult decision involves how the measurement can best be done. Some alternative measurement devices include: audio-tapes, video-tapes, rating scales, questionnaires, interviews, telephone calls, client file check, record-keeping, schedule books, etc. Again, the device to be used must fit the variable to be measured.

As the data on each goal are being collected, the practitioner can organize the results so that they are understandable and useful. Functionally organizing the results involves using either a pass-fail standard or an improvement standard or a comparative standard. Essentially, practitioners can either compare their performance to a previously determined expected level, to their own previous performance, or to the performance of other practitioners. Practitioners can then profile the results to determine their strengths and deficits, tendencies, trends, and relative performance on the various variables.

In order for practitioners to use this new understanding of personal performance, they must develop and implement a plan promoting such usage. The plan to use the results depends on the practitioners' reasons for using the results. Basically, there are three reasons for using evaluation results. Practitioners are motivated to: 1) improve their delivery to clients, 2) meet an administrative demand, or 3) develop their own career. The reason or combination of reasons dictates the specific outcomes desired from using the evaluation results (e.g., get in-service training or redefine expectancy levels) and how the results can best be used to achieve the desired outcomes.

The plan to use the evaluation results should reflect these initial objectives. The following are the questions that need to be answered by the practitioner's plan to use the evaluation results:

1. What is the evaluation result? (Description of the result to be used)

2. Why is the result going to be used? (Reason for using the results)

3. What are the outcomes desired from use of the results? (Specific outcomes)

4. With whom is the result to be shared?

5. How are the results to be used? (Specific mode or way of using)

Table 9-1 presents one practitioner's plan to use three of the evaluation results which were previously prioritized and operationalized. As can be seen in Table 9-1, the *result* column is essentially a summary of these evaluation results which the practitioner chooses to use. The decision regarding which results to act on first depends upon the importance of the variable. The importance of the variable is based on the priority of its corresponding outcome goal. For example, the highest priority outcome goal for this practitioner was "to increase the number of clients placed in competitive employment." A related process goal was to reduce client cancellations. Therefore, the results of the evaluation of the practitioner's performance on the "client cancellation" variable would be more important to act on than the results on some other lower priority variable.

The *reason* for using the evaluation results relate to the practitioner's evaluation objectives. In the majority of cases, the reason will be either to improve his or her delivery to clients or to meet an administrative demand. When the practitioner's performance is clearly "desirable," the reason may be to develop the practitioner's career (e.g., get promoted).

The desired outcomes in using the result are those specific changes which the practitioners hope to effect by their use of the result. When the reason for using the result is *to improve the delivery to clients*, the types of outcomes desired by practitioners will primarily be: 1) to set and achieve a specific level of performance on a delivery goal; 2) to request and receive in-service training; 3) to add a new delivery goal or, 4) to evaluate and improve their performance on a more basic process goal. When the motivation for using the results is to *meet an administrative demand*, the practitioner's desired outcomes will most likely be: 1) to receive positive recognition or reinforcement; 2) to change

the definition of expected performance levels; 3) to change his or her job description (e.g., type or size of caseload) or, 4) to request and receive in-service training. The setting of new specific levels of performance on a delivery goal may be based on the existing expectancy levels. For example, a new goal for the practitioner illustrated in Table 9-1 might be to increase the number of clients she sees weekly from the "undesirable level" (16 clients) to at least the "acceptable level" (18 clients).

The decision about *who is to share in* the evaluation results depends on the reason for using the result and the desired outcomes. For example, to obtain the desired outcome of positive recognition or reinforcement, the practitioner will need to share the result with someone who can provide the reinforcement or rewards (e.g., a supervisor, co-worker or administrator). Practitioners will probably not share any result that they can act on independently to improve their rehabilitation delivery to clients.

The method of presenting the results should be functional in terms of the reason for using the results and the desired outcome. The important point is that a method must be selected and used. When practitioners are using the results independently to improve their own performance, the preferred mode of presentation is the one which will provide the most information as often as possible. The more immediate and detailed the feedback, the easier it will be for the practitioner to obtain the desired outcome. When the practitioner decides to share the results, the best mode of presentation is the one that clearly makes the point with as little extraneous information as possible.

The time schedule for beginning to use the results and the deadline for achieving the desired outcome depend on the specific results and outcomes. Again, the important point is that a timeline be set and followed.

Implementing the plan to use the evaluation results requires the practitioner to use those same program development and implementation skills primarily described in Chapter V. The desired out-

TABLE 9-1

PRACTITIONER'S PLAN TO USE THE EVALUATION RESULTS

I. Result	II. Reason	III. Outcome	IV. With Whom	V. Mode	VI. When
1) Low percentage of clients placed in competitive employment	1) Improvement with clients 2) Administrative demand	1) Receive additional training and supervision from practitioner with the highest percentage	Supervisor	Profile Monthly	1) Begin by: 1st of next month 2) Outcomes by: Half year from now
2) Very undesirable level of client cancellation	1) Improvement with clients	1) New performance level on delivery goal of reducing weekly client cancellations — cut average from 2.6 cancellations to less than 2.0 cancellations 2) Add delivery goal of follow-up on client cancellations (e.g., encourage to come in, explore with client, or contract regarding cancellations).	Self	Profile Monthly	1) Begin by: Immediately 2) Outcomes by: End of next quarter
3) Caseload desirable	1) Administrative demand 2) Improvement with clients	1) Positive reinforcement.	Supervisor	Comparative Profile	1) Share next supervision session
4) Undesirable percentage of caseload seen weekly	1) Improvement with clients	1) New specific goal of increasing percent of caseload seen weekly from 25% to at least 50% 2) In-service training in use management skills 3) Change expectancy scale levels	Self Supervisor Supervisor	1) Weekly charts and monthly profile 2) Verbal Report 3) Profile Monthly	1) Begin by: Immediately Outcomes by: End of next quarter 2) Share next supervision session 3) Hold until after next quarter

comes become the practitioner's goals. The practitioner systematically develops and implements the steps to reach these goals.

As practitioners implement the plan, they focus on the continued evaluation of their performance on the same evaluation variables. In most cases, the plan should improve their performance. It is suggested that practitioners continue to focus on the same evaluation variables until they are satisfied with their performance on these variables. When practitioners reach the point where they are satisfied with their performance, it is time to recycle the evaluation process.

The evaluation process is continual.

The practitioner's improved performance on the evaluation variables points toward new evaluation variables, procedures and results. Remember that in the initiation of the evaluation procedures *many* delivery and administrative outcome goals are determined and prioritized. For reasons of time, only *some* of the highest priority outcome goals and related process goals are operationalized into evaluation variables. Initially, only a *few* of the evaluation variables are naturally evaluated, the results organized, and a plan to use the results developed. In an ongoing evaluation process more and more of the remaining outcome goals can eventually be focused upon.

USING THE SKILLS OF SELF-EVALUATION

Case Illustration 9-2

Reggie pinned the chart to the bulletin board which took up space on one wall of her office and stepped back to admire the results.

"Not bad," she murmured. "Not bad at all!"

"Oh yeah?" The voice behind her was cheerful but skeptical. "Listen, lady, you may think that's the hottest bit of original art since the Mona what's-her-face, but I'm here to tell you it just ain't so."

Reggie turned to confront Peter, the practitioner whose office adjoined hers. She was about to protest but he held up his hand, regarding her with mock gravity.

"I know this must hurt," he said mournfully. "But I'm here to testify that you'd get a lot of competition from any three-year-old with a crayon and a paper bag!"

"I wasn't talking about the artistic quality of the thing," Reggie told him, fighting off laughter. "If you must know, I was talking about the job I'm doing. I was giving myself a little pat on the back. Anything wrong with that, Mr. Art Critic?"

"Not if you deserve it . . ." Peter was drifting over to examine Reggie's chart. "What is this thing, anyway?"

"That happens to be nothing less than an outline of the progress which yours truly has made during the last quarter in

reaching some very definite goals." She regarded Peter who, for his part, seemed fascinated by the outline. "Impressed to the point of wordlessness, huh?"

"I might be," Peter said. "Why don't you explain just what it means."

"You really want to know?"

Peter looked at her somewhat sheepishly. "Yes, I do. I mean, I know I play the wise guy a lot. But I really am interested in learning as much as I can — and I've got a feeling maybe you can teach me something."

So Reggie launched into a careful explanation of the results which she had plotted only that morning — results of her own evaluation.

"These are outcome goals, see? And these, they're process goals — the things that have to be achieved before the outcome goals can be taken care of . . ." She explained each goal and told Peter the manner in which each had been operationalized so that progress toward it could be measured. Finally, she outlined the way in which she had interpreted the results in terms of the 'pass-fail,' 'improvement,' and 'comparative' methods.

"You mean that's how you figured out what — oh, say your 10%-recidivism-rate-after-one-year result really meant?"

Reggie nodded. "Uh huh. Among other

things, I found out that's the lowest recidivism rate for any practitioner in the whole psychiatric rehab program — which may tell you why I was patting myself on the back so immodestly when you came in."

"It sure does . . ." Peter was clearly impressed. "Listen, do you think maybe you could teach some of the rest of us how to do this kind of evaluation? I could speak to my supervisor and see if we could set something up . . .?"

Reggie agreed readily and Peter left, promising to take the matter up with his supervisor. That was good news as far as Reggie was concerned. She had been pleased by Peter's obvious admiration. And she also had some very definite ideas about where she wanted to go in terms of her own carrer. An informal session along the lines that Peter had in mind could help Reggie move up to a regular position as an in-service trainer.

She checked her "Goal Sheets" again, reviewing once more where she was in terms of all her outcome and related process goals. She'd reached her goal in the area of recidivism. A full 90% of her clients were making it on their own a year after getting out of the state-run program for which she worked. She wanted to maintain this level. She also wanted to move toward some other goals — her employment outcome goal, for example. This would mean recycling the evaluation process.

Reggie was ready for that. In fact, at that moment she felt ready for just about anything.

SOME ADDITIONAL CONSIDERATIONS

Program evaluation procedures must become an integral part of any psychiatric rehabilitation facility and program. It is the theme of this chapter that the only way for this to occur is for each individual practitioner to be trained in program evaluation skills. Obviously, this is a long-range approach to the problem. In the interim, evaluations will have to be conducted by program evaluation specialists. However, if evaluation efforts are ever to receive their appropriate emphasis, individual practitioners must be completely involved in the process and not feel that the evaluation is being imposed and pressured upon them. Caution must also be exercised. Self-evaluation efforts, as well as evaluations performed by others, may be manipulated to imply client benefit when in fact none occurs. Walker (1972) has identified some of the more common methods of misconstruing the actual outcome:

"Perhaps the most popular is to be highly selective concerning who receives services. By careful avoidance of recidivist-prone clients, such as drug addicts, alcoholics, or public offenders, many programs appear to be scoring high on program benefits. The task of the program evaluator is to require management to specify target populations in such a way that benefit gains are not obtained through changes in client selection. A second alternative sometimes employed by result-oriented organizations is to reduce the volume of clients served, thereby saturating the service recipients with professional staff. This can be controlled by defining volume requirements (i.e., the number of clients to be served in relation to the capacity of the system) or, better yet, by holding the program accountable for cost. A third method of obtaining spurious benefits involves the point in time when benefit measures are applied. For example, one program solved its performance problem by not formally enrolling clients until they had passed the high dropout period. With dramatic suddenness the program became an overnight success. A similar strategy involves measuring outcomes before the client loses them. This is often used in some manpower programs that measure the stability of employment after thirty days. An opposite approach is to measure benefits as late as possible, in hopes that the environment will achieve the goal. A final method used to obtain spurious benefits is to manipulate goal setting. For those organizations that use gain scores based on pre- and post-measures, setting goals that are easy to

achieve or defining client status-at-entry as lower than it actually is can spuriously increase program benefits" (page 53).

In the training of individual practitioners and their supervisors and administrators, one must be made aware of these potential manipulations. If everyone is knowledgeable about these potential problems, the possibility of surreptitious manipulation of the evaluation data can be cut down.

Besides the training of individual practitioners in program evaluation skills, it is equally as important to train the supervisors in how to reward or reinforce their staff for engaging in program evaluation activities. Supervisors have often been reminded of the importance of reinforcing their staff for the achievement of excellent outcome. However, in a self-evaluation system, supervisors should also reward their staff for engaging in program evaluation activities, *independent of how well the evaluation indicates that they are doing!* Of course the actual outcomes achieved by individual practitioners can also be differentially rewarded. Those practitioners whose self-evaluation indicates that they need improvement should rarely be directly punished. Such supervisory action will probably encourage deception, withholding, or manipulation of the data. Rather, supervisors should have more successful practitioners teach the less successful, provide additional skill training opportunities, modify the job in line with the practitioners strong points, or change the practitioner to a different position.

The ultimate test of any evaluative program is whether or not the results are used to improve the program, so that increased client benefits do in fact occur. Unfortunately, many program evaluation efforts are either ignored or rejected. A study by Bigelow (1975) suggested that evaluative feedback has influence on decision makers in terms of stimulating further exploration and communication, but that evaluative information is not reflected in improved program performance. Walker (1972) has recounted how the results of early demonstration program evaluation projects were both ignored and re-

jected. Walker (1972) recounts how the program evaluation results did not improve the agency functioning, and that the two projects that showed positive results were discontinued while the program which was evaluated most negatively was expanded! Another example of the rejection of program evaluation findings has been provided by Thomander (1976) in his report of Ward and Kassebaum's (1972) five-year-study on the effectiveness of group counseling among prison inmates:

"Contrary to the expectations of the treatment theory, there were no significant differences in outcome (arrest record 2 years after release) between various treatment groups or between the treatment groups and the control group. Furthermore . . . participation in group counseling and community living did not lessen endorsement of the inmate code, and did not result in a desirable decrease in frequency of prison discipline problems for the inmates in counseling as opposed to controls" *(Ward & Kassebaum, 1972, pp. 306-307).*

Yet in spite of this negative evaluation ". . . the Department of Corrections made group counseling programs part of the program of every person in the department and made participation compulsory in some institutions" (Thomander, 1972, p. 225).

These evaluations were done prior to more recent developments in program evaluation technology. However, they do serve to highlight the difficult problem of getting the agencies to actually use the results of evaluations. This difficulty presents a strong case for the development of practitioner self-evaluation skills. In this instance the evaluation is a continual ongoing component of the practitioner's job. Thus, there really is no end point to the evaluation process. The most important stimulus to using the evaluation results continues to be the *individual practitioner's direct involvement in the evaluation process.*

MAKING THE EVALUATION MORE COMPREHENSIVE

One additional concern has permeated the issue of rehabilitation program evaluation; that is, the issue of what specific criteria are most reflective of rehabilitation outcome. Chapter II of this book evaluated the overall efficacy of rehabilitation by focusing on two outcome variables: recidivism and employment. This chapter has recommended that practitioners who engage in self-evaluation procedures focus on two types of outcome measures: real-life client skill outcome and real-life client benefits. In this scheme the outcome criteria of recidivism and employment would be classified as measures of real-life client benefits.

A recent article has suggested using an even more comprehensive approach on evaluating psychiatric rehabilitation programs (Anthony, Cohen & Vitalo, 1978). Specifically, these authors recommended that evaluative procedures attempt to include measures of the following four types of rehabilitation outcome: (a) skill gain, (b) client/society benefits, (c) client quality of life, and (d) client satisfaction with services. These categories are by no means discrete; rather the categories are used to ensure that the outcome evaluation effort is as comprehensive as is needed.

Client Skill Gain

As discussed in Chapter IV, research studies have reported the positive correlation between client level of skilled activities and the outcome criteria of recidivism and employment. In addition, most of the treatment programs which have had a positive effect on rehabilitation outcome have used a skills training approach as an important component of their treatment. The primary focus of the rehabilitation approach is either on building skills or modifying the environment so that the client can function more effectively at her or his present skill level. Thus, it would make sense to diagnose the client's critical skill areas at the start of the rehabilitation intervention and to re-evaluate these critical skill areas at the conclusion of services. Measures of client skill gain can provide an immediate and direct assessment of whether or not the rehabilitation program has had a direct impact on client behavior. Obviously, in order for an evaluation of client skill gain to occur, rehabilitation practitioners must know how to objectively diagnose the specific client skills which the client needs to more effectively function in his or her particular environment.

Client/Society Benefits

A rehabilitation intervention, in addition to affecting client skill level, should also bring about benefits both to the client and society. A benefit means some change in the client's living, learning, or working environment brought about by the rehabilitation program.

The traditional outcome criteria of recidivism and employment are measures of patient and society benefits. Other examples might be number of days hospitalized, number of times needed agency services, cost of treatment, source of financial support, number of weeks employed, earnings per week, percent of coursework still needed to achieve training or educational objective, number of contacts with police and so forth. It is crucial that evaluation data be collected on measures which clearly indicate the benefits to society of a rehabilitation approach. The growth of a rehabilitation model within the mental health system is in a large part dependent on the taxpayers and the politicians who represent the taxpayers. If rehabilitation evaluation procedures avoid outcome measures which indicate the benefits to society of a rehabilitation approach, the proponents of rehabilitation will be hard pressed to justify the importance of increased public support.

Client Quality of Life

Recent developments in the mental health field have focused increased attention on the psychiatrically disabled person's quality of life. The process of deinstitutionalization, ostensibly designed to improve client and society benefit criteria (e.g., number of days hospitalized, cost of treatment, etc.), has been extensively criticized for not focusing on improvements in the client's quality of life. Popular magazines and newspapers periodically detail the deleterious environments of many discharged patients, just as in past years these same media revealed the nightmare of institutionalization.

Quality-of-life measures are useful to ensure that any society benefits that might occur as a result of a rehabilitation intervention do not occur at the expense of the client's quality of life. Some examples of various quality-of-life measures are: number of hours per week spent alone, number of social contacts per week, number of club or organizational meetings attended, number of recreational sports activities attended per month, number of conversations per week, number of new items of clothing per year, number of hot meals eaten per week, etc.

Client Satisfaction with Services

Encouraged by the advent of the civil rights and consumer rights movements, the outcome criterion of client satisfaction has developed increasing credibility as an important outcome area. It is now common practice in many agencies to obtain *client* estimates of program efficiency and effectiveness. Information of this type can be used to identify problem areas as viewed from the client's perspective with the obvious goal being to remove the sources of dissatisfaction. In addition, the rehabilitation practitioners' knowledge that client satisfaction is important and will be monitored may have an effect on the manner in which services are delivered to clients.

Client satisfaction is typically assessed by asking the helpee questions related to specific elements of the rehabilitation program. Rather than a simple yes-no answer, the usual procedure is to have the client indicate his or her degree of satisfaction with each area. Some examples of client satisfaction measures are: practitioner understood my feelings and viewpoints; helped me identify my rehabilitation goal; helped me identify what I must do to reach the goal, etc.

No doubt the most relevant study of client satisfaction with rehabilitation treatment is an investigation of the comparative impact of vocational rehabilitation and psychotherapy on psychiatrically disabled poverty clients (Smith & Hershenson, 1977). All ninety subjects studied were unemployed and evidenced emotional problems of sufficient severity to preclude immediate job placement. The results indicated that the clients were more satisfied with the rehabilitation treatment than with the psychotherapeutic treatment, specifically in terms of the reported impact of the rehabilitation program on such items as their self-confidence, public image, and chances for success.

Measures of client satisfaction provide a completely different source of data than do measures of skill gain, client and society benefits, and quality of life. Taken together, these four categories of rehabilitation outcome can provide an extremely comprehensive assessment of rehabilitation effectiveness. Even more importantly, the outcome criteria employed should provide a detailed diagnosis of the rehabilitation program, so the program strengths can be publicized and program deficiencies corrected.

Clearly, rehabilitation programs should be evaluated on those outcome criteria which the program was specifically designed to affect. Yet, it also makes sense to evaluate a program in a more comprehensive manner, so that some of the unintended effects of a rehabilitation program might be evaluated. In addition, a comprehensive evaluation will be more likely to generate outcome data that can be used in comparing studies done at different times and in different places.

ENDNOTE

[1]Adapted in part from an article by Anthony, Cohen and Vitalo (1978).

REFERENCES

Anthony, W. A., Cohen, M. R. and Vitalo, R. The measurement of rehabilitation outcome. **Schizophrenia Bulletin,** 1978, in press.

Bigelow, D. A. Impact of therapeutic effectiveness data on community mental health management: Systems evaluation project. **Community Mental Health Journal**, 1975, *11*: 64-74.

Burck, H. D. and Peterson, G. W. Needed: More evaluation not research. **Personnel and Guidance Journal**, 1975, *53*: 563-569.

Campbell, D. T. and Stanley, J. C. **Experimental and quasi-experimental designs for research**. Chicago: Rand McNally, 1963.

Cohen, M. R., Pierce, R. M., Anthony, W. A. and Vitalo, R. **Psychiatric rehabilitation practice: The skills of rehabilitation evaluation**. Amherst, Mass.: Carkhuff Institute of Human Technology, 1977.

Cooper, M. and Parker, L. Accountability and the future of rehabilitation. **Journal of Rehabilitation**, 1975, *41*: 18-21.

Evaluation. Volumes 1-6, 1972-1977.

Glaser, T. E. and Backer, T. E. Outline of questions for program evaluators utilizing the clinical approach. **Evaluation**, 1972, *1*: 56-59.

Lacks, P. B. and Plax, K. The need for an honest look. **Journal of Rehabilitation**, 1972, November-December, 19-22: *41*.

Smith, H. C. and Hershenson, D. B. Attitude impact of vocational rehabilitation and psychotherapy on black poverty clients. **Journal of Applied Rehabilitation Counseling**, 1977, *8*: 33-38.

Suchman, E. **Evaluative research principles and practice in public service and social action programs**. New York: Russell Sage Foundation, 1967.

Thomander, D. Researching psychotherapy effectiveness in mental health service agencies. **Journal of Community Psychology**, 1976, *4*: 215-238.

Walker, R. A. The accountability game. **Journal of Rehabilitation**, 1971, July-August, 34-36.

Walker, R. A. The ninth panacea: Program evaluation. **Evaluation**, 1972, *1*: 45-53.

Ward, D. and Kassebaum, G. G. On biting the hand that feeds: Some implications of sociological evaluations of correctional effectiveness. In C. M. Weiss ed. **Evaluating action programs: Readings in social action and education**. Boston, Mass: Allyn & Bacon, 1972.

CHAPTER X

Applications
of The Principles of
Psychiatric Rehabilitation
Programming[1]

During the last five years there has been an increased acceptance of the need for a skills-oriented approach in psychiatric rehabilitation and other helping professions. The basic assumption is that psychiatric rehabilitation clients have problems because they lack the living, learning, or working skills needed to function independently in their lives. The goal then becomes diagnosing the client's skill strengths and deficits and providing the client with the opportunity to learn and use the needed skills in his or her life. The following chapter describes some applications of the principles of psychiatric rehabilitation programming in a variety of rehabilitation settings. The first section presents a research study comparing the differential effects of a "medication" versus "medication plus a skills-oriented psychotherapeutic approach" to helping aftercare clients. Drs. Vitalo and Ross demonstrate a clear impact of the learning of skills on client incidences of employment, development of new friendships, and level of recreational activities. All of these impacts suggest a greater quality of life for these clients and their increased potential for community adjustment and reduced recidivism. The second section describes an interesting application of rehabilitation programming by Green-

berg (1976) to an activity therapy program within a psychiatric facility offering short-term inpatient services. Within a relatively brief amount of time during their hospitalization, psychiatric patients were able to learn skills needed to live more productively in the community. The Greenberg study represents an initial effort deserving replication. In the third section, three studies of the efficacy of psychiatric rehabilitation programming as a way of helping improve marital communication and overall marital functioning (Pierce, 1973; Santantonio, 1977; Valle and Marinelli, 1975) are discussed. These studies used similar methodology, outcome measures, and obtained similar results. Together, they represent an encouraging beginning in the development, use, and evaluation of a skills-oriented approach to marital communication problems. Lastly, in section four, an innovative study by Cohen and Greenberg (1975) is described and discussed. The study applied psychiatric rehabilitation programming to mental health intervention in a crisis in an inner-city elementary school. The implications of the findings point to the role psychiatric rehabilitation programming can have on preventative efforts in mental health.

AN APPLICATION IN AN AFTERCARE SETTING [2]

OVERVIEW

A total of eighty-eight clients were involved in this treatment study. Clients were residents of a predominantly urban-suburban area who had been referred to their community mental health center for outpatient aftercare supportive services. As a group, the clients were predominantly female (75%), almost equally divided in their marital status (46% married, 54% unmarried), averaged 47.19 years of age with two-thirds of the group having a history of three or more psychiatric hospitalizations (66%). In essence, the group appeared to represent a population of moderately chronic post-hospitalized psychiatric patients.

Clients were assigned to one of two

conditions: Chemotherapy only or chemotherapy plus skills-oriented psychotherapy. The provision of chemotherapy alone as a treatment system was a new development at the mental health center. Previously, all psychotically diagnosed aftercare clients received a combination of chemotherapy and psychotherapy. The initiation of this new treatment system was partly a product of the high demand of service in excess to staffing and partly at the insistence of the medical staff.

The medication-only treatment condition (MOTC) was administered by two certified psychiatrists each with over four years of experience working with chronic psychiatric client populations. Both psychiatrists were committed to the "medical model" approach to treating "mental illness" and both voiced confidence in the sufficiency of chemotherapy in meeting aftercare client needs. Each psychiatrist determined his or her drug regimens and rate of client contact. Prescribed drug regimens predominantly used the phenothiazine derivatives and fluphenazine decanoate. The average rate of client contact varied between psychiatrists. Psychiatrist A saw his active clients on a once-per-month schedule. Psychiatrist B saw her clients on a once-per-two-month schedule. In each instance, the psychiatrist was the assigned case manager for the clients and solely responsible for meeting their needs. Naturally, the remaining resources of the mental health center were available to assist them. Anecdotal verbal reports by the psychiatrists supported the continuance of their experience of MOTC as sufficient and effective in meeting the clients' needs. Indeed, the psychiatrists' work was acclaimed by the nurse and several other staff in the center.

The skills-oriented treatment condition (SOTC) followed the Human Resource Development Model (Carkhuff, 1969; 1969a; 1976). This approach emphasizes building the treatment delivery from the client's frame of reference. The client is progressively facilitated through exploration, understanding, and action culminating in a teaching-learning delivery which capacitates the client by equipping him or her with skills which the client has defined as needed in order to function more effectively and satisfyingly in his or her life. While the process is individualized for each client, it incorporates all the essential components of patient care. The practitioner implementing the procedure required mastery of a set of special skills including: pre-helping skills of attending, observing, and listening; and helping skills of responding, personalizing, and programming (Carkhuff, 1974; 1976). Many of these skills are mentioned in Chapters IV and V which describe rehabilitation diagnostic and programming skills. The therapist implementing the skills-oriented Human Resource Development approach was a licensed clinical psychologist who

had been trained in the above described skills. In addition, this psychologist had approximately three years of previous experience treating chronic psychiatric clients. Clients receiving the skills-oriented Human Resource Development approach also received adjunctive chemotherapy. The medications used paralleled those used in the medication-only treatment conditions with a predominance of and use of the phenothiazine derivatives and fluphenazine decanoate. Contacts for medication renewal were on a once-per-ten-week average. Face-to-face treatment contacts averaged once per week.

TREATMENT ASSESSMENT

Two forms of assessment indices were used: process and outcome indices. Process indices focused on the characteristics of the two treatment conditions. Process indices can verify the differential effect of the treatment conditions. It was hoped that process measures might also allow partialing out of the elements in the treatment conditions which account for their differential impact if, indeed, such impact was found to exist.

Outcome indices focused on assessing changes in the client's personal world. Ultimately, treatment should impact the client's life in ways that facilitate a more stable base of community adjustment and personal satisfaction. It was hoped that the outcome measures would allow us to draw inferences about the impact of treatment on the quality of community adjustment of the aftercare clients.

In this treatment study, process measures focused on the presence of treatment components which appear to define effective rehabilitation. Additionally, process measures include assessing the presence of skill gain in clients, including the number of different skills learned by clients. The instrument used to obtain the data was the outpatient treatment follow-up questionnaire (Vitalo, 1977). This is a fifteen-item inventory which elicits information on the client's experience of treatment outcome, therapist relationship characteristics, treatment components and treatment organizational and situational variables. The outpatient treatment follow-up questionnaire is a face-valid instrument which has been standardized by over four years of use with over five hundred out-patient clients (Vitalo, 1977). Specific to this study, item 6 on the questionnaire lists twelve components of rehabilitation treatment delivery and asks clients to check off each component which he or she experienced during outpatient care. Item 7 on the questionnaire elicits client feedback concerning whether as a result of treatment they are "able to do something" that they previously could not do, and to label that "something." This item provided feedback on skills learning.

Outcome indices were of two types: the traditional sympton relief dimension and the use of three indices of life base enhancement. The life base enhancement measures were included especially since the likelihood of aftercare clients recidivating to hospitalization status appears at least partially a product of their inability to establish a stable and rewarding base of living in the community. Also, a recent study has focused on the "dumping" of patients out of state facilities into the communities and the apparent resulting impoverished existence of such post-hospitalized patients who are maintained in the community. Thus, the life base enhancement indices also serve to assess the quality of life of aftercare clients as facilitated by the two treatment conditions. Life base enhancement indices include: employment record, incidence of new friendships, and the incidence of new recreational activities initiated since the onset of treatment. Information on clients' number of weeks of employment, number of new social relationships, and number of new recreational activities was obtained by a separate single-page questionnaire. The assessment of experienced symptomatic relief used client response to Item 11 of the outpatient treatment follow-up questionnaire.

Of the eighty-eight clients involved in this treatment study, thirty-three were assigned to skills-oriented treatment condition and fifty-five were assigned to the medication-only treatment condition.

Assignment was based on the availability of care. Those aftercare clients referred for treatment at a time when case openings existed in the skills-oriented treatment condition were assigned to that treatment. When no such openings existed, assignment was made to the medication-only treatment condition. Treatment for all clients began during the second quarter 1976 (April through June). At the time of data collection (second quarter, 1977), all clients had been in treatment for approximately twelve months. In order to standardize the forms for the outcome variables of employment, socialization, and new activities — clients were directed to answer these questions in terms of events since June, 1976. Thus, the outcome assessed on these dimensions was for a period of twelve months. Each client was sent a copy of the survey measures and an introductory letter that explained the purpose of a follow-up. Those who had not mailed back their forms within two weeks were followed up via a telephone.

RESULTS

The evaluation of the study concentrated on the following measures and resulted in the following findings.

COMPARABILITY OF CLIENTS ASSIGNED TO TREATMENT CONDITIONS

Table 10-1 presents a summary of the age, sex distribution, marital status, admission, and process-reactive score of clients assigned to the medication-only and the skills-oriented treatment conditions. No significant differences were found between the experimental and control groups on any of the dimensions. As a whole, both groups represent a single population of aftercare clients who can be described as middle-aged, predominantly female, equal numbers married and unmarried, the majority of whom have had three or more hospitalizations. The additional use of the self-report process reactive scale (Ullman and Giovannani, 1963) revealed that the two groups were highly comparable with both scoring slightly toward the process end of the scale. In essence, both groups were composed of moderately chronic aftercare clients.

TABLE 10-1

COMPARABILITY OF CLIENT ASSIGNED TO TREATMENT CONDITIONS ON DIMENSIONS OF AGE, SEX, MARITAL STATUS, NUMBER OF PSYCHIATRIC ADMISSIONS AND PROCESS-REACTIVITY

DIMENSION	MOTC CLIENTS	SOTC CLIENTS	STATISTIC	SIGNIFICANCE
Age (Mean)	47.96 (S.D.=14.16)	43.00 (S.D.=11.98)	t=.13 (df=86)	n.s.
Sex	38F 17M	28F 5M	X^2=2.90 (df=23)	n.s.
Marital Status	17 married[1] 24 unmarried	17 16	X^2=.79 (df=3)	n.s.
Psychiatric Admissions	0=0 1=4 2=6 3=4 3+=24[2]	=1 =3 =8 =1 =13[3]	X^2=3.5 (df=9)	n.s.
Process/ Reactive Mean	11.44	12.00	t=.70	n.s.
S.D.	(S.D.=3.92)	(S.D.=2.91)	(df=71)[4]	

[1] Data obtainable for only 41 out of 55 clients
[2] Data obtainable for only 38 out of 55 clients
[3] Data obtainable for only 26 out of 33 clients
[4] Data obtainable for only 73 out of 88 clients

Differential Effect of Treatment Approach

Of the eighty-eight clients surveyed for outcome data, a total of sixty-seven, or 76%, returned the assessment questionnaires. As indicated previously, the differential effect of treatment conditions was assessed according to the client's reports of the presence of the components of rehabilitation, that is, the experience of skill learning and the number of skills learned. This check on the differential nature of the treatment is important since research suggests that therapist reports of providing distinctive treatment modalities have not been supported by objective findings (Fielder, 1950). Thus, the assumption that clients assigned to skills-oriented treatment would actually receive such treatment is not automatically tenable. Similarly, the assumption that clients assigned to medication-only treatment would only receive prescriptions for medication is similarly not automatically tenable. Since the program of treatment is the source of outcome variance under question here, it must be established that these treatment programs (SOTC, MOTC) did indeed differ.

Table 10-2 provides a comparison of

the programs of treatment for the two treatment conditions. Relative to the components of care, SOTC clients reported receiving, on the average, 7.23 out of the 12 defined components of a skills-oriented treatment delivery. Essentially, SOTC clients received approximately 60% of a full skills-oriented treatment delivery. MOTC clients reported receiving, on the average, 3.97 or 33% of the components of a skills-oriented delivery. Clearly, on the basis of client reports, the skills-oriented treatment condition was not a full human resource development treatment delivery and the medication-only treatment condition was not simply the dispensing of medication. In order to analyze whether the difference that did exist between treatment conditions was significant, the data were subjected to a median test (Dixon & Massey, 1955). The median test was selected since the data displayed a marked rectilinear distribution. The results of this analysis are reported in Table 10-3. The findings support the distinctiveness of the two treatment conditions. More clients receive more components of a skills-oriented treatment delivery with significantly greater than expected frequency ($X^2 = 6.94$, df = 2, p < .01) in the SOTC group than in the MOTC group. Additionally, 86% of the SOTC clients reported skill learning as compared to 38% of the MOTC clients (Table 10-2). Table 10-4 lists examples of the kinds of skills reported as learned. Chi square analyses of the frequencies of skills learning as reported by clients between the two treatment conditions proved significant ($X^2 = 15.05$, df = 3, p < .005). Further analysis of the reports by clients of the number of skills learned in the SOTC treatment as compared to the MOTC condition also revealed statistically reliable differences ($x^2 = 13.51$ df = 1, p < .005). SOTC treated clients label learning 1.62 skills on the average as compared to an average of .38 skills labeled as learned by MOTC counseled clients (Table 10-2). Again, these data were analyzed by the median test due to the extreme non-normality of its distribution (See Table 10-5).

TABLE 10-2

COMPARISON OF THE MOTC AND SOTC TREATMENTS IN TERMS OF NUMBER OF REPORTED TREATMENT COMPONENTS PROVIDED AND THE INCIDENCE AND EXTENT OF CLIENT SKILL ACQUISITION

DIMENSION	MOTC CLIENT REPORTS	SOTC CLIENT REPORTS
Mean number of Treatment Components Experienced	3.97 (S.D.=3.66)	7.23 (S.D.=3.65)
Skill Learning	yes=13 no=24[1]	yes=25 no=4[2]
Mean Number of Skills Learned	.38 (S.D.=.49)	1.62 (S.D.=1.08)

[1] 37 out of 55 clients responded to the item.
[2] 29 out of 33 clients responded to the item.

TABLE 10-3

MEDIAN TEST ANALYSIS OF CLIENT REPORTS OF NUMBER OF TREATMENT COMPONENTS RECEIVED

TREATMENT CONDITION	N ABOVE MEDIAN	N BELOW MEDIAN
MOTC	13	24[1]
SOTC	20	10[2]

[1] 37 out of 55 clients responded to the item.
[2] 30 out of 33 clients responded to the item.

TABLE 10-4

EXAMPLES OF SKILLS LABELED BY CLIENTS AS BEING LEARNED AS A RESULT OF TREATMENT

TREATMENT CONDITIONAL	SKILLS LABELED AS LEARNED
SOTC	how to relate to people
	how to control my weight
	how to make decisions on own
	how to label and express my feelings
	how to swim
	how to relax myself
	how to control drinking
	how to attend
	how to listen
	how to drive a car
	how to be polite
	how to read
	how to write
MOTC	how not to listen to others
	how to face problems more
	how to sleep

Thus, the analysis of client feedback does support the distinctiveness of the SOTC and MOTC treatments quantitatively (number of treatment components) and qualitatively (degree of skills acquisition). The medication-only treatment provided fewer service steps and, in general, did not culminate in skills acquisition.

TABLE 10-5

MEDIAN TEST ANALYSIS OF CLIENT REPORTS OF THE NUMBER
OF SKILLS LEARNED AS A RESULT OF TREATMENT

TREATMENT CONDITION	N ABOVE MEDIAN	N BELOW MEDIAN
MOTC	10	24[1]
SOTC	22	7[2]

[1] 34 out of 55 clients labeled the skills they learned thus permitting the analysis

[2] 29 out of 33 clients labeled the skills they learned thus permitting the analysis

Differential Effect of Treatment Outcome

The impact of treatment on aftercare clients was assessed relative to symptomatic relief and life base enhancement including employment facilitation, socialization facilitation, and activity facilitation. Table 10-6 summarizes the symptomatic relief data. Relative to symptom relief, both SOTC and MOTC appear equally effective in eliciting client reports of symptomatic benefit. On the average, both groups of clients report being "helped very much" by their respective treatment modalities.

TABLE 10-6

COMPARISON OF CLIENT REPORTS OF SYMPTOMATIC
BENEFIT FOR MOTC AND SOTC TREATMENTS

TREATMENT CONDITION	MEAN LEVEL OF BENEFIT REPORTS	STANDARD DEVIATION	t
MOTC	3.97[1]	.75	
SOTC	4.05	.64	
Comparison			t=.66[2]

[1] Scale range from 1-5 with level 1 = hurt by treatment; level 2 = not helped; level 3 = helped slightly; level 4 = helped very much; and level 5 = helped fully.

[2] Not significant at .05 level.

Relative to life enhancement measures, SOTC clients reported higher gains than the MOTC clients on all dimensions with two of the differences achieving statistical significance and a third approaching significance (see Table 10-7). SOTC clients reported, on the average, 8.93 weeks of work (S.D. = 16.08) as compared to 5.14 weeks of MOTC clients (S.D. = 12.53). Because the distribution was skewed, the data was analyzed by chi square. Although 38% of the SOTC clients attained employment as compared to 21% of MOTC clients, this difference only approached, but did not achieve, significance (X^2 = 4.43, df = 3, p < .15 < .10). A possible confounding variable to this analysis was the higher ratio of female to male clients in the SOTC group with their attendant lower probability of employment background and, therefore, less likelihood of attaining new employment.

TABLE 10-7

COMPARISON OF CLIENT REPORTS OF GAIN ON LIFE ENHANCEMENT MEASURES AS A RESULT OF MOTC AND SOTC TREATMENTS

LIFE ENCHANCEMENT INDEX	MOTC CLIENT REPORTS	SOTC CLIENT REPORTS
Employment (weeks worked)	5.14 (S.D.=12.53)	8.93 (S.D.=16.08)
Employment (% clients achieving employment)	21%	38%
Socialization % reporting new friends	50%	83%
% reporting no new friends	50%	17%
Activities (New Activities)	.34 (S.D.=78)	1.38 (S.D.=1.15)
% reporting new activities	23%	69%
% reporting no new activities	77%	31%

Relative to socialization facilitation, 83% of SOTC clients reported developing new friendships as compared to 50% of the MOTC clients. Chi square analysis of the frequencies proved significant ($X^2 = 8.43$, df = 3, p < .05). Thus, skills-oriented-treated clients had a significantly higher rate of socialization facilitation than clients treated by medication only.

On the third life enhancement index, SOTC clients reported both a higher number of new activities and as a group evidenced greater incidence of engaging in new activities (See Table 10-8). SOTC clients reported, on the average, engaging in 1.38 new recreations (S.D. = 1.15) as compared to .34 (S.D. = .78) for the MOTC clients. A t-test for heterogeneous samples supported the significance of these findings (t = 4.28, df = 46, p < .01). Additionally, 69% of the SOTC clients initiated new recreations (See Table 10-8 for examples) concommitant to treatment as opposed to just 23% of the MOTC clients ($X^2 = 13.44$, df = 3, p < .01). Thus, SOTC treatment appeared to have both a more potent absolute effect on the initiation of new activities as well as a greater spread of effect across clients.

TABLE 10-8
EXAMPLES OF NEW ACTIVITIES INITIATED BY SOTC CLIENTS
ACTIVITIES

fishing

walking

night school

church attendance

bowling

YWCA

playing cards

voice lessons

volunteer for Senior Citizen Program

volunteer at hospital

dancing

ceramics

In summary, the outcome assessment supports a conclusion of equal potency between the MOTC and SOTC treatments in producing symptomatic relief as measured by client self-report. If this were the only index used, the addition of a rehabilitation approach to medication treatment would appear to be superfluous. However, relative to life base enhancement measures, the skills-oriented treatment did appear to be associated with a greater incidence of employment, a significantly greater frequency of new friendship development, and a significantly greater absolute level and general incidence of new activity initiation.

Discussion

Before discussing the findings of this treatment study, several limitations inherent in this investigation should be addressed. First, considerable research supports the relationship skills of a therapist as a significant contributor to client outcome (Carkhuff, 1969; 1969a; 1976; Truax & Mitchell, 1971). In this study it was not possible to control for this variable. The basic difficulty rested with the inability to locate a psychiatrist functioning at high enough levels on the research-supported relationship dimensions (Carkhuff & Berenson, 1976) to be comparable to the level of skills functioning required by a practitioner charged with the proper implementation of a skills-oriented

human resource development treatment. Future studies might attempt prior training of willing psychiatrists so that their interpersonal functioning could be brought to the level of functioning needed to implement the SOTC treatment. A second limitation of this study is the singular emphasis on client self-report. While client self-report is indeed a legitimate outcome index, such reports would support still stronger conclusions if objective assessments could also be included. Finally, the absence of inclusion to the SOTC of any skills delivery specific to employability may have negatively biased the treatment's ability to demonstrate clear impact on that dimension. These limitations render the findings of this study suggestive.

Notwithstanding this caution, several potentially critical results emerge. First, the MOTC and SOTC treatments appear to have essentially the same level of impact on symptomatic relief as reported by clients. Essentially, the addition of skills-oriented treatment to medication regimens does not markedly enhance clients' subjective report of benefit from treatment. Obviously, if the goal of aftercare treatment delivery were solely client subjective reports of benefits, then medication-only treatment would be the most cost-effective mode of the two investigated.

However, the central goal of aftercare treatment is to successfully sustain the post-hospitalized helpees' community adjustment, thereby reducing recidivism. Furthermore, professional and community consciences have been aroused by the emerging picture of social desolation which surrounds many recently discharged hospital patients. In both regards, that is, sustaining successful community adjustment and minimal quality of community living, such issues as employment, level of socialization within the community, and level of community involvement become relevant. It seems reasonable to entertain the principle that the more successfully engaged the aftercare client is in the community to which he or she is discharged, the more likely he or she will remain in the community. In this regard, the results of this study suggest a differential effectiveness between the MOTC and SOTC conditions. The skills-oriented treatment approach appeared to be associated with both a personal and environmental enrichment of the clients served. SOTC clients reported developing significantly more skills or competencies as a result of care. The positive impact of such learning on client self-esteem — though not directly assessed — seems highly reasonable. Further, the greater incidence of employment, the greater development of new friendships, and the higher level of new recreational activities all demonstrate a qualitative enhancement in these clients' community adjustment. All of these impacts suggest a greater life base enhance-ment effect via SOTC treatment. Given prevailing clinical logic and some initial research findings (Buell & Anthony, 1973; Franklin et al. 1975) such life base enhancement should be predictive of low recidivism. Thus, SOTC treatment may be a necessary ingredient in aftercare services if recidivism is to be minimized.

Future research should focus on further elucidating the different effects of medication-only treatment and skills-oriented treatment with aftercare clients. In addition to incorporating the control measures identified previously, such research should also attempt the implementation of SOTC with a placebo control in order to partial out what contribution, if any, the medication makes to this skills-oriented treatment process. Recent research suggests that psychotropics may be an "indispensable" treatment component for only 30% to 40% of clients experiencing psychotic disorders. Thus, for some 60% to 70% of aftercare clients, skills-oriented treatment plus a placebo might well suffice (Davis et al. 1976; Gardos & Cole, 1976; Tobias & MacDonald, 1974). The use of a placebo would appear to be necessary since post-hospitalized clients are generally conditioned to believe that medication is essential to their treatment. Nonetheless, if supported in its effectiveness, SOTC plus placebo would be far more cost-effective than SOTC and medication or medication-only treatment.

AN APPLICATION TO AN INPATIENT SETTING[3]

Greenberg (1977) described an interesting application of psychiatric rehabilitation programming to an activity therapy department within a one-hundred-fifty-five-bed state psychiatric facility offering short-term inpatient services. The activity therapy department of the hosptial had as its goal both patient adjustment in the hospital and the learning of the everyday living skills needed for social interaction, home maintenance, recreation, and self-help. The department's facilities, programs and staff reflected a caring for patients. Staff displayed a commitment to patients by the contextual and spatial arrangements of rooms, their work activity level, and the offering of afternoon discussion sessions (45 minutes) for personal exploration of feelings and problems, and a conceptual learning of skills.

At a conference sponsored by the local community mental health center, the activity department staff was exposed to the psychiatric rehabilitation programming model (Anthony, 1977). The very brief encounter with the model led to a request for additional training. Fortunately, the local community mental health center had staff capable of offering the training. The outcome goal for the training was a successful living skills program as measured by patient participation, patient learning, and patient benefits.

A two-part training program was designed to provide activity therapy staff with the skills necessary to develop living skills training modules and to deliver them effectively to patients. The first part of training focused on the acquisition of interpersonal skills necessary for the effective diagnosing and teaching of skills. Trainees learned basic attending, responding, and personalizing skills (Carkhuff & Berenson, 1976). Three all-day workshops (24 hours) were spent on didactic presentations and modeling of skills by the trainer, and experiential practice incorporating feedback by the trainees. Homework assignments were made including reading of the *Art of Helping* (Carkhuff, 1972). Follow-up sessions were held at the hospital to allow for on-the-job observation of the trainees' use of these skills with patients.

The second part of training focused on the acquisition of curriculum development skills necessary for designing a living skills training program. Training was based on the teaching skills described by Carkhuff, Berenson, Berenson & Carkhuff (1978); Carkhuff, Berenson & Pierce (1975) and highlighted in Chapter V of this text. Trainees learned how to facilitate and incorporate trainee input to write a skill module, and to evaluate skill delivery. Eighteen hours were spent in lectures, demonstration, and practice. Training hours were spread across three workshop days. Homework assignments were made including reading *The Trainer's Guide to The Art of Helping* (Carkhuff & Pierce, 1976). Two follow-up sessions were held at the hospital to allow for on-the-job observation of the trainees' delivery of a skill module to patients.

In order to evaluate the effectiveness of the two-part training program, a number of questions were raised. These questions were directed at gains made in training, gains made on-the-job, and gains made by patients.

RESULTS OF THE TRAINING PROGRAM

1. Did the trainees learn the skills?

Objective pre-/post-measurement of individual skills yielded positive and significant gains. Table 10-9 presents pre- and post- mean scores on each skill, difference scores, and levels for significance of the difference between means. Scores reflect ratings of trainee skills performance on Likert-type scales presented by Carkhuff and Pierce (1976). These were adopted to accommodate evaluation of each individual skill. The scales represent five levels of functioning. Each level is concrete and behaviorally defined. However, for the sake of comparability, level 1 is conceptualized as very ineffective, level 2 as ineffective, level 3 as minimally effective, level 4 as effective, and level 5 as very effective.

Subjective reports by trainees of gains on skills confirmed objective evaluation. Trainees reported significant gains in attending, observing, listening, responding, and personalizing skills. Self-reports of input development, module development, and evaluation were not made. In general, trainee ratings were higher than trainer ratings. However, trainee and trainer scores were positively correlated ($r = .51$).

2. How did trainees assess the training experience?

Trainees were asked to evaluate training on fourteen criteria. Again, a five-point rating scale was employed. Level 1 represented a measure of dissatisfaction, level 3 a measure of acceptable satisfaction, and level 5 a measure of great satisfaction. The mean rating across all criteria was 4.3. The training materials were rated extremely high at 4.85. All the trainees strongly expressed the desire to go on for additional training (5.0) and recommended that other colleagues participate (5.0).

3. Did trainees use their skills on the job?

Pre- and post- ratings were made on the use of interpersonal skills on the job. Using the scales mentioned above, objective ratings of attending and responding skills were done. As with the acquisition of skills, trainees demonstrated significant gains in the use of interpersonal skills. Table 10-10 shows the pre- and post- mean ratings, and levels of significance for the application of interpersonal skills.

TABLE 10-9
MEAN PRE-/POST- SCORES AND DIFFERENCES

SKILL	PRE-	POST-	DIFFERENCE
Attending	1.5	4.3	2.8*
Observing	1.8	4.1	2.3**
Listening	1.6	3.9	2.3**
Responding	1.3	4.2	2.9*
Personalizing	2.0	3.3	1.3***
Input Development	1.1	3.5	2.4**
Module Development	1.7	3.7	2.0**
Evaluation	2.1	3.2	1.1***

* $p < .001$
** $p < .01$
*** $p < .05$

TABLE 10-10
PRE-/POST- MEAN RATINGS FOR THE APPLICATION OF INTERPERSONAL SKILLS

SKILL	PRE-	POST-
Attending	1.1	4.1*
Responding/ Personalizing	1.0	2.78**

* $p < .01$
** $p < .05$

In assessing the use of curriculum development skills, trainees were measured by the presence or absence of the following components of a skill module: gathering and using patient input; the use of "tell, show, do" modes of learning; and evaluation including feedback to the patient. For the presence of each element, one point was awarded. A scale of 7 was the highest score achievable. The mean on-the-job score for the group before training was 2.3. The mean on-the-job score for the trainees after training was 7.0.

4. **Did patients learn and use skills?**

Following the staff training, living skills training groups were initiated for patients. These groups focused on the acquisition and application of interpersonal skills in the hospital. Co-trainers worked with mixed male and female patient groups of eight to ten. Patients for the group were the same as those attending the previously offered afternoon "discussion" groups. A six-month follow-up of the training groups yeilded some striking findings. Again, questions were raised about skill acquisition, application, and patient benefit. Trainers report that the mean percentage of trainees learning skills to the criterion of a successful trial in training was 91%. Self-report by trainees of their use of skills in the hospital as measured by completed homework assignments was 85%. In addition, 40% reported application of skills with visitors to the hospital.

5. What have been the benefits for patients?

Trainer reports of comparisons between discussion groups and skill training illustrate significant patient and staff benefit of training. The most frequently and intensely cited advantage to skill training was the amount of patient participation. The trainers reported that training presented a non-threatening atmosphere for patients. As opposed to discussion groups, training offered a more structured learning experience that was conducive to patient understanding of expectations. The result was significantly increased participation. As can be seen in Table 10-11, patients in skill training participated at higher levels than patients in the discussion group.

TABLE 10-11

PERCENTAGES OF LEVELS OF PATIENT PARTICIPATION FOR DISCUSSION GROUP VERSUS SKILLS TRAINING

SCALE LEVELS	PERCENTAGES	
	Discussion Group	Skills Training
1.0 Detractor	20	0
2.0 Observer	50	10
3.0 Participant	30	70
4.0 Contributor	0	20
5.0 Leader	0	10

Particularly relevant given the level of functioning of the patient population was the involvement of withdrawn patients. The trainers reported being able to involve depressed and withdrawn patients who had previously been passive if not "invisible" discussion group members.

Another significant indicator of patient involvement was the attendance of patients for skill training in a voluntary unit of the hospital. A 90% show rate was calculated for skills-training patients.

To assess longer term patient benefits, six-month readmission rates were examined for skills-trained patients. Twenty percent of the trained patients were readmitted within six months. The six-month readmission rate for the hospital was not available. However, Anthony and Buell (1973) report a 30% to 40% six-month readmission rate. Interestingly, the 20% rate for patients trained on an inpatient basis is comparable to the rate reported for ex-psychiatric patients who chose to attend aftercare clinics.

1. What have been the benefits for staff?

Staff benefits have paralleled patient benefits. The staff experienced a feeling of "success" and "professional accomplishment." All trainers involved felt that skill training as a mode of treatment had become a "natural" and integrated part of their delivery repertoire. This was a significant change from earlier reports of feelings of "awkwardness." It also lends support for staff modeling of behaviors for patients.

Also cited was the staff's satisfaction with the flexibility of the training model for patients with different symptoms and levels of chronicity. The training approach provided a structure within which personalized responses could be made for individual patients.

Staff also were pleased with the transferability of the training approach. Interpersonal skills as well as training skills became useful tools in other situations, such as individual patient meetings, working with other staff, staff meetings, and patient assessments.

As a result of the success of skill training, the Activity Therapy Unit has undergone significant program changes. For one, the skills-training approach has been extended from interpersonal skills to a full range of functional skills including hygiene, appearance, first aid, budgeting, buying, cooking, meal planning, and others. The effectiveness of the psychiatric programming model for patients and for staff is supported. Significant gains in acquisition of skills, applications of skills, and transfer of skills were documented. In addition, patient benefits were assessed in terms of participation and readmission.

The present study has implications for other inpatient settings. In a relatively brief amount of time (approximately four hours) patients were able to learn emotional-interpersonal skills. The study represents an initial effort at using psychiatric programming in an inpatient setting. Replications with a more structured research design are needed to confirm and understand these initial results. Specifically, more patient demographic data (e.g., previous patient admissions) is needed. Also needed is more emphasis on the follow-up of the patients' use of skills after leaving the hospital.

AN APPLICATION TO A SPECIFIC SKILL AREA[4]

Although there have been an increasing number of efforts to apply psychiatric rehabilitation programming to specific problem or skill areas (e.g., parenting, dieting, etc.), these initial efforts have been isolated. The most complete efforts thus far appear to exist in the area of helping couples with marital problems stemming from poor interpersonal functioning. There have been three related studies (Pierce, 1973; Santantonio, 1977; Valle and Marinelli, 1975) of the efficacy of training couples in interpersonal skills as a way of helping improve marital communication and overall marital functioning. These studies used similar methodology, outcome measures, and obtained similar results. Together they represent an encouraging beginning in the development, use, and evaluation of a skills-oriented approach to marital communication problems.

The setting for the Valle and Marinelli (1975) and Pierce (1973) research studies were private counseling clinics. The Santantonio (1977) study was conducted at an outpatient department of a community mental health center. In all the studies, the couples had requested help for marriage problems and were diagnosed as possessing poor communication skills. The interpersonal skills training program used in all three studies was based on the systematic didactic and experiential group approach developed by Carkhuff (1972). The couples were trained in attending, observing, listening, and responding skills. The length of training ranged from twenty-five hours (Pierce, 1973) to fifty hours (Valle and Marinelli, 1975). The training resulted in significant improvement in interpersonal skills in all the studies as measured by comparison of pre-/post- interview ratings (Pierce, 1973), and pre- and post- responses to written stimuli (Santantonio, 1977; Valle & Marinelli, 1975). In both the Pierce (1973) and Valle and Marinelli (1975) studies the growth in interpersonal skills was significantly greater than in a treatment control group receiving traditional insight-oriented therapy. Additionally, the Pierce study confirmed similar results when compared with a time-control group.

A meaningful extension in the Valle and Marinelli (1975) and Santantonio (1977) studies was to assess the overall marital functioning of the couples based on their improved interpersonal functioning. Valle and Marinelli set aside time within the training for having the couples process problem areas using their newly learned communication skills in order to explore and understand specific conflict areas in the marriages. Using perceptions of self and spouse functioning in the relationship, as measured by the Interpersonal Relationship Rating Scale (Hipple, 1972) and a self-rating of overall functioning, Valle and Marinelli found a significant improvement in overall marital functioning as compared to traditional insight therapy group participation. Santantonio extended the Valle and Marinelli work by adding training in goal-setting skills and evaluation of the achievement of specific marital communication goals outside of the training group (e.g., increased number of daily conversations, increased number of kind or thoughtful actions). Santantonio found significantly increased levels of satisfaction with the marriage, the spouse's level of communication skills, and achievement of real-life communication goals.

An interesting aspect of the Valle and Marinelli (1975) and Santantonio (1977) studies was the use of ratings reflecting spouses' perceptions of the interpersonal skills of their partners. The findings that the spouses' perceived a higher level of interpersonal skills in their partners than the individuals perceived in themselves (Valle and Martinelli, 1975) suggest the importance of using the perceptions of significant others when assessing rehabilitation outcome.

There are a number of implications for other rehabilitation practitioners working with clients with marital communication problems that flow from these studies:

1. Direct systematic training programs can significantly raise the level of interpersonal skills between spouses of a deteriorated marriage in a relatively brief time.

2. Systematic objective ratings of marital interpersonal skills reflect the couples perceived experience of marital communication skills and overall marital functioning.

3. The unique benefits of training as compared to traditional insight therapy may lie: 1) in the combination of both telling, showing, and having the couples heavily practice specific skill behaviors; and 2) the advantages of multiple helpers generated by a group of couples trained in interpersonal skills.

4. The additional component of relating the learning of interpersonal skills to real-life communication goals facilitate motivation to learn the skills and improvement in overall marital functioning.

Although the results of these studies are extremely encouraging, the need for further study remains. Specifically, an assessment of the effects of transferring the learning of interpersonal skills in a marital context to the interpersonal functioning in other relationships needs to be done. Expanding training to include how to use these skills in other life contexts is suggested. Also the continued use and evaluation of this approach applied to other specific skill areas (e.g., parenting, job retention, and others) is strongly indicated.

AN APPLICATION TO A PREVENTION SETTING[5]

The present crisis in our schools is well documented. The schools are described as not only failing to achieve their educational goals, but destructive to the emotional well-being of the students. Yet little has been done to offer concrete solutions to the crisis, or help to the students. The result is a frustrating predicament for our educators who are criticized, aware of failure, offered theories, but not offered the help they need. The result for the students is the lack of the skills needed to live, learn, and eventually work productively. Without these skills the students cannot experience pride, satisfaction, and the good feelings associated with mental health. Instead, out of every hundred children it is predicted that two will commit major crimes and serve time in jail, ten will become severely mentally ill, four will be too retarded to be self-supporting, and fifty will be sufficiently maladjusted to add to the ranks of the petty criminals, the marital failures, and the emotionally unstable; and for those that make it through school, 15 to 30% will not be able to find work (Cohen & Greenberg, 1975).

Psychiatric rehabilitation programming is unique in that it offers the means not only to resolve the crisis, but also to begin guaranteeing the physical, emotional, and intellectual growth of our students. Cohen and Greenberg (1975) have described the application of psychiatric rehabilitation programming to a mental health intervention in a crisis in an inner-city elementary school. The history of mental health intervention in the schools has been a difficult one, due to the stigma of mental illness and the resistance to intervention by professionals outside the educational system.

In the Cohen and Greenberg study, contact between the consultation and education department and the school was initiated by a guidance counselor who had received previous training by the mental health department.

DESCRIPTION OF NEEDS

During an initial meeting between mental health staff, the guidance counselor, fourth-grade teachers, and the school principal, the problems of the schools two fourth-grade classes were described. The educators began by expressing their concern that the sixty fourth-grade students were having unusually severe behavioral problems as evidenced by continual fighting and unruly behavior. Additionally, the students' academic skills were described as exceptionally weak. Aside from the students' poor reading, writing, and math skills, the teachers shared their frustrations about the students' overall lack of ability to answer questions correctly, complete assignments, or participate in class.

A comprehensive needs assessment was planned as the initial step toward a larger rehabilitation program. The needs assessment focused on diagnosing the physical, emotional, and intellectual skill deficits of the key people (students, teachers, building administrators, and parents), and key programs (educational, physical, environmental, parental, etc.). The result of subjective (e.g., interviews) and objective (e.g., test results) measurements was a needs assessment matrix that summarized the numerous data collected, and outlined a minimum of three recommendations for each of the people populations. Using a decision-making matrix to explore and select the most appropriate program goals based on values such as benefits to students, students' expressed interest, staff expertise, staff time, the quantity of resources needed, and chances of success, a direction began to concretely emerge. Two

significant goals were defined: first, to increase student participation in class as measured by teacher and outside observer ratings; and second, to reduce the incidences of discipline problems and inappropriate behavior in school as measured by teacher and principal reports.

Using the principles of psychiatric rehabilitation programming, a program for systematic training for students and teachers was developed and implemented. The students were trained in basic "learning-to-learn" skills including paying attention to the teacher, presenting to the class with pride, and listening in class. In addition, mental health staff were prepared to train both simpler and more complex skills as needed. The teachers were trained to respond to the unique needs and wants of their students, to make the classroom environment a place where students would want to behave appropriately, and to participate in student training.

Training was offered to students grouped according to their initial skills diagnosis (e.g., academic functioning). Two large groups of thirty students each composed the basic training groups. Additionally, small practice groups of eight to ten students each were formed based upon their shared needs or interests (e.g., high scores on interpersonal behavior but low scores on classroom listening). The curricula for the student training program was developed using the skills of teaching outlined by Carkhuff (Berenson, Berenson & Carkhuff, 1978; Berenson & Pierce, 1975). Student training sessions lasted approximately forty-five minutes to one hour. There were a total of six sessions for each group, totaling approximately six hours of training. Two key principles for skill practice were *flexibility* and *repetition*. Exercises for each small group were developed to fit the particular student's interest and future aspirations (e.g., football). Once the skill was acquired, the student's skill ability was systematically applied from an area of interest to the actual school setting (e.g., listening for football plays to listening to the teacher). When needed, more elementary skills were first offered. For example, the students with more severe behavioral problems required training in such "decency" skills as being silent when someone is talking, as a prerequisite to training in listening skills.

The training provided the students with the skills needed to participate in the learning process. Research on outcome in rehabilitation and education has clearly spelled out the role of the helper/teacher in the learning process. Teachers equipped with the necessary interpersonal and curriculum development skills as well as the academic content knowledge can facilitate physical, emotional, and intellectual gains in students. Teachers not equipped with these skills and knowledge do not facilitate and may, in fact, retard student growth.

The teacher training program consisted of three stages. The first stage of training centered on the acquisition and application of basic interpersonal skills for the classroom based on the curricula designed by Carkhuff (1975). Teachers were trained in contextual and physical attending, observing and responding skills. During the second stage of the training, teachers were familiarized with the student training procedures and curricula, and taught to participate in the student training program. Also, a reinforcement system was developed for the teachers to use in order to reward student performance of skills in class. The third stage of training for the teachers consisted of systematically teaching the teachers to develop and implement skill modules and "learning-to-learn" curricula. The teachers learned psychiatric rehabilitation programming skills including student skill assessment, goal setting, program development, and program evaluation. In total, teacher training lasted approximately forty hours. Sessions included all-day workshops as well as after-school meetings. Training included application to the classroom immediately following acquisition, with emphasis on continued follow-up and feedback in the classroom.

Evaluation of the program included many objective and subjective measures. The findings of the evaluations were:

1. Pre- to post- student gains on attending, presenting proud, and listening to the teacher *showed significant student learning of the skills*. Also when students were asked how much they had learned, 68% reported learning *all* of what was taught and another 28% reported they learned most of what was taught.

2. The students and teachers were asked to assess the *students' use of training skills in the classroom*. The students reported significant gains in their abilities to attend, listen to the teacher, and present themselves proudly when speaking in class. More importantly, the teachers reported significant gains in the students' attending, listening, and presenting proud in the daily classroom situation. Also mental health staff ratings of the students' use of the skills in class showed significant pre- to post- gains.

3. Teacher and mental health staff observations and ratings of student behavior in class indicated *more student participation in class*. It appeared to the teachers that the use of "learning to learn" skills in class seemed to greatly contribute to student participation and the elusive dimension of student "motivation."

4. Using eleven behavioral indicators reflecting discipline, school involvement, attitudes toward school, responsibility as students, and participation in extracurricular activities, the teachers' ratings yielded significant growth for students. Most importantly, *the teachers reported changes in behaviors reflecting student control and relationships with other students*. The number of disciplinary problems weekly, the number of fights weekly, and the number of referrals to the principal were reduced significantly. The reduction in undisciplined behavior was supported by the principal's rating as well. Also, positive changes in the students' attitude toward the teachers were indicated. In addition, the teachers noted greatly increased participation by students in extracurricular activities. A follow-up assessment one year later confirmed the maintenance of reduction in student behavioral problems.

5. *Most dramatically, the training programs appeared to affect absenteeism and tardiness records.* The trained students on the average attended school 33% more frequently than a control group of untrained students. Additionally, trained students came to school on time 46% more frequently than untrained students.

6. *Student evaluation of the "learning-to-learn" program found that students very much liked the training.* Ninety-four percent of the students felt they learned "most" or "all" of the skills, 86% liked the training "very much," 84% liked the trainers, and 72% wanted to have more training in "learning-to-learn" skills.

Training the students and teachers had made a difference — but what did it all mean? The implications that flow from this study are:

1. **Rehabilitation can provide an entrance that can make preventative work possible.**

Typically, mental health efforts have been supported because of their treatment and rehabilitation efforts. The community has seen mental health programs as caring for the mentally ill. Prevention programs in mental health, which theoretically touch the lives of all individuals, are more difficult to understand and therefore get less support. In the Cohen and Greenberg study, the need for rehabilitation initiated a mental health program that not only could be designed to meet the immediate student problems, but also to prevent future difficulties.

2. **Rehabilitation can provide skill growth that can lead to prevention.**

Both the fourth-grade teachers and the school were aware of significant behavioral changes in the students. Fighting decreased as did other behaviors that would require disciplinary action. The skills (e.g., presenting proud) appeared to provide the students with a functional alternative to fighting. Cohen and Greenberg drew the connection between the skills and their implications for the students' future mental health. Potentially serious intra- and interpersonal problems appeared to be attended to by the students. Also, the Cohen and Greenberg study seems to make the point that the students' so-called poor attitude toward school that led to absence and tardiness was really the students' lack of the "learning-to-learn" skills needed to be active in their education. These skills and the resulting improved student attitude, attendance, and classroom ability can help prevent school problems in the future.

3. **Rehabilitation can provide knowledge that may be transferred to new populations for prevention.**

The Cohen and Greenberg study began as a rehabilitation program for the fourth-grade students. In addition to the helping of the students, the study provided the impetus for new directions. The learning that came from the needs assessment, development of training curricula, the actual training, and the evaluation of the program was used to develop an effective preventative "learning-to-learn" program for first graders. The skills that the fourth graders lacked appeared to be those that students need to learn in school.

4. **Rehabilitation can lead to the training of teachers/practitioners who can then use the skills for rehabilitation or prevention.**

The teachers in the Cohen and Greenberg study represent "front-line" helpers, people who are in a position as teachers/practitioners to help students daily. Their training was important because their education may not have included the necessary skills to enable them to fully help their students. If "front-line" teachers/practitioners are better able to deliver necessary skills, then the emergence of serious problems and subsequent need for treatment will be reduced. The teachers in the Cohen and Greenberg study were left prepared to deliver "learning-to-learn" skills to future students with skill deficits, or to those students for whom the learning of these skills might help prevent future problems.

ENDNOTES

[1] This chapter was authored by Drs. Mikal Cohen, Bernard Greenberg, Christopher Ross and Raphael Vitalo.

[2] This section of the chapter was written by Drs. Raphael Vitalo and Christopher Ross and is based on the research reported in: **The Differential Effects of Medication and Medication Plus Counseling with Aftercare Clients**, Springfield, Mass., 1977.

[3] This section of the chapter was written by Dr. Bernard Greenberg and is based on the research reported in: **The Development of An Inpatient Skills Training Program**, unpublished manuscript, 1977.

[4] This section of the chapter was written by Dr. Mikal Cohen, Amherst, Mass.

[5] This section of the chapter was written by Dr. Mikal Cohen and is based on the research reported in: Cohen, M. and Greenberg, B. **The Money Tree: Franklin School Consultation Project**, unpublished manuscript, Amherst, Mass., 1975.

REFERENCES

Anthony, W. A. Psychological rehabilitation: A concept in need of a method. **American Psychologist**, 1977, *32*: 658-662.

Anthony, W. A. and Buell, G. J. Psychiatric aftercare clinic effectiveness as a function of patient demographic characteristics. **Journal of Consulting and Clinical Psychology**, 1973, *41*: 116-119.

Berenson, D. H., Berenson, S. R. and Carkhuff, R. R. The skills of teaching: Lesson planning skills. Amherst, Mass.: Human Resource Development Press, 1978.

Buell, G. J. and Anthony, W. A. Demographic characteristics as predictors of recidivism and post-hospital employment. **Journal of Counseling Psychology**, 1973, *20*: 361-365.

Carkhuff, R. R. Helping and human relations — Vol. I, New York: Holt, Rinehart & Winston, 1969.

Carkhuff, R. R. **Helping and human relations** — Vol. II. New York: Holt, Rinehart & Winston, 1969a.

Carkhuff, R. R. **The art of helping**. Amherst, Mass.: Human Resource Development Press, 1972.

Carkhuff, R. R., Berenson, D., and Pierce, R. **The skills of teaching: Interpersonal skills**. Amherst, Mass.: Human Resource Development Press, 1975.

Carkhuff, R. R. and Berenson, B. G. **Teaching as treatment**. Amherst, Mass.: Human Resource Development Press, 1976.

Carkhuff, R. R. and Pierce, R. **The trainer's guide to the art of helping**. Amherst, Mass.: Human Resource Development Press, 1976.

Cohen, M. and Greenberg, B. **The money tree: Franklin School Consultation Project**. Unpublished manuscript, Amherst, Mass., 1975.

Davis, J., Gosenfeld, L. and Tsai, C. Maintenance anti-psychotic drugs do prevent relapse: A reply to Tobias and MacDonald. **Psychological Bulletin**, 1976, *83*: 441-447.

Dixon, W. and Massey, F. **Introduction to statistical analysis.** New York: McGraw Hill, 1957.

Fielder, F. Factor analysis of psychoanalytic, non-directive and Adlercin therapeutic relationships. **Journal of Consulting Psychology**, 1950, *14*: 436-445.

Franklin, J., Kittredge, L. and Thrasher, J. A survey of factors related to mental hospital readmissions. **Community Psychiatry**, 1975, *26:11*, 749-751.

Gardos, G. and Cole, J. Maintenance of anti-psychotic therapy: Is the cure worse than the disease? **American Journal of Psychiatry.** 1976, *133*:7, 32-36.

Greenberg, B. The development of an inpatient skills training program. Unpublished manuscript, Oberlin, Ohio, 1977.

Hipple, J. L. The interpersonal relationship rating scale. In Pfeiffer, W. J. and Jones, J. F. **The 1972 Handbook for Group Facilitators.** Iowa City: University Associates, 1974, pp. 69-74.

Pierce, R. M. Training in interpersonal communication skills with the partners of deteriorated marriages. **The Family Coordinator,** 1973, *21*: 223-227.

Santantonio, D. An interpersonal skills training approach to marital counseling. Unpublished manuscript, Austintown, Ohio, 1977.

Tobias, L. and MacDonald, M. Withdrawal of maintenance drugs with long-term hospitalized mental patients: A critical review. **Psychological Bulletin**, 1974, *81*: 107-125.

Truax, C. and Mitchell, K. Research on certain therapeutic interpersonal skills in relation to process and outcome. In A. Bergin and S. Garfield, eds. **Handbook of Psychotherapy and Behavior Change.** New York: Wiley, 1971.

Ullman, L. and Giovannani, J. The development of a self-report method of the process-reactive continuum. **Journal of Nervous and mental diseases,** 1964, *138*: 38-41.

Valle, S. K. and Martinelli, R. P. Training in human relations skills as a preferred mode of treatment for married couples. **Journal of Marriage and Family Counseling,** 1975, 359-365.

Vitalo, R. Three methods of outcome evaluation. Paper presented at Conference on Evaluation in Community Mental Health, Southwest CMHC, Columbus, Ohio, 1977.

CHAPTER XI
Professional Training For Psychiatric Rehabilitation Practitioners[1]

Almost fifty years after professional training programs formally emerged in America, the debate concerning a preferred training mode is still unresolved. For many years the controversy could be summarized, on the one hand, as teaching the student, or, on the other, as treating the student (Truax & Carkhuff, 1967). The didactic or teaching approach is seemingly born from the assumption that traditional educational methods are an effective means of shaping an individual's behavior. In contrast, the treatment or experiential approach sought instead to develop in the trainee feelings of safety and freedom which promote an openness to experience and a willingness to experiment. In essence, the didactic approach emphasized the learning of theories and concepts, while the experiential approach emphasized the trainee's personal growth and development.

More recently, however, the controversy over training procedures has been fueled by other concerns. Increasingly, those involved in professional training programs have been questioning what specific training efforts translate into constructive client change. The response to that inquiry has been unsettling. During the twenty-five years since Eysenck (1952, 1962, 1972) first challenged the helping professions to demonstrate their efficacy, little concrete evidence of their effectiveness exists.

In terms of rehabilitation outcome, measures of rehabilitative success for the juvenile and adult justice system (Lipton, Martinson & Wilks, 1975), drug and alcohol centers (Emrick, 1975; Nietzel, Winett, MacDonald & Davidson, 1977; Viamontes, 1972), vocational and employment services (Bolles, 1977) as well as psychiatric hospitals (Anthony, Buell, Sharratt, Althoff, 1972) have all yielded distressingly similar results. Professionally trained helpers have on the average been unable to provide constructive alternatives to the specific life crises confronting their clients.

At a very basic level those involved in the preparation and development of helping professionals bear the responsibility of this failure. One of the traditional explanations suggested to defend the current status of our helping effectiveness has been that we represent a young profession. As such, we are only beginning to identify the dimensions of facilitative interactions (Goldstein, Heller & Sechrest, 1966). Another is that the qualities of the "effective helper" were until recently too poorly and variously defined to be of functional value (Krasner, 1966). Although still other explanations have been offered in defense of traditional training efforts, they offer little meaning or solace to those whom we are paid to help!

HISTORY OF SUPERVISION AND TRAINING: AN OVERVIEW

In retrospect, it seems that essentially two basic models of supervision have dominated the training of professional helpers; the medical model (didactic) and the social work model (experiential). In general, the medical model developed a rather rigid teacher-student process (Lester, Gussen, Yamomoto & West, 1962; Romans, 1961; Schwartz & Abel, 1955; Wolberg, 1954). In contrast, the social work model typically was less authoritarian and therefore tried to emphasize the relationship between the supervisor and supervisee. This process called for the student's own development and awareness (Austin, 1963; Boehm, 1961; Ekstein & Wallerstein, 1958; Moore, 1969;

Towles, 1961; Wessel, 1961). Boyd (1978) recognizes the central element of this latter approach to be the belief that the core of supervision resides in the relationship and interaction between the supervisor and supervisee as they investigate the trainee's interactions with clients, consultees, and supervisors.

Ultimately, other professional disciplines (psychiatric nursing, rehabilitation counseling, occupational therapy, clinical and counseling psychology) accepted one or the other paradigm (Carkhuff, 1966). Sone educators (Arbuckle, 1963; Mueller & Dell, 1972; Lister 1966; Patterson, 1964; Rogers 1957) looked to the social work model, that is, the one with an experiential base. Others were much more closely linked to a strong didactic approach (Krasner, 1963; Korner & Brown, 1952; Krumbolt 1966). Carkhuff (1966) writes that in an historical sense "one cannot help but conjecture that the attitudes and orientations found in the literature reflect the dominant and assertive disposition of the medical profession, the passive and submissive disposition of social work, and the intensified role conflicts of applied psychology."

Based on this perspective it is perhaps understandable why so few attempts at developing adequate models of supervision have tried to integrate these two basic models. Most of the early efforts were timid and not carefully researched. For example, in 1958, Fleming and Hamburg developed a role-playing situation in which the instructor became the patient and the counselor-trainee the therapist. The authors felt this had several advantages. It offered the counselor-trainee first-hand experience while avoiding possible injurious consequences to a real patient. Second, it provided a maximal learning experience because it occurred in the classroom before other students. Although this was a modification of previous strategies for counselor training, it was hardly a radical innovation.

This is not to suggest, however, that the various theories of counseling and psychotherapy underlying those two models have failed to provide learning experiences for their trainees. In fact, a clear example of an iatrogenic impact that a supervisor's theoretical stance may have on developing counselors is provided by Pasaminick, Dinitz and Lefton (1959):

". . .(research) findings provide concrete statistical affirmation for the view that despite protestations that their point of reference is always the individual patient, clinicians in fact may be so committed to a particular school of thought that the patients' diagnosis and treatment is largely predetermined" (p. 131).

More specifically, as a consequence of training experiences, helpers may selectively perceive and attend to only those characteristics and behaviors of clients which are congruent to their preconceived system of thinking. Thus, counselors are rarely trained to attend, observe, listen or respond to those thoughts, beliefs, or behaviors which most concern the *patient!*

A GENERATION OF VICTIMS

The objective rehabilitation consequences of traditional therapeutic training programs have been documented across the broad spectrum of human service agencies. Professionals in the helping field have worked with problems in the schools, the juvenile justice system, adult corrections, drug abuse and alcoholism, unemployment, and psychiatric hospitals. Yet, research efforts document that professionally trained helpers have been insufficiently prepared to respond to the crises of their clients. In a sense, both are victims of a society and a profession that has recognized the urgent need for effective human beings to help others but one which is unable to produce them!

This inability to affect rehabilitation outcomes is certainly not limited to psychiatric rehabilitation. For example, there is an increasing national concern over the steady rise of serious crime in America. The FBI's recent Federal Crime Reporting Document reports the annual increase in murder, forceable rape, robbery, aggravated assault, burglary, theft, and motor vehicle theft to be up 110% from 1965 to 1975. Although the expense and extent of crime is incalculable (Netter, 1974), the cost to the federal, state, and local justice systems is reported to be in excess of approximately four billion dollars annually. Over 2.5 million criminals go through our correctional systems per year (President's Commission, 1967). Nearly one-fifth of all male youths between fourteen and sixteen in one midwestern city have at least one official police contact (Davidson, 1975).

In response to this serious and growing problem, professional trained practitioners have been employed to help rehabilitate the criminals. Unfortunately, the outcome of these efforts are as distressing as they are consistent (Nietzel et al. 1977). Recidivism is reported to be approximately 75% (Clark,

1970) with approximately 90% of the recidivism occurring in the three years immediately following release. According to Robinson and Smith (1971), there is no evidence to support any of the current correctional alternatives as reducing recidivism. In an analysis of 231 studies on the effectiveness of correctional treatment, Lipton, Martinson, and Wilks (1975) reviewed various strategies affecting recidivism of criminals including individual counseling and psychotherapy, group counseling and milieu therapy (or therapeutic community). Again, previous research attesting to the inability to produce rehabilitation outcome was corroborated. These authors concluded that counseling may be harmful if it is administered to "Nonamenable or younger male or female offenders, particularly in cases of unenthusiastic therapists with a psychoanalytic orientation" (p. 581). An additional tragedy for everyone involved is that recidivists tend to be increasingly more violent and their crimes more carefully calculated.

Related to the area of adult and juvenile corrections is alcoholism and drug abuse. Kittrie (1971) reports almost 50% of convicted felons were in some measure acting under the influence of alcohol during their crime. Alcohol and homocide has been significantly correlated (Goodwin, 1973) and the connection between drug addiction and crime is now clearly linked (Lindesmith, 1965). Unfortunately, the effectiveness of psychologically based treatment for these two client populations is also dismal. Emerick (1975) reviewed 384 studies of psychologically oriented alcoholism treatments and found that they did not significantly obtain long-term results. In effect, no mean difference in abstinance existed between treated and untreated alcoholics. While group psychotherapy has been believed to be a preferred mode of treatment for alcoholics (Blum & Blum, 1967; Cahn, 1970), there is little empirical evidence to support this assumption (Glasscote, 1967). Equally ineffective has been the various drug-induced treatments of alcoholism (Mottin, 1973).

The various psychological treatment modalities for drug addiction are similarly discouraging (Gay, Metzger, Bathhurst & Smith, 1971). Although some chemically based treatments have emerged as preferred alternatives in helping drug addicts, they are still highly controversial treatments (Lennard & Allen, 1973). For example, methadone hydrochloride, a synthetic opiate, is one of the major treatment approaches for heroin addicts (Dupont, 1974). Methadone itself, however, is addictive and once methadone is withdrawn the desire for narcotics returns almost immediately (Dole, 1970).

As mentioned in Chapter II, the area of psychiatric rehabilitation is also plagued with a discouraging history of failure. Major reviews of the literature (Anthony, Buell, Sharratt & Althoff, 1972; Anthony, Cohen, & Vitalo, 1978) have revealed that traditional psychologically based treatments do not differentially affect the outcome measures of recidivism and post-hospital employment. Three to five years after hospital discharge, between 65-75% of the patients return to psychiatric facilities and only 25% are able to work in full-time employment! As mentioned in Chapter V the advent of drug-based treatments has not changed these rehabilitation outcome measures for discharged psychiatric patients.

Each of these client populations (offenders, alcoholics, drug abusers, and the psychiatrically disabled) has subtle and distinctive characteristics or psychopathologies which confound efforts to equate them. Yet the outcome studies reviewed are similar in that they examined the effects of professionally trained helpers. All are similar in the high rates of failure as measured by recidivism or by a return to their pathological conditions which existed before the treatment intervention. Essentially, professionally trained helpers fail to rehabilitate their clients between 50% to 75% of the time.

The alarming results are not necessarily limited to outcomes with severely disturbed individuals. For instance, professionally trained employment counselors working with "normal" clients have equally poor results. Private employment agencies are reported to have a successful placement rate of only 5% (Bolles, 1977)! The U.S. government's employment service was able to place only 46% of the 9.9 million Americans who used its vocational placement services. In one area surveyed, 57% of those who were successfully placed by the Employment Service were not working in those jobs just thirty days later (Bolles, 1977)!

In general, it would appear that the traditional strategies for training and supervision have not effectively equipped our rehabilitation professionals with the skills they need to constructively rehabilitate their helpees.

A PREFERRED MODEL FOR PSYCHIATRIC REHABILITATION TRAINING

As suggested previously, initial attempts at developing a successful model of training and supervision were traditionally either didactic or experiential in nature. However, the research has not strongly supported the unique efficacy of those training models as they relate to constructive client change.

In response to the deficit of this dichotomous reasoning in traditional helper preparation, Carkhuff attempted to integrate the didactic and experiential approaches (Carkhuff, 1969; Carkhuff & Truax, 1965). Although previous attempts at such an integration (Fleming & Hamburg, 1958) were unsystematic and simply descriptive, Carkhuff attempted to develop a solid research base for his training approach.

Historically, it has been from this base of research that the overall efficacy of graduate school training for developing professionals was challenged (Anthony & Carkhuff, 1968; Carkhuff, 1967; Truax & Carkhuff, 1967). It was also from this research base that Truax and Carkhuff (1965) reported that, in approximately one hundred hours of systematic training, lay personnel could be brought to the same level of interpersonal functioning in a helping situation as the professional! It was also from this research base that other studies emerged showing the effects on individuals who come into contact with interpersonally skilled or unskilled significant others (Carkhuff, 1969). Furthermore, it was from this base of research that a full model for training and supervision has been developed and implemented (Carkhuff, 1966; 1971b, 1972c, Carkhuff & Berenson, 1976).

It is Carkhuff's research and development with respect to the training of human service providers that forms the foundation for the approach used to train psychiatric rehabilitation practitioners. Carkhuff's skill training approach has developed out of fifteen years of training experience, representing over 10,000 hours of training with over 50,000 people in all kinds of helper and helpee populations (Carkhuff & Pierce, 1977). It is a guaranteed way of teaching helpers many of the complex skills needed to increase their helping effectiveness. It is a training method that combines both the didactic and experiential phases of learning, in combination with extensive skill practice and feedback. In most simple terms the Carkhuff training approach incorporates a tell-show-do method of teaching professional helping skills. The training approach itself is very similar to the approach used to teach new skills to rehabilitation clients. The major difference, of course, being that the particular skills that must be mastered by the helper are much more complex than those skills learned by the helpee.

The remainder of the chapter will focus first on the *content* of a psychiatric rehabilitation training approach, and then on the *teaching process*, the means by which this content is mastered. A final section of the chapter addresses the issue of training uncredentialed helpers (paraprofessionals, volunteers, etc.) in the practice of psychiatric rehabilitation.

THE CONTENT OF PSYCHIATRIC REHABILITATION TRAINING

As mentioned in Chapter I, helpers from a number of different professions practice psychiatric rehabilitation. Each of those professionals contribute their own unique expertise to the field. Over and above these unique contributions, however, a specific content area for psychiatric rehabilitation practitioners has begun to be defined (Anthony, Cohen, & Vitalo, 1978). This content area has developed out of an increased understanding of what constitutes a psychiatric rehabilitation model of treatment (Anthony, 1977). In addition, the content area has emerged from a growing recognition of the unmet needs of the psychiatrically disabled helpee (NIMH, 1976), as well as an awareness of some of the ingredients capable of improving the outcome of psychiatric rehabilitation (Chapters III-X).

The content of a psychiatric rehabilitation training program is a unique combination of professional skills and knowledge. At present this combination of skills and knowledge is neither comprehensively nor routinely taught in any traditional human service discipline. However, the content is capable of being mastered by any professional, regardless of the professional discipline in which she or he has been trained.

In terms of the psychiatric rehabilitation *knowledge component*, the type of material with which the professional needs to become familiar is fairly obvious, that is, all the psychiatric rehabilitation research and writing which has been done in this decade. The problem in mastering this material is that it has appeared in books and articles written for a variety of professional disciplines. Thus, the best method of acquiring the knowledge of psychiatric rehabilitation would be to read material which provides an overview (with bibliography) of various aspects of the field. The practitioner can then consult first hand the references which seem most important to his or her specific interest.

The most difficult part of conquering the knowledge component of psychiatric rehabilitation is staying abreast of current writing and research. Innovative ideas, research, and applications occur monthly in various professional journals. Thus, the practitioner must peruse the table of contents of the major journals of psychology, nursing, rehabilitation, social work, psychiatry, and occupational therapy. In addition, the practitioner should use the services of the federal government to run computer searches of specific psychiatric rehabilitation interest areas. Regardless of the methods employed, the practitioner

must keep his or her knowledge of psychiatric rehabilitation current. Unlike some highly specialized fields, however, this means being aware of the developments in a number of different disciplines. The practice of psychiatric rehabilitation is the exclusive province of no one profession, nor is it dominated by any one profession. Thus, the psychiatric rehabilitation practitioner must have a broad base of knowledge.

Although an awareness of the knowledge of psychiatric rehabilitation is important, it is the mastery of the *skills component* of psychiatric rehabilitation which truly defines the psychiatric rehabilitation practitioner. The gradual emergence of a comprehensive set of psychiatric rehabilitation skills is an even more recent development than the identification of a body of psychiatric rehabilitation knowledge. Obviously the current skills of psychiatric rehabilitation practice will be continually added to and modified. However, at present the following skills seem to best characterize the unique competencies of psychiatric rehabilitation practitioners:

1. Diagnostic planning skills
2. Rehabilitation programming skills
3. Rehabilitation evaluation skills
4. Career counseling skills
5. Career placement skills
6. Community coordinating skills.

The first two skill areas enable the psychiatric rehabilitation practitioner to become more expert in diagnosing and improving the skills which the client needs to function more effectively in his or her particular community (Chapters IV and V). The skills of rehabilitation evaluation provide the practitioner with the abilities necessary to evaluate the outcome of his or her rehabilitation efforts (Chapter IX). Career counseling and career placement skills are practitioner skills which have been the historical concern of the psychiatric rehabilitation practitioner (Chapter VII). The final set of skills — community coordinating — prepare the practitioner to be better able to evaluate, modify, and use the resources of the community to better accommodate the client's present abilities and programming needs (Chapter VIII).

The following several pages present a slightly more detailed overview of these psychiatric rehabilitation skills. More details may be found in various chapters of this book. Still greater detail may be found in the training books specifically written to teach practitioners each of these skill areas. Each of these training manuals is referenced on the following pages.

1. **Diagnostic planning skills.**

Rehabilitation diagnostic skills involve both *interviewing* and *assessment* skills. These skills enable the rehabilitation practitioner to explore the client's strengths and deficits, understand how these strengths and deficits affect the client's ability to function in specific environments, and assess in an objective and observable manner the level of client skill performance in relation to what is needed to function in these specific environments. The outcome of the rehabilitation diagnostic planning process is a diagnostic picture of the psychiatrically disabled client which *implies a treatment plan;* for the purpose of a rehabilitation diagnosis is to improve the efficacy of treatment services eventually provided to the client (Anthony, Pierce & Cohen, 1977a).

Two principles underlying the entire diagnostic process are *comprehensiveness* and *comprehensibility*. That is, the diagnostic process should be broad in scope, as well as presented in such a way that maximizes the client's understanding of the diagnosis. To the greatest extent possible, the client should be involved in developing the diagnostic picture, as this will improve the probability of the client becoming involved in the rehabilitation treatment procedures which flow out of the diagnosis. Client comprehension as well as diagnostic comprehensiveness can be facilitated by using the simple categorization process of physical, intellectual, and emotional skills by living, learning, and working environments (See Chapter IV).

It must also be pointed out that the rehabilitation diagnostic process demands a highly skilled diagnostic interviewer. Psychiatrically disabled clients typically do not readily acknowledge their most crucial strengths and deficits. The client often begins the interview with a victimized exploration of past events, and must be guided by the rehabilitation diagnostician to an understanding of his or her personal responsibility in terms of future rehabilitation activities. In essence, the rehabilitation diagnostic process develops from an external exploration of past situations to the client's more personal awareness of his or her responsibility for actively *learning* and *doing* specific skill behaviors in present and future situations (Anthony, Pierce, and Cohen, 1977a).

2. **Rehabilitation programming skills.**

It is not enough to identify exactly what skills are needed by the client, as few clients can acquire these skills on their own. The most efficient way to teach new skills is through a systematic program. Rehabilitation is not complete unless the psychiatrically disabled clients can act skillfully to enable themselves to grow from where they are to where they need to be (Anthony, Pierce, and Cohen, 1977b). Mastery of programming skills enables the practitioner to write a series of behavioral steps, arranged in a hierarchy, which the client can do in order to learn these living, learning, and working skills which he or she needs in order to function in the community.

3. **Practitioner evaluation skills.**

The need for improvement of psychiatric rehabilitation services has been documented in previous sections. Improvement can only occur if the effectiveness of present efforts are documented and intelligibly organized in such a way as to suggest better alternative modes of intervention. Each individual psychiatric rehabilitation practitioner must be able to assess and evaluate his or her own rehabilitation efforts (Cohen, Anthony, Pierce, and Vitalo, 1977). By mastering evaluation skills, the practitioner can assess the attainment of client rehabilitation goals and communicate these measurements to the staff for the purpose of program improvement.

4. **Career counseling skills.**

Vocational concerns have been the historical emphasis of the psychiatric rehabilitation practitioner. The mastery of these skills will enable the practitioner to teach the psychiatrically disabled the skills necessary to plan their careers systematically rather than haphazardly or fortuitously (Pierce, Anthony, and Cohen, 1977). Practitioners must be able to use their career counseling skills in order to first expand the client's career alternatives, then narrow those alternatives down to the most favorable, and finally to assess the client's ability to meet the career's requirements.

5. **Career placement skills.**

It is not enough for the client to plan and decide on a career. The practitioner must often teach the skills of career placement which allow the client to achieve complete vocational rehabilitation (Pierce, Cohen, Anthony, and Cohen, 1977). Career placement skills enable the practitioner to teach psychiatrically disabled clients the skills necessary to obtain a job, retain the job, and to advance on the job.

6. **Community coordinating skills.**

Obviously, if the rehabilitation goal is to improve community functioning, the rehabilitation practitioner must have the skills necessary to work in the community (Cohen, Pierce, Anthony and Cohen, 1977). Community coordinating skills include the ability of the practitioner to systematically evaluate and decide upon the specific environment or community resource which will best allow the patient to overcome deficits or accommodate existing strengths and deficits; the ability to get the commitment of the environment or resource to provide specific services needed by the patient; or the ability to develop and implement a program to overcome potential patient or environmental problems in using the environment or resource.

THE PSYCHIATRIC REHABILITATION TRAINING (TEACHING) PROCESS

These major skill content areas of psychiatric rehabilitation cannot be conquered by simply reading about these skills. A simple didactic type of presentation of these skills does not engage the trainee in a learning process which clearly results in an observable, measurable improvement in the practitioner's skilled performance. In order for the practitioner to master the skills and knowledge of psychiatric rehabilitation, she or he must be engaged in a skill-learning process quite different from the typical helping profession training model. First of all, the teaching emphasis must be on observable and measurable changes in practitioner skills. It is upon these measures of the trainee's skill improvement that the training program and training personnel are judged. Although increased knowledge of psychiatric rehabilitation facts and concepts is important, the ultimate criteria is practitioner skill gain. That is, can the practitioner perform these rehabilitation skills with psychiatrically disabled clients?

Traditionally, professional training programs in the human services have focused the bulk of their assessments of training outcome on the knowledge component. Changes in the professionals' skills, although expected, were rarely evaluated with the same intensity. This omission was typically due to the fact that these skills were seldom operationalized, and thus careful and objective evaluation of these vague performance criteria was almost impossible.

In contrast, the major psychiatric rehabilitation skills are capable of being observably measured. Because of the operationalization of these skills, it is possible to assess a trainee's performance. Even more importantly, because these psychiatric rehabilitation skills have been operationalized, it is now possible to systematically train practitioners in these necessary skills.

The actual procedure for training each of these skills is the same. The skill to be learned is observably defined and then broken down into the smaller subskills which comprise the overall skill. The trainees are told what each skill involves, shown examples of the skill, and then practice the skill in a classroom setting. During the classroom practice sessions, feedback is given to each trainee with respect to his or her skill performance. Once the trainee has mastered the skill in class, he or she will be given an assignment to try the skill in his or her fieldwork or job setting.

Thus, the content of the training program is essentially taught in a tell-show-do procedure. The trainee is *told* about the skill through a lecture or reading material, *shown* examples of the skill through classroom demonstrations or reading material, and *does* the skill, first in the class and then on the job or in his or her field placement.

For example, one of the subskills of program evaluation is the ability to prioritize rehabilitation goals. The trainee is told what this skill involves; for example, the ability to identify and rank order the agency's most important goals, and then weigh these goals in terms of their overall value to the practitioner or the agency. Additional reading material and lecture-discussion supplement this tell or didactic step. The show step involves the teacher presenting an example of how this might be done in a typical rehabilitation agency. The in-class do step directs the trainees in helping each other to prioritize goals for their home environments. The in-field do step directs the trainees to prioritize the rehabilitation goals of their particular agency or agency department, and to bring their results to class for feedback and discussion. This tell-show-do teaching approach successfully integrates the contributions of both the didactic and experiential approaches. The didactic phase is addressed by means of defining the skill, indicating the steps involved in learning the skill, and in developing the rationale, or how the skill works and why it is important. At this time the knowledge base underlying each particular skill can be introduced through lectures, discussions, and supplementary readings. For example, if the trainees are learning basic responding skills in order to encourage client self-exploration during the diagnostic planning process, they might read some of the research which found a positive relationship between the practitioners' responding skills and client self-exploration (Carkhuff, 1969).

The show step provides the practitioner with additional insights into the skill. The trainer can arrange for the skill to be demonstrated, simulated, shown on tape, or in a book. For many trainees the chance to see the skill modeled is an important component of the learning process.

The do step(s) provides the trainee with an opportunity to experience the skill, practice the skill, and receive feedback on his or her performance. The trainees experience the skill by practicing on one another; they become each other's clients. For example, when the trainees are learning how to categorize client strengths and deficits, they first learn how to categorize their own strengths and deficits. Every skill is first practiced on oneself or one's peers before the skill is used with clients. A trainee does not use the skill with clients until he or she first successfully experiences and demonstrates the skill. Not only does this provide an additional opportunity for practice and feedback, it also provides the trainees a chance to learn more about themselves. Additional practice and feedback sessions prior to skill use with clients can be provided by having the trainee further practice the skill on family and friends.

The skill learning outcome of each of these training sessions is an observable, measurable cluster of practitioner skills. As mentioned in Chapter I, these psychiatric rehabilitation practitioner skills are not meant to replace the skills of the various disciplines currently involved in the practice of psychiatric rehabilitation. Rather, these skills are seen as complementary to the professional's current unique skills. The mastery of these rehabilitation skills can play an extremely important role in improving the present outcome of psychiatric rehabilitation.

THE CONTRIBUTIONS OF THE FUNCTIONAL PROFESSIONAL[2]

The term *functional professional* has has been coined by Carkhuff (1971b) to identify those individuals who heretofore have been called non-professionals, para- professionals, companions, volunteers, lay professionals, and sub-professionals. Groups of individuals who have been referred to by these labels include college students, psychiatric aides, community workers, parents, and mental health technicians. Underlying these different terms is the commonality of functions which binds these various groups and labels together into a single entity. Thus, the functional professional in the mental health field may be defined as a person who, lacking formal credentials, performs those functions usually reserved for credentialed mental health professionals. In addition, individuals who have credentials in other fields, such as education and corrections, may be appropriately referred to as functional mental health professionals when they are engaging in tasks designed to have an effect on various mental health outcome criteria.

THE RESEARCH BASE

In 1968, Carkhuff reviewed over eighty articles concerned with the use and effectiveness of functional professionals (Carkhuff, 1968). Based on those studies, Carkhuff (1968) arrived at the following three conclusions:

1. Extensive evidence indicates that functional professionals can be trained to function at minimally facilitative levels of conditions related to constructive client change over relatively short periods of time.

2. Functional professionals can effect significant constructive changes in the clients whom they see.

3. In directly comparable studies, selected lay persons with or without training and/or supervision have patients who demonstrate change as great or greater than the patients of professional practitioners.

In the past decade, no significant body of data has emerged which can seriously challenge those conclusions which were based on the research of the early and mid-sixties. Although there are still professionals who criticize either the methodologies or conclusions of the functional professional research (McArthur, 1970; Rosenbaum, 1966; Sieka, Taylor, Thomason & Muthard, 1971), these same critics have been notably unsuccessful in designing and undertaking their own research in this field.

What apparently has occurred within recent years, however, has been a shift in focus in the functional professional movement. The trend in the literature indicates far less concern with the effectiveness of the functional professional; instead, more attention has been directed toward descriptions of how to develop and use functional professionals within different agency settings (e.g., Christmas, 1969; Christmas, Wallace & Edwards, 1970; Collins, 1971; Hartog, 1967; Levenson, Beck, Quinn & Putnam, 1969; Oppliger, 1971; Rioch, 1966).

Directly comparative outcome studies between functional mental health professionals and credentialed mental health professionals have remained a rare commodity. In the last decade, the few studies that have been done have all found the same results. Regardless of the client outcome criteria studied, in all cases the clients of functional professionals did as well or better than the clients of credentialed professionals (Poser, 1966; Truax & Lister, 1970; Zunker & Brown, 1966).

Various criticisms of these comparative studies have been outlined (McArthur, 1970; Rosenbaum, 1966; Sieka et al. 1971), and generally focused on the researcher's failures to control for functional professional/credentialed professional differences in age, sex, and motivation. Concerning sex differences between therapist and client, Zunker and Brown (1966) did use only same sex pairs and found the same results. The critics' suggestion that the relatively greater effectiveness of functional professionals could be due to their younger ages and hypothesized higher levels of motivation is in reality a harsh indictment of professional education. Why spend so many years of school learning about therapeutic treatment modalities if the main therapeutic effects are due to the age and motivation of the therapist?

Regardless of the research criticisms, it is simply amazing that no empirical studies exist which are in opposition to these findings. While few in number, these studies represent a broad sampling of clients, credentialed professionals, and outcome criteria. The unanimity of their results is indeed impressive.

In contrast to the dearth of directly comparative studies there has been a number of investigations of the effectiveness of functional professional interventions with both inpatients and outpatients (Anthony & Carkhuff, 1978). The results have by no means been consistent; for example, some studies have reported a positive effect on a variety of client outcome data (Carkhuff & Truax, 1965; Ellsworth, 1968; Hetherington & Rappaport, 1967; Holzberg, Knapp & Turner, 1967; Katkin, Ginsburg, Rifkin & Scott, 1971; Katkin, Zimmerman, Rosenthal & Ginsburg, 1975; Sines, Silver & Lucero, 1961; Verinis, 1970; Weinman, Sanders, Kleiner & Wilson, 1970) while other studies have reported negligible effects (Gruver, 1971; Spiegal, Keith-Spiegal, Zirgulis & Wine, 1971; Stevenson, Viney & Viney, 1973).

In general, while this more recent research supports the three major conclusions of Carkhuff's (1968) earlier review, some additional principles have emerged.

1. **The "psychiatric aide" (mental health worker) can have a beneficial effect on psychiatric patients only when he or she is given additional training and responsibility.**

It does not make sense to merely "turn the psychiatric aide loose" with only a minimum of supervision to do what the aide considers to be of therapeutic value for the patient. Aides can provide a valuable source of functional professionals, but only if properly trained and utilized.

2. **Unselected and untrained lay personnel have not consistently demonstrated their therapeutic effectiveness.**

It would seem that in some instances the credentialed professionals' well-intentioned rush to get on the functional professional "bandwagon" has led them to employ as functional professionals anyone who shows up at their door. Merely because the person has no credentials, is indigenous to the community, and is similar in appearance to the clients being serviced does not guarantee that the person can be an effective functional professional. Although those characteristics may give the functional professional an "edge" (Cark-

huff, 1968), these attributes do not translate directly into constructive client change.

3. **The functional professional housewife volunteer has consistently shown herself to have a constructive impact on both psychiatric patients and outpatients.**

These results are so convincing that if the treatment goal is simply to increase the patients' chances of being discharged or staying out of the hospital, the use of the functional professional housewife would appear to be a preferred mode of treatment.

4. **The treatment approaches in which functional professionals are most adept would appear to be the ability to develop a friendly supportive relationship with the patient and the ability to train the patient in the skills necessary to function productively in the community.**

Obviously, these abilities are not mutually exclusive and could both comprise a part of the functional professionals' contribution to the rehabilitation process.

ISSUES IN THE SELECTION AND TRAINING OF FUNCTIONAL PROFESSIONALS

The goal of selection and the goal of training are synonymous — the development of effective functional professionals. Despite the rapid growth of functional professionalism, there has been limited research on how best to select and train this new source of practitioners. While descriptions of selection and training procedures abound, there is a paucity of hard data.

In general, it would appear that with some notable exceptions (Carkhuff, 1971b) the selection and training of functional professionals has not developed much past the early conceptualizations of Pearl and Riessman (1965). On-the-job training and didactic presentations, augmented by individual and group supervision or discussions, remains the traditional approach to training functional professionals. Variations of this training approach, while seldom researched, have been described periodically (Baker, 1972; Christmas et al.

1970; Collins & Cavanaugh, 1971; Euster, 1971; Lynch & Gardener, 1970). In essence, it seems that credentialed professionals are teaching functional professionals to do and think in a manner similar to themselves, thus replicating to a great extent, the theories and practices which historically have not been tremendously successful in documenting their effectiveness (Anthony et al. 1972; Eysenck, 1952, 1972; Levitt, 1957).

Although it may be true that the backgrounds and experiences of the indigenous functional professionals are similar to that of the client and may provide them with some inherent advantages over the typical credentialed professional (Carkhuff, 1968), it has *not* been shown that these differential background and experiential characteristics are the characteristics which relate to outcome. It seems that similarities between client and care-giver, although helpful in developing a positive first impression, are not the crucial determinants of helping outcome.

The research evidence suggestive of the initial impact of client-counselor social similarities has been summarized by Carkhuff (1972a). Although a black counselor working with a black client has an initial advantage over a white counselor, this advantage can be overcome to a great extent by the interpersonal and speciality skills of the counselor (Banks, 1971; Banks, Carkhuff & Berenson, 1967; Carkhuff & Banks, 1970; Carkhuff & Pierce, 1967). The negative effects of racial differences are mitigated by the helper's skills, and it is the helper's skills which consistently have been shown to relate to helping outcome.

Thus, the proponents of functional professionalism cannot consider their job to be done once they have selected functional professionals with characteristics similar to the clients. Client-counselor similarity may be a first step toward effectiveness, but not much more. Nor can the trainers of functional professionals assume their job to be done once the functional professional has received on-the-job experience, didactic presentations, and opportunities for group discussions. No research exists which suggests that this training approach makes a difference in terms of observable criteria of client change.

Logically, the training of functional professionals must occur on those variables which past research has shown to be related to helping outcomes. Likewise, the selection of functional professionals must be based on those variables which past research has shown to be related to training outcome.

Outcome research on functional professionals in mental health, corrections, and education converges on one indisputable finding — mental health outcome is a function of the helpers' skills or the activities in which the helper engages. In terms of helper skills, the skills are typically interpersonal skills and program development skills; in terms of helper activities, the activities are usually either supportive, friendship-type activities, or direct skills-training of clients in those skills which they need in order to live most effectively.

Interpersonal skills are those diagnostic planning skills (Chapter IV) which are also referred to as attending, observing, listening, and responding skills. In terms of the functional professional activity of providing a friendly, supportive relationship in which the client can function, it would appear that the functional professionals' ability to provide this type of environment could be improved through interpersonal skills training.

The mastery of rehabilitation programming skills (Chapter V) can increase the functional professionals ability to teach the clients the skills they need to more effectively live, learn, and work in the community. A functional professional trained in interpersonal and programming skills can not only teach the client skills, but also can model the skills, modify the teaching program as needed, monitor the client's behavior, and selectively reward the client's skill performance.

In addition to learning interpersonal and programming skills, functional professionals could also be trained in various aspects of community coordinating skills (Chapter VIII). Often the functional professional acts as an advocate for the client.

The functional professionals' community decision-making, marketing, and programming skills can be extremely helpful when performing this advocacy role.

In essence, it would be possible to train selected functional professionals in all the skills of psychiatric rehabilitation. However, it makes most sense to train functional professionals in those skills which they specifically need in order to function effectively. Will they be engaging in supportive activities with the clients? Will they be involved in the skill-teaching process? Will they be acting as advocates for the clients? Answers to these and similar questions will help structure the content of the functional professional training program. No matter what the content, however, the outcome of the training program should be an observable measurable cluster of skills.

Once the outcome of training has been identified as a certain level of skilled behavior, the selection process loses much of its mystery. In contrast to the selection procedures in graduate education, which have been notably unsuccessful in predicting either future clinical or research expertise (Anthony, Gormally & Miller, 1974), research into the selection of functional professionals has developed several empirically based principles upon which to guide the selection effort. This success in selection is a direct result of the ability of functional professional trainers to define the goals of the training in objective, behavioral terms. Without this empirical specificity, there could be no effective selection procedures. It is only when we know exactly what criteria we want the training to achieve, that trainee selection can become a legitimate and meaningful activity.

A number of research studies have investigated how to select those individuals most likely to profit from skills training, and in particular, interpersonal skills training. The findings unanimously converge on one fundamental selection principle — the best index of a future criterion is a previous index of that criterion (Anthony & Wain, 1971; Anthony et al. 1974; Carkhuff 1971b; Carkhuff & Griffin, 1970,

1971). The application of that selection principle to functional professional training is as follows: The best index of whether a functional professional can profit from a training experience is an index of the prospective functional professional's present ability to profit from a training-analogue experience.

In essence, selection involves allowing prospective trainees to experience a representative sample of the training program for which they are being considered, and determining the effects of this brief part of the training program through pre- and post-testing of their functioning on the relevant criterion. To achieve this selection goal, brief standardized training-analogue procedures need to be constructed. Anthony et al. (1974) have recently developed a written analogue experience (the Trainability Index) which has accounted for up to 70% of the variance in interpersonal skills training outcome (Carkhuff, 1971b, 1972b). The Trainability Index consists of having the subject read a brief (2-1/2 pages) explanation of the concept of empathy, along with examples of various helper responses rated on a five-point empathy scale (Carkhuff, 1969). Following the description, the subject is asked to respond in writing to five written helpee statements and to rate his or her own responses on the five-point empathy scale. A trainability - communication score is obtained by means of trained judges' ratings of the subjects' responses on the same five-point empathy scale (Carkhuff, 1969). The trainability - self-discrimination score is obtained by computing the absolute deviation between the subject's ratings of his or her responses and the ratings of the trained judges.

Additional training outcome variance can also be studied by correlating various pre-training functional professional behavior with the observable training outcome criteria. For example, Collingwood (1973) has consistently found that measures of physical fitness account for a significant proportion of variance in Carkhuff's (1971b, 1972b) interpersonal skills training approach.

THE SELECTION AND TRAINING
OF FUNCTIONAL PROFESSIONALS:
SOME PRINCIPLES

1. **Functional professional training goals must be defined in observable, measurable terms.**

Without an observable measure of training outcome, there can be no valid assessment of training effectiveness. Thus, the result will be a continued plethora of training program descriptions and a dearth of training program evaluations.

2. **The functional professional training process should be designed to increase the trainees' skills in areas that previous research has shown to relate to mental health outcome.**

Defining the training goal in terms of increased functional professional skills will also result in the definition of training goals that are observable and measurable. Because skills training outcome is observable, the trained functional professional will have documented evidence of the attainment of criteria relevant to his or her performance as a functional mental health professional. In fact, criteria which assess a person's level of skills are much more relevant to helping outcome than the criteria presently used for completion of advanced course-work. The functional professional's demonstration of a certain level of skilled behavior should become his or her credentials certifying his or her ability to have a positive impact on the clients with whom the functional professional comes in contact.

3. **The selection of functional profession-** als should be based on a training-analogue experience.

Future ability to profit from training may be most efficiently predicted from the functional professionals' present ability to profit from a brief aspect of that training. In contrast to the above selection principle, many of the selection procedures currently operating are really no more than screening procedures, just as many of the current training procedures are more similar to orientation tasks rather than systematic training programs.

ISSUES IN TRAINING:
A SUMMARY STATEMENT

The importance of training to the future growth of the field of psychiatric rehabilitation must be continually emphasized. Equally important is the continued development of new rehabilitation treatment settings. Also important is the development of new legislation which mandates a rehabilitation treatment approach. However, if additional rehabilitation environments are created and additional rehabilitation services mandated, there must be trained personnel to perform these functions in these settings. The skills of psychiatric rehabilitation are too complex and too important to be learned by trial and error or "on the job." Mastery of the skills and knowledge of psychiatric rehabilitation must be an integral part of both professional and functional professional training programs. Skilled and knowledgeable psychiatric rehabilition practitioners *can* make a difference.

ENDNOTES

[1] This chapter was written in conjunction with Dr. Keith Hume.

[2] This section is adapted in part from Anthony and Carkhuff (1978).

REFERENCES

Anthony, W. A. Psychological rehabilitation: A concept in need of a method. **American Psychologist**, 1977, *32*: 658-662.

Anthony, W. A., Buell, G., Sharratt, S. and Althoff, M. E. The efficacy of psychiatric rehabilitation. **Psychological Bulletin**, 1972, *78*: 447-456.

Anthony, W. A. and Carkhuff, R. R. The effects of rehabilitation counselor training upon trainee functioning. **Rehabilitation Counseling Bulletin,** 1970, *13*: 333-342.

Anthony, W. A. and Carkhuff, R. R. The functional professional therapeutic agent. In Gurman, A. S. and Razin, A. M. eds., **Effective psychotherapy: A handbook of research.** Oxford, Pergamon Press, 1978.

Anthony, W. A., Cohen, M. R. and Vitalo, R. The measurement of rehabilitation outcome. **Schizophrenia Bulletin,** 1978, in press.

Anthony, W. A., Gormally, J. and Miller, H. The prediction of human relations training outcome by traditional and non-traditional selection indices. **Counselor Education and Supervision,** 1974, *14*: 105-111.

Anthony, W. A., Pierce, R. M. and Cohen, M. R. **Psychiatric rehabilitation practice: The skills of diagnostic planning. Book one.** Amherst, Mass.: Carkhuff Institute of Human Technology, 1977(a).

Anthony, W. A., Pierce, R. M. and Cohen, M. R. **Psychiatric rehabilitation practice: The skills of rehabilitation programming. Book two.** Amherst, Mass.: Carkhuff Institute of Human Technology, 1977(b).

Anthony, W. A. and Wain, H. J. Two methods of selecting prospective helpers. **Journal of Counseling Psychology,** 1971, *18*: 155-156.

Arbuckle, D. The learning of counseling: Process not product. **Journal of Counseling Psychology,** 1963, *10*: 163-168.

Baker, E. J. The mental health associate: A new approach in mental health. **Community Mental Health Journal,** 1972, *8*: 281-291.

Banks, G. The effects of race on one-to-one helping interviews. **Social Service Review,** 1971, *45*: 137-146.

Banks, G., Carkhuff, R. R. and Berenson, B. G. The effect of counselor race and training upon counseling process with Negro clients in initial interviews. **Journal of Clinical Psychology,** 1967, *23*: 70-72.

Blum, E. and Blum, H. **Alcoholism: Modern psychological approaches to treatment.** San Francisco: Jossey Bass, 1967.

Boehm, W. Social work: Science and art. **Social Service Review,** 1961, *36*: 144-151.

Bolles, R. N. **What color is your parachute? A practical manual for job hunters and career changes.** Berkley, Calif.: Ten Speed Press, 1977.

Boyd, J. D. **Counselor supervision approaches, practices, and preparation.** Muncie, Ind.: Accelerated Development, 1978.

Cahn, S. **The treatment of alcoholics: An evaluation study.** New York: Oxford University Press, 1970.

Carkhuff, R. R. Training in counseling and psychotherapy. **Journal of Counseling Psychology,** 1966, *13*: 360-367.

Carkhuff, R. R. The differential functioning of lay professional helpers. **Journal of Counseling Psychology,** 1968, *15*: 117-126.

Carkhuff, R. R. **Helping and human relations. Volumes 1 and 2.** New York: Holt, Rinehart & Winston, 1969.

Carkhuff, R. R. Principles of social action in training for new careers in human services. **Journal of Counseling Psychology,** 1971, *18*: 147-151, (a).

Carkhuff, R. R. **The development of human resources.** New York: Holt, Rinehart & Winston, 1971, (b).

Carkhuff, R. R. Black and white in helping. **Professional Psychology,** 1972, *3*: 18-22, (a).

Carkhuff, R. R. **The art of helping.** Amherst, Mass.: Human Resource Development Press, 1972, (b).

Carkhuff, R. R. The development of systematic human resource development models. **The Counseling Psychologist,** 1972, *3*: 4-11, (c).

Carkhuff, R. R. and Banks, G. P. Treatment as a preferred mode of facilitating relations between races and generations. **Journal of Counseling Psychology,** 1970, *17*: 413-418.

Carkhuff, R. R. and Berenson, B. G. **Beyond counseling and therapy.** New York: Holt, Rinehart & Winston, 1967.

Carkhuff, R. R. and Berenson, B. G. **Teaching as treatment: An introduction to counseling and psychotherapy.** Amherst, Mass.: Human Resource Development Press, 1976.

Carkhuff, R. R. and Griffin, A. H. The selection and training of human relations specialists. **Journal of Counseling Psychology,** 1970, *17*: 443-450.

Carkhuff, R. R. and Griffin, A. Selection and training of functional professionals for concentrated employment programs. **Journal of Clinical Psychology,** 1971, *27*: 163-165.

Carkhuff, R. R. and Pierce, R. M. Differential effects of therapist race and social class upon patient depth of self-exploration in the initial clinical interview. **Journal of Consulting Psychology,** 1967, *31*: 632-634.

Carkhuff, R. R. and Pierce, R. M. **The art of helping trainer's guide.** Amherst, Mass.: Human Resource Development Press, 1977. 1977.

Carkhuff, R. R. and Truax, C. B. Lay mental health counseling. The effects of lay group counseling. **Journal of Consulting Psychology,** 1965, *29*: 426-432.

Christmas, J. J. Sociopsychiatric rehabilitation in a black urban ghetto. **American Journal of Orthopsychiatry,** 1969, *39*: 651-661.

Christmas, J. J., Wallace, H. and Edwards, J. New careers and new mental health services: Fantasy or future? **American Journal of Psychiatry,** 1970, *126*: 1480-1486.

Clark, R. **Crime in america.** New York: Simon & Schuster, 1970.

Cohen, M. R., Anthony, W. A., Pierce, R. M. and Vitalo, R. L. **Psychiatric rehabilitation practice: The skills of rehabilitation evaluation. Book three.** Amherst, Mass.: Carkhuff Institute of Human Technology, 1977.

Collingwood, T. The human resource development model and physical fitness. Chapter 5. In D. W. Kratochvil ed. **The Human Resource Development Model in Education**. Baton Rouge, La.: Southern Louisiana University Press, 1973.

Collins, J. A. The paraprofessional: I. Manpower issues in the mental health field. **Hospital and Community Psychiatry**, 1971, *22*: 362-367.

Collins, J. A. and Cavanaugh, M. The paraprofessional: II. Brief mental health training for the community health worker. **Hospital and Community Psychiatry**, 1971, *22*: 367-370.

Davidson, W. S. The diversion of juvenile delinquents: An examination of the process and relative efficacy of behavioral contracting and child advocacy. Unpublished doctoral dissertation, University of Illinois, 1975.

Dole, V. Research on methadone maintenance treatment. **International Journal of Addictions**, 1970, *5*: 359-369.

Dupont, R. L. **The future of the federal drug abuse program**. Paper presented at the 36th Annual Scientific Meeting of the Commission on Problems of Drug Dependence. Mexico City, 1974.

Eckstein, R. and Wallerstein, R. S. **The teaching and learning of psychotherapy**. New York: Basic Books, 1958.

Emerick, C. D. A review of psychologically oriented treatment of alcoholism: The relative effectiveness of different treatment approaches and the effectiveness of treatment versus no treatment. **Quarterly Journal of Studies on Alcohol**, 1975, *36*: 88-108.

Euster, G. L. Mental health workers: New mental hospital personnel for the seventies. **Mental Hygiene**, 1971, *55*: 283-290.

Eysenck, H. J. The effects of psychotherapy: An evaluation. **Journal of Consulting Psychology**, 1952, *16*: 319-324.

Eysenck, H. J. The effects of psychotherapy. In H. J. Eysenck ed., **Handbook of Abnormal Psychology**. London: Pitmans, 1960.

Eysenck, H. J. New approaches to mental illness: The failure of a tradition. In H. Gottesfeld ed., **The Critical Issues of Community Mental Health**. New York: Behavioral Publications, 1972.

Fleming, J. and Hamburg, D. A. An analysis of methods for teaching psychotherapy with a description of a new approach. **Archives of Neurological Psychiatry**, 1958, *79*: 179-200.

Gay, G., Metzger, A., Bathhurst, W. and Smith, D. Short-term heroin detoxification of an outpatient basis. **The International Journal of Addictions**, 1971, *6*: 241-264.

Glasscote, A. M., et al. **The treatment of alcoholism**. Washington, D.C. Joint Information Service of the American Psychiatric Association and the National Association of Mental Health, 1967.

Goldstein, A. P., Heller, K. and Sechrest, L. B. **Psychotherapy and the psychology of behavior change**. New York: Wiley, 1966.

Goodwin, D. Alcohol in suicide and homicide. **Quarterly Journal of Studies on Alcohol,** 1973, *34*: 144-156.

Gruver, G. G. College students as therapeutic agents. **Psychological Bulletin,** 1971, *76*: 111-127.

Hartog, J. Nonprofessionals as mental health consultants. **Hospital and Community Psychiatry,** 1967, *18*: 223-225.

Hetherington, H. and Rappaport, J. Homecoming: A volunteer program to rehabilitate chronic patients. **Hospital and Community Psychiatry,** 1967, *18*: 171-174.

Holzberg, J. D., Knapp, R. H. and Turner, J. L. College students as companions to the mentally ill. In E. L. Cowen, E. A. Gardner, and M. Zax eds., **Emergent Approaches to Mental Health Problems.** New York: Appleton-Century-Crofts, 1967.

Katkin, S., Ginsburg, M., Rifkin, M. J. and Scott, J. T. Effectiveness of female volunteers in the treatment of outpatients. **Journal of Counseling Psychology,** 1971, *18*: 97-100.

Katkin, S., Zimmerman, V., Rosenthal, T. and Ginsburg, M. Using volunteer therapists to reduce hospital readmissions. **Hospital and Community Psychiatry,** 1975, *26*: 151-153.

Kittrie, H. N. **The right to be different.** Baltimore: The John Hopkins Press, 1971.

Korner, I. N. and Brown, W. H. The mechanical third ear. **Journal of Consulting Psychology,** 1952, *16*: 81-84.

Krasner, L. The therapist as a social reinforcement machine. In H. H. Strupp and L. Luborsky eds., **Research in Psychotherapy.** **Vol. 2.** Washington, D.C.: APA, 1962.

Lennard, H. and Allen, S. The treatment of drug addiction: Toward new models. **The International Journal of Addictions,** 1973, *8:* 521-536.

Lester, B. K., Gussen, J., Yamamoto, J. and West, L. J. Teaching psychotherapy in a longitudinal curriculum. **Journal of Medical Education,** 1962, *37*: 28-32.

Levenson, A. I., Beck, J. C., Quinn, R. and Putnam, P. Manpower and training in community mental health centers. **Hospital and Community Psychiatry,** 1969, *20*: 37-40.

Levitt, E. E. The results of psychotherapy with children. **Journal of Consulting Psychology,** 1957, *71*: 189-196.

Lindesmith, A. **The addict and the law.** Bloomington: Indiana University Press, 1965.

Lipton, D., Martinson, R., and Wilks, J. **The effectiveness of correctional treatment: A survey of treatment evaluation studies.** Chicago: Praeger Press, 1975.

Lister, J. L. Counselor experiencing: Its implications for supervisors. **Counselor Education,** 1966, *5*: 55-60.

Lynch, M. and Gardener, E. A. Some issues raised in the training of paraprofessional personnel as clinic therapists. **American Journal of Psychiatry,** 1970, *126*: 1473-1479.

McArthur, C. C. Comment on "Effectiveness of counselors and counselor aides." Journal of Counseling Psychology, 1970, 17: 335-36.

Moore, M. The client's voice in expression. The Art and Science of Psychotherapy, 1969, 5: 76-78.

Mottin, J. L. Drug-induced attenuation of alcohol consumption. Quarterly Journal of Studies on Alcohol, 1973, 34: 444-472.

Mueller, W. J. and Kell, B. L. Coping with conflict. New York: Appleton-Century-Crofts, 1972.

National Institute of Mental Health. Deinstitutionalization: An analytical review and sociological perspective. DHEW Publication No. (ADM) 76-351, Superintendent of Documents, U. S. Government Printing Office, Washington, D.C. 20402, 1976.

Netter, G. Explaining crime. New York: McGraw Hill, 1974.

Nietzel, M., Winett, R. A., MacDonald, M. L. and Davidson, W. S. Behavioral approaches to community psychology. New York: Pergamon Press, 1977.

Oppliger, S. Volunteers in community programs. Hospital and Community Psychiatry, 1971, 22: 111-112.

Pasaminick, B., Dinitz, S. and Lefton, M. Psychiatric orientation and its relationship to diagnosis and treatment in a mental hospital. American Journal of Psychiatry, 1959, 116: 127-132.

Patterson, C. H. Supervising students in the counseling practicum. Journal of Counseling Psychology, 1964, 11: 47-53.

Pearl, A. and Riessman, F. New careers for the poor. New York: The Free Press, 1965.

Pierce, R. M., Anthony, W. A. and Cohen, M. R. Psychiatric rehabilitation practice: The skills of career counseling. Book four. Amherst, Mass.: Carkhuff Institute of Human Technology, 1977.

Pierce, R. M., Cohen, M. R., Anthony, W. A. and Cohen, B. F. Psychiatric rehabilitation practice: The skills of career placement. Book five. Amherst, Mass.: Carkhuff Institute of Human Technology, 1977.

Poser, E. G. The effects of therapists' training on group therapeutic outcome. Journal of Consulting Psychology, 1966, 30: 283-289.

President's Commission on Law Enforcement and the Administration of Justice. Task Force Report: Juvenile Delinquency and Youth Crime. Washington, D.C.: Government Printing Office, 1967.

Rioch, M. Changing concepts in the training of therapists. Journal of Consulting Psychology, 1966, 30: 289-292.

Robinson, J. and Smith, G. The effectiveness of correctional programs. Crime and Delinquency, 1971, 17: 67-80.

Rogers, C. R. The necessary and sufficient conditions of therapeutic personality change. Journal of Consulting Psychology, 1957, 21: 95-103.

Romans, F. Teaching psychiatry to medical students. **Lancet**, July, 1961, 93-95.

Rosenbaum, M. Some comments on the use of untrained therapists. **Journal of Consulting Psychology**, 1966, *30*: 292-294.

Schwartz, E. K. and Abel, T. M. The professional education of the psychological therapist. **American Journal of Psychotherapy**, 1955, *9*: 253-261.

Sieka, F., Taylor, D., Thomason, B. and Muthard, J. A critique of "Effectiveness of counselors and counselor aides." **Journal of Counseling Psychology**, 1971, *18*: 362-364.

Sines, L., Silver, R. J. and Lucero, R. J. The effect of therapeutic intervention by untrained therapists. **Journal of Clinical Psychology**, 1961, *17*: 394-396.

Spiegal, D., Keith-Spiegal, P. K., Zirgulis, J. and Wine, D. G. Effects of student visits on the social behavior of regressed schizophrenic patients. **Journal of Clinical Psychology**, 1971, *27*: 396-400.

Stevenson, G. The paraprofessionals. **Occupational Outlook Quarterly**, 1973, *17*: 3-9.

Towles, C. Roles of the supervisor in the union of cause and function in social work. **Social Services Review**, 1961, *35*: 144-151.

Truax, C. B. and Carkhuff, R. R. The experimental manipulation of therapeutic conditions. **Journal of Consulting Psychology**, 1965, *34*: 119-124.

Truax, C. B. and Carkhuff, R. R. **Toward effective counseling and psychotherapy**. Chicago: Aldine Press, 1967.

Truax, C. B. and Lister, J. L. Effectiveness of counselors and counselor aides. **Journal of Counseling Psychology**, 1970, *17*: 331-334.

Verinis, J. S. Therapeutic effectiveness of untrained volunteers with chronic patients. **Journal of Consulting and Clinical Psychology**, 1970, *34*: 152-155.

Viamontes, J. A. Review of drug effectiveness in the treatment of alcoholism. **American Journal of Psychiatry**, 1972, *12*: 120-121.

Walz, G. and Roeber, E. Supervisor reaction to a counseling interview. **Counselor Education and Supervision**, 1962, *2*: 2-7.

Weinman, B., Sanders, R., Kleiner, R. and Wilson, S. Community based treatment of the chronic psychotic. **Community Mental Health Journal**, 1970, *6*: 12-21.

Wessell, R. Social work education and practice. **Social Service Review**, 1961, *35*: 151-160.

Wolberg, L. R. **The technique of psychotherapy**. New York: Grune and Stratton, 1954.

Zunker, V. G. and Brown, W. F. Comparative effectiveness of student and professional counselors. **Personnel and Guidance Journal**, 1966, *44*: 738-743.

CHAPTER XII
The Promise of Psychiatric Rehabilitation

The history of the mental health movement in the United States is dotted with strong changes in treatment emphasis, some of which were briefly mentioned in Chapter III. Such "breakthroughs" included the construction of large mental hospitals, the popularity of psychoanalytic theorizing, the development of modern chemotherapy, and the construction of community mental health centers. However, these historical contributions contributed only minimally to the goals of rehabilitation.

In retrospect, the greatest shortcomings of each of these approaches is that they promised too much. To be sure each of these approaches has made a significant contribution to the mental health movement. Unfortunately, some of the more vocal adherents of each of these approaches has hailed these breakthroughs as either cures for "mental illness" or, at a minimum, they suggested that these new approaches heralded a breakthrough in the eradication of "mental illness." In essence, the public was led to believe that these breakthroughs were capable of effecting more outcome than they were subsequently able to produce. In short, *these breakthroughs promised more than they delivered*. The developing field of psychiatric rehabilitation cannot afford to repeat such a mistake.

A related failure of these historical innovations is in the area of cost. At times, each of these new approaches was considered capable of reducing the cost of treatment over a client's lifetime, either by providing more humane care at less expense, or by bringing about total cure. Promises of decreased cost have typically come up as empty promises; at present few people even take such promises seriously.

Concerning the issue of cost, it is interesting to note that there may not be a relationship between cost of treatment and treatment success. One variable contributing to this finding is the fact that expensive forms of psychotherapy may not produce more clinical improvement than can be achieved by chemotherapy alone. When psychotherapy is given to chronic patients, it may increase the cost of treatment but not necessarily the outcome (Grinspoon, Ewalt & Shader, 1972). A related study of the social disability of patients one month after discharge from a number of different hospitals found no relationship between hospital per diem costs and the patient's social adjustment. As a matter of fact, ex-patients of the hospital with the highest per diem rate were less adjusted socially than ex-patients from the hospital with the lowest per diem rate (Walker, 1972).

It would seem that, based on what can be learned from history, proponents of a rehabilitation model within the mental health system should not cite reduced costs as a reason for adopting a rehabilitation approach. A comprehensive well-run rehabilitation approach should produce additional helpee benefits, but it might also produce additional or at least different types of costs. Cost projections at this stage of our knowledge are difficult if not impossible. Indeed, the real per patient cost of the community-based-treatment approach has yet to be determined. Schwartz and Epps (1974) have cautioned that errors are being made with respect to the data evaluating the cost of community mental health care. These authors point out that the data-gathering systems have not caught up with the new diversified treatment modalities. For example, a patient may first be treated in the community, then hospitalized in a general hospital, transferred to a state hospital, and then seen again in the community. Such a situation could be incorrectly interpreted as four different poeple instead of one, resulting in the total treatment cost being divided by four and thereby inaccurately estimating the cost per patient as much less than if the cost had been correctly estimated for one person.

In summary, the development of a rehabilitation model within the mental health system can promise neither reduced costs nor a cure for mental illness. What then can be the promise of psychiatric rehabilitation?

The rehabilitation model advanced in this book is in a developmental stage, reflective of the present state of our knowledge. It represents a tentative direction in need of much future research and conceptualizing. At this early stage of development a rehabilitation model holds the following promise for the field of mental health:

1. **A promise of an increasing level of independence for those psychiatrically disabled helpees who are treated by a rehabilitation approach.**

The goal of a psychiatric rehabilitation approach is to increase those physical, emotional, or intellectual skills which the helpee needs to live, learn, or work in the community, given the least amount of support necessary from agents of the helping professions. Based on past and current research, it is a reasonable, achievable goal for rehabilitation to pursue. Many psychiatrically disabled helpees can be taught to function at higher skill levels than the levels at which they are currently functioning. The benefits of this increased skill level can be a more independent level of community functioning.

2. **A promise of treatment goals directed at health induction rather than symptom reduction.**

The rehabilitation model is viewed as complementary to most of the current treatment approaches which are primarily aimed at symptom reduction. In particular, drug therapy and rehabilitation treatment are seen as complementary. Future research might investigate whether in fact there may be a reciprocal effect between drug therapy and rehabilitation. That is, the symptom reduction brought about by drug therapy should increase the helpees' ability to learn and use their skills. Likewise, health induction brought about by rehabilitation might lessen the helpees' dependence on drugs and increase the helpees' chances of successful withdrawal from maintenance medication.

3. **A promise of a diagnostic system relevant to the rehabilitation goal.**

The immediate goal of rehabilitation is skill gain and improved community functioning. Thus the diagnostic process assesses the helpee's present level and the skill level demanded by the helpee's unique community. The helpee's diagnosis results not in a diagnostic label but in a functional description of what relevant behavior the helpee can and cannot perform. The rehabilitation diagnosis is in actuality the first step in the rehabilitation treatment process. In essence it is the beginning formulation of a rehabilitation treatment plan.

4. **A promise to communicate to both the helpee and significant others the diagnostic goals and rehabilitation program in terms that are as understandable as possible.**

The rehabilitation approach attempts to maximize the involvement of the helpee and significant others. As a result, the language and model of rehabilitation must be as understandable as possible to these lay persons. Attempts must be made to minimize the sometimes mysterious and esoteric jargon which is characteristic of most mental health theorizing and treatment. Unfortunately, there may be concern on the part of some professionals that if the treatment process is demystified, they will lose their role as "expert." Yet mental health professionals should achieve expertise on the basis of what they are capable of *doing*, not saying. Furthermore, just because something (in this case the rehabilitation approach) is relatively straightforward and simple to explain does not mean that it is relatively simple to *do*.

5. **A promise of a comprehensive approach to the psychiatrically disabled helpee.**

The rehabilitation approach diagnoses and treats (or arranges for treatment) the helpee's physical, emotional, and intellectual spheres of functioning. The rehabilitation approach assumes that growth or deterioration in one area of functioning may influence growth or deterioration in another area of functioning. A rehabilitation approach is particularly congnizant of the physical aspects of a helpee's functioning. Psychiatric rehabilitation practitioners must make deliberate attempts to increase the helpee's physical fitness skills and to mitigate any fortuitous negative physical effects resulting from other types of mental health treatments or settings.

6. **A promise of systematic effective programs designed to reduce society's negative attitudes and behavior toward the psychiatrically disabled.**

If rehabilitation practitioners attempt to reintegrate the helpee into the community, then it is also incumbent upon practitioners to positively influence the behavior of society toward the helpee. One effective method is to equip the helpees themselves with stigma reduction skills. In this way each helpee is prepared to overcome as best he or she can any negative behavior which the helpee directly confronts. Another method of changing society's negative attitude is to make contact with and provide informational experiences for groups of lay persons who are or will be coming in contact with psychiatrically disabled persons.

7. **A promise of newly trained people equipped with newly developed programs.**

In the past the mental health system has focused too much of its energies and finances on where and in what type of building treatment should occur. Without a concomitant emphasis on the people and programs that functioned in these new buildings, these new treatment settings were handicapped in achieving their hoped-for success. The probability of a rehabilitation model becoming an accepted component of the mental health treatment system will be enhanced by a reduced emphasis on architecture and an increased focus on the rehabilitation personnel and their rehabilitation programs.

8. **A promise of a personnel selection and training program relevant to the goals of psychiatric rehabilitation.**

The promise of psychiatric rehabilitation will be achieved only by the efforts of highly competent personnel. The particular skills identified in Chapter XI can form the nucleus of skills needed to practice psychiatric rehabilitation. The practice of rehabilitation is not so simple or so natural as to be learned by trial and error. Nor is rehabilitation so similar to the practice of other human service professions that other professionals can simply switch into psychiatric rehabilitation positions without additional training. The practice of psychiatric rehabilitation is the exclusive province of no one profession. However, the practice of psychiatric rehabilitation does demand a unique set of skills and knowledge, over and above that which is currently taught in the other helping professions.

9. **A promise of using rehabilitation personnel based on their rehabilitation expertise and not their professional credentials.**

In the past the mental health system has overemphasized the particular educational credentials for certain jobs and underemphasized the requisite skills demanded of the job holder. In contrast, psychiatric rehabilitation positions must be defined by a certain set of practitioner skills designed to achieve certain types of client outcomes. Any type of human service professional can be trained in rehabilitation skills and aspire to various levels of rehabilitation positions. In particular, rehabilitation must explore the various uses of noncredentialed lay persons, many of whom can be trained in a variety of rehabilitation skills.

10. **A promise of an ongoing evaluation of the field in general as well as specific rehabilitation techniques and programs.**

If the field of psychiatric rehabilitation is going to develop past its present stages, it can do so only by learning from its current efforts. The history of mental health is plagued by new treatment orientations and techniques which have never been evaluated. Recently there have been questions regarding the cost effectiveness and treatment effectiveness of the community mental health center (Lego, 1975; Schwartz & Epps, 1974; Smith, 1975; Smith & Hart, 1975). One interesting aspect of these articles is not the fact that these questions are being asked, researched, and evaluated; rather, what is amazing is that it took so long for the field to try and find answers to these questions of effectiveness. In retrospect, an evaluation component should have been an integral part of each mental health center from the very beginning of its operation. In order for psychiatric rehabilitation not to replicate this failure, the evaluation process needs to be viewed as the means by which rehabilitation efforts can continue to improve their effectiveness and not as a one-shot test out of which a person or program receives a pass-fail grade. To ensure the prominence of evaluation within the rehabilitation model, each individual professional practitioner needs to be trained in rehabilitation evaluation skills.

FUTURE TRENDS IN PSYCHIATRIC REHABILITATION

The future direction of any field rests to a great extent on its past and current accomplishments. Previously there has really been no well-recognized body of rehabilitation knowledge and techniques in the mental health system. However, the monumental efforts aimed at developing supportive living, learning, and working environments for the psychiatrically disabled helpee have laid the groundwork for the development of the field of psychiatric rehabilitation. The future growth and direction of psychiatric rehabilitation rests on the programs to be developed and research to be conducted within the next decade.

The author of this text traces the conceptual beginning of the science of psychiatric rehabilitation to the writings of Carkhuff, in which he first formulated and researched the idea of "training as a preferred mode of treatment" (Carkhuff, 1969, 1971). At that time Carkhuff suggested that training clients directly in the skills which they need to function in society could be a potent treatment method. This training as treatment concept forms the basis for the psychiatric rehabilitation model. The earlier studies of this concept trained psychiatric patients in the emotional-interpersonal area of functioning (Pierce & Drasgow, 1969; Vitalo, 1971). Specifically, these two studies found that psychiatric patients (some chronic and all with symptoms) could be trained to function at higher levels of interpersonal skills, independent of their particular symptomatology and diagnostic labels. Since that time a number of studies have evaluated a variety of skills-training approaches for psychiatrically disabled persons (see Chapter V).

Carkhuff has since refined his training as treatment model into a "teaching as treatment" model, so as to more accurately reflect the intricacies of skill training (Carkhuff & Berenson, 1976). The diagnostic programming and evaluation sections of this text reflect much of Carkhuff's later research and model building. It would be expected that the practice of psychiatric rehabilitation would likewise move into a more educational approach. As psychiatric rehabilitation practitioners move from training individual helpees into teaching groups of helpees, the practitioner must be more knowledgeable about the learning process and the teaching skills needed to facilitate the skills-learning process of groups of clients. Too often in the past, clients have learned certain skills simply because *those skills were the only skills the practitioner knew how to teach*, and not because the skills were the most critical for the clients to learn. To a great extent this inappropriate learning has occurred because the practitioner has lacked a systematic and comprehensive diagnostic approach or the ability to develop new skills-teaching programs.

The future of psychiatric rehabilitation is based to a great extent on the ability of rehabilitation practitioners to develop better teaching methodologies, both for individual cases and group situations. The teaching process is much more than, for example, giving a lecture, playing a videotape, and providing feedback. It is a highly interpersonal, motivational yet systematic method (Carkhuff, Berenson & Pierce, 1977). If rehabilitation practitioners wish to improve their abilities to get their clients fully involved in the learning process, they must continue to develop their teaching skills. Thus rehabilitation practitioners must remain aware of the ongoing developments in the field of education.

The key to the development of the field of psychiatric rehabilitation, however, is the skill level of the psychiatric rehabilitation practitioner (Anthony, 1977). The promise of rehabilitation can only be achieved by individual practitioners who continually evaluate and refine their own professional skills. In the past the emphasis has been on *where* people get treated. Yet the research suggests that rehabilitation approaches and outcome can be effectively instituted in both inpatient and outpatient settings. In psychiatric rehabilitation the emphasis now must be on *what outcome* the rehabilitation intervention brings about. Most of the variance in rehabilitation outcome is most affected by how skillfully the helpee is treated and not where the helpee is treated. The focus of psychiatric rehabilitation must be on the skillful functioning of people, including both the rehabilitation helpee and the rehabilitation practitioner.

REFERENCES

Anthony, W. A. Psychological rehabilitation: A concept in need of a method. **American Psychologist**, 1977, *32*: 658-662.

Carkhuff, R. R. **Helping and human relations. Volumes 1 and 2.** New York: Holt, Rinehart & Winston, 1969.

Carkhuff, R. R. Training as a preferred mode of treatment. **Journal of Counseling Psychology**, 1971, *18*: 123-131.

Carkhuff, R. R. & Berenson, B. G. **Teaching as treatment: An introduction to counseling and psychotherapy.** Amherst, Mass.: Human Resource Development Press, 1976.

Carkhuff, R. R., Berenson, D. and Pierce, R. M. **The skills of teaching: Interpersonal skills.** Amherst, Mass.: Human Resource Development Press, 1977.

Grinspoon, L., Ewalt, J. R. and Shader, R. E. **Schizophrenia: Pharmacotherapy and psychotherapy.** Baltimore, MD: Williams and Wilkins, 1972.

Lego, S. The community mental health center: Is it an improvement over the old system? **Perspectives in Psychiatric Care**, 1975, *8*: 105-112.

Schwartz, D. A. and Epps, L. D. The numbers myth in community mental health. **Psychiatric Quarterly**, 1974, *48*: 320-326.

Smith, W. G. Evaluation of the clinical services of a regional mental health center. **Community Mental Health Journal**, 1975, *11*: 47-57.

Smith, W. G. and Hart, D. W. Community mental health: A noble failure? **Hospital and Community Psychiatry**, 1975, *26*: 581-583.

Walker, R. Social disability of 150 mental patients one month after hospital discharge. **Rehabilitation Literature**, 1972, *33*: 326-329.

APPENDIX A

AN EXAMPLE OF AN APPLICATION PROGRAM

Skill: Using Community Resources

Skill Operationalized: Number of days after hospital discharge client arrives for scheduled appointment at outpatient clinic

Assessment of Present Level: 30 days

Assessment of Needed Level: 5 days

Step No.: 1   PROGRAM DEVELOPMENT AND IMPLEMENTATION SHEET   Name: Bob K.

Time Limit: July 31   Reinforcements: Play one hour of pool

Major Step: List 3 reasons for attending the clinics

Time	Secondary Steps	Check Steps
8)		After: During: Before:
7)		A: D: B:
6)		A: D: B:
5)		A: D: B:
4)		A: D: B:
3)		A: D: B:
2)	Choose the three reasons I like the best	A: Have I checked off three? D: Am I looking at it? B: Do I have the list?
1)	Ask other patients and staff why they think attendance is important	A: Have I written it down? D: Are they answering the question? B: Have I identified who to ask?

238

PROGRAM DEVELOPMENT AND IMPLEMENTATION SHEET

Step No.: 2

Name: Bob K.

Time Limit: August 1

Reinforcements: Dessert after evening meal

Major Step: List possible obstacles to clinic attendance and a method for overcoming each

Time	Secondary Steps	Check Steps
1)	Write down situations that might prevent attendance (e.g., no bus fare)	A: Do I understand each obstacle? D: Am I listing these obstacles? B: What prevents me from keeping appointments?
2)	Ask staff for possible solutions to each obstacle	A: Do I have a solution for each obstacle? D: Am I listing solutions? B: What staff would be helpful?
3)		A: D: B:
4)		A: D: B:
5)		A: D: B:
6)		A: D: B:
7)		A: D: B:
8)		After: During: Before:

239

PROGRAM DEVELOPMENT AND IMPLEMENTATION SHEET

Step No.: 3 Name: Bob K.

Time Limit: August 5

Reinforcements: Extra meeting with practitioner to talk about call

Major Step: Telephone for appointment within 5 days after projected hospital release

Time	Secondary Steps	Check Steps
		After:
		During:
		Before:
8)		
7)		A:
		D:
		B:
6)		A:
		D:
		B:
5)		A:
		D:
		B:
4)		A:
		D:
		B:
3)		A:
		D:
		B:
2) Place telephone call		A: Did I write appointment time down?
		D: Am I talking to correct person?
		B: Do I have calendar and pencil?
1) Ask treatment coordinator for expected discharge date		A: Is an appointment time available?
		D: What dates are within 5 days?
		B: Do I have a calendar?

240

PROGRAM DEVELOPMENT AND IMPLEMENTATION SHEET

Name: Bob K.

Time Limit: August 6

Reinforcements: Go to basketball game with brother

Major Step: Write a travel itinerary for trip from apartment to clinic

Time	Secondary Steps	Check Steps
		After: How long will it take?
		During: Is this most direct route?
		Before: Do I have clinic address?
8)		A: / D: / B:
7)		A: / D: / B:
6)		A: / D: / B:
5)		A: / D: / B:
4)		A: / D: / B:
3)		A: / D: / B:
2)		A: / D: / B:
1)		A: / D: / B:

Step No.: 5   PROGRAM DEVELOPMENT AND IMPLEMENTATION SHEET   Name: Bob K.

Time Limit: On date of appointment   Reinforcements: Visit with friends at local bar

Major Step: Arrive for appointment 5-15 minutes early

Time	Secondary Steps	Check Steps
		After: What time did I arrive?
		During: Am I following itinerary?
		Before: Have I checked appointment time?
8)		
7)		A: D: B:
6)		A: D: B:
5)		A: D: B:
4)		A: D: B:
3)		A: D: B:
2)		A: D: B:
1)		A: D: B:

242

APPENDIX B

Skill:	Stigma Reduction
Skill Operationalized:	Number of positive and negative statements client can make about self in response to questions about psychiatric hospitalization when asked by an employment interviewer
Assessment of Present Level:	0 positive comments 2 negative comments
Assessment of Needed Level:	2 positive comments 0 negative comments

Step No.: 1   PROGRAM DEVELOPMENT AND IMPLEMENTATION SHEET   Name: Sue C.

Time Limit: July 31   Reinforcements: Watch T.V. movie

Major Step: Read material on stigma reduction

Time	Secondary Steps	Check Steps
8)		After: During: Before:
7)		A: D: B:
6)		A: D: B:
5)		A: D: B:
4)		A: D: B:
3)		A: D: B:
2)	Underline any points that might apply to my situation	A: Have I underlined? D: Am I concentrating? B: Do I have a pen?
1)	Ask practitioner for needed material	A: Do I have what I wanted? D: Does he/she understand my request? B: Is he/she listening?

244

Step No.: 2　　　PROGRAM DEVELOPMENT AND IMPLEMENTATION SHEET　　　Name: Sue C.

Time Limit: August 1 – August 5　　　Reinforcements: Go to a movie this weekend

Major Step: Ask persons in similar situations what they have said

Time	Secondary Steps	Check Steps	
	8)	After:	
		During:	
		Before:	
	7)	A:	
		D:	
		B:	
	6)	A:	
		D:	
		B:	
	5)	A:	
		D:	
		B:	
	4)	A:	
		D:	
		B:	
	3)	A:	
		D:	
		B:	
Aug. 3, 4 or 5	2) Tell volunteer my problem and goal	A: Have I written down the points?	
		D: Is problem being addressed?	
		B: Is volunteer listening?	
Aug. 1	1) Ask staff to make an appointment with volunteer from Recovery Incorporated	A: Have I written appointment down?	
		D: Did I tell my reason?	
		B: Who knows about these volunteers?	

245

PROGRAM DEVELOPMENT AND IMPLEMENTATION SHEET

Step No.: 3

Time Limit: August 8

Name: Sue C.

Reinforcements: See next step

Major Step: List all possible statements that could be made

Time	Secondary Steps	Check Steps
	8)	After: During: Before:
	7)	A: D: B:
	6)	A: D: B:
	5)	A: D: B:
	4)	A: D: B:
	3)	A: D: B:
	2) Write down possible responses from the volunteer on the same sheet of paper	A: Are there any other points? D: Do I understand each point? B: Do I have volunteer's responses?
	1) Write down possible responses from my reading on a sheet of paper	A: Have I included all underlines? D: Do I understand what I've written? B: Do I have reading materials?

246

PROGRAM DEVELOPMENT AND IMPLEMENTATION SHEET

Step No.: 4 **Name: Sue C.**

Time Limit: August 8

Reinforcements: Treat self to a chocolate milkshake

Major Step: Rank the statements based on how I like them

Time	Secondary Steps	Check Steps
		After: Does each have a number?
		During: Have I numbered the best & worst?
		Before: Do I have all the statements?
	8)	A: D: B:
	7)	A: D: B:
	6)	A: D: B:
	5)	A: D: B:
	4)	A: D: B:
	3)	A: D: B:
	2)	A: D: B:
	1)	A: D: B:

Step No.: 5 PROGRAM DEVELOPMENT AND IMPLEMENTATION SHEET **Name: Sue C.**

Time Limit: August 9 Reinforcements: Buy a new record

Major Step: Write a script containing the best sentences

Time	Secondary Steps	Check Steps
8)		After: / During: / Before:
7)		A: / D: / B:
6)		A: / D: / B:
5)		A: / D: / B:
4)		A: / D: / B:
3)		A: / D: / B:
2) Sequence the remaining phrases		A: Can I actually say this? / D: Where do they fit? / B: Are there any more good points?
1) Identify from the list of best sentences what should be said first and last		A: Do I have a beginning and ending? / D: What will I say first and last? / B: Do I have my list?

248

Time Limit: August 12 and 13   Reinforcements: Read latest Cosmopolitan

Major Step: Say from memory the best statements

Time	Secondary Steps	Check Steps
8)		After: During: Before:
7)		A: D: B:
6)		A: D: B:
Aug. 3	5) Repeat process for entire script	A: Was I accurate? D: Can I say it without looking? B: Have I read it over?
Aug. 2	4) Repeat process for any other sentence	A: Have I done every sentence? D: Am I saying without looking? B: Are there other sentences?
Aug. 2	3) Repeat until can say it 3 times without looking	A: Was that 3 times? D: Am I accurate each time? B: Is sentence out of sight?
Aug. 2	2) Cover up first sentence and say it aloud	A: Was I accurate? D: Am I not looking? B: Is sentence out of sight?
Aug. 2	1) Read first sentence aloud	A: Can I remember it? D: Can I say it? B: Do I have completed script?

PROGRAM DEVELOPMENT AND IMPLEMENTATION SHEET

Step No.: 7 Name: Sue C.

Time Limit: August 14 and 15 Reinforcements: Join practitioner for coffee break

Major Step: Role-play best statements

Time	Secondary Steps	Check Steps
	8)	
	7)	After: During: Before:
	6)	A: D: B:
	5)	A: D: B:
		A: D: B:
Aug. 15	4) Say script from memory to interviewer from personnel in response to his/her question about hospitalization	A: Did I answer the question? D: Am I listening? B: Am I attending?
Aug. 15	3) Say script from memory to interviewer from personnel department of hospital	A: Did I ask for feedback? D: Am I looking at the practitioner? B: Have I introduced myself?
Aug. 14	2) Say script from memory to the practitioner in response to a question about hospitalization	A: Did I answer the question? D: Am I listening to the question? B: Am I looking at the practitioner?
Aug. 14	1) Say script from memory to the practitioner	A: Did I ask for feedback? D: Am I looking at the practitioner? B: Is script out of sight

Step No.: 8   PROGRAM DEVELOPMENT AND IMPLEMENTATION SHEET   Name: Sue C.

Time Limit: On date of interview   Reinforcements: Sleep in on the next day

Major Step: Say statements in real interview

Time	Secondary Steps	Check Steps							

Check Steps

After:
During:
Before:

8)

7) A:
    D:
    B:

6) A:
    D:
    B:

5) A:
    D:
    B:

4) A:
    D:
    B:

3) A:
    D:
    B:

2) Say statement to real interviewer if question is asked   A: Was it the same as the script?
    D:
    B:

1) Say script from memory 3 times on the day of the interview   A: Was I accurate?
    D: Am I looking straight ahead?
    B: Do I have the script?

251

Author Index

Abel, T.M., 213, 231
Alexander, M., 109, 121
Allen, D.B., 74, 215
Allen, S., 229
Allport, G., 103, 121
Althoff, M.E., 6, 17, 71, 98, 213, 215, 225
Anderson, R., 110, 122
Angrist, S., 26, 36
Anthony, W.A., 2, 5, 6, 16, 17, 39, 43, 44, 45, 46, 47, 55, 65, 71, 72, 79, 82, 87, 91, 98, 100, 105, 106, 122, 129, 132, 134, 137, 150, 151, 156, 157, 166, 171, 172, 181, 190, 191, 192, 202, 205, 211, 213, 215, 216, 217, 218, 219, 222, 223, 224, 225, 226, 227, 230, 236
Arbuckle, D., 213, 226
Arnet, C., 109, 122
Arthur, G., 6, 18, 40, 71
Aspy, D.N., 51, 71, 82, 100, 111, 122

Bachrach, L.L., 6, 16, 17, 132, 150
Backer, T.E., 180, 192
Baker, E.J., 222, 226
Baker, F.M., 100
Baker, R.L., 51, 71, 77, 100
Banks, G., 109, 122, 223, 226, 227
Barbee, M.S., 9, 17
Barofsky, I., 91, 100
Barry, A., 110, 111, 113, 122
Barton, W.E., 12, 20
Bathhurst, W., 215, 228
Bayer, C., 15, 17
Beard, J.H., 12, 17
Beck, A.T., 38, 71, 74
Beck, J.C., 221, 229
Becker, P., 15, 17
Bell, M., 152
Bell, R.L., 95, 100
Bellack, A.S., 95, 101, 151
Berenson, B.G., 55, 77, 109, 110, 122, 124, 201, 203, 208, 211, 216, 226, 227, 235, 236
Berenson, D.H., 51, 72, 208, 211
Berenson, S.R., 203, 208, 211
Berkman, V.C., 12, 17, 21
Berry, K.L., 9, 41, 46, 74
Biddulph, L., 108, 110, 122
Bigelow, D.A., 189, 192
Blanchard, K.H., 136, 151

Black, D.S., 150
Bloom, L.B., 6, 7, 18
Blum, E., 215, 226
Blum, H., 215, 226
Blumenthal, R.L., 13, 20
Boblitt, E.W., 10, 19
Boehm, W., 213, 226
Bohn, M.J., 133, 152
Bolles, R.N., 213, 216, 226
Bolton, B., 108, 122
Botwinick, W.I., 12, 18
Boucher, L., 150
Boudewyns, P.A., 18
Boudreau, L., 150
Bourestom, N.C., 155, 171
Boyd, J.D., 213, 226
Braginsky, B.A., 157, 171
Braginsky, D., 157, 171
Brahn, J., 126
Brand, F., 108, 125
Brand, R.C., 156, 171
Bratton, K.M., 16, 20, 155, 172
Breen, J., 107, 122
Brown, B., 111, 122
Brown, B.S., 133, 150
Brown, W.F., 221, 231
Brown, W.H., 214, 229
Brunswick, L.K., 95, 101
Buell, G.J., 6, 17, 39, 43, 44, 45, 46, 47, 71, 98, 202, 205, 211, 213, 215, 225
Bugle, G., 95, 102
Burck, H.D., 177, 192
Burley, L., 110, 122

Caffey, E.M., 11, 18
Cahn, S., 215, 226
Cameron, R., 136, 151
Campbell, D.T., 177, 192
Campbell, M., 95, 102
Carkhuff, R.R., 10, 13, 16, 18, 33, 36, 51, 54, 55, 59, 64, 71, 74, 92, 96, 100, 103, 105, 106, 109, 110, 111, 112, 113, 120, 121, 122, 124, 138, 150, 194, 201, 203, 206, 208, 209, 211, 213, 214, 216, 220, 221, 222, 223, 224, 225, 226, 227, 231, 235, 236
Carmichael, D.D., 11, 19
Carpenter, J.O., 155, 171
Carron, A., 108, 122
Cattell, R., 103, 108, 122

Forsyth, R.P., 6, 41, 72
Francis, R.J., 110, 124
Friedman, I., 7, 19
Form, W.H., 145, 150
Foster, L., 6, 18
Franklin, J.L., 45, 72, 90, 101, 155, 172, 202, 212
Frantz, T.T., 82, 101
Freeman, H.E., 7, 8, 9, 17, 19, 40, 41, 46, 72
Friel, T.W., 33, 36, 137, 138, 150
Frost, E.S., 9, 21

Galbrecht, C.R., 11, 18
Gansereit, K.H., 46, 73
Gardener, E.A., 223, 229
Gardos, G., 91, 101, 202, 212
Garfield, S.L., 58, 72
Gay, G., 215, 228
Gebhard, M.E., 18, 72
Gergen, K.J., 150
Ginsburg, M., 12, 19, 155, 172, 222, 229
Giovannani, J., 195, 212
Glaser, T.E., 180, 192
Glasscote, A.M., 215, 228
Goertzel, V., 12, 17, 19
Goffman, E., 134, 150
Goldberg, N., 11, 20
Goldenberg, I.I., 135, 151
Golding, L., 113, 114, 124
Goldsmith, J.B., 95, 101
Goldstein, A.P., 213, 228
Goodwin, D., 215, 229
Gormally, J., 224, 226
Gosenfeld, L., 91, 100, 212
Goss, A.M., 41, 42, 49, 73
Gottheil, G., 108, 127
Green, W., 107, 123
Green, H.J., 41, 42, 46, 73
Greenburg, B., 193, 202, 207, 208, 210, 211, 212
Gregory, C.C., 40, 41, 73
Griffin, A.H., 122, 224, 227
Grinspoon, L., 232, 236
Grob, S., 41, 74
Groenendijk, H., 110, 112, 114, 124
Gruber, J., 110, 124
Gruver, G.G., 222, 229
Gurel, L., 33, 36, 39, 43, 44, 46, 47, 73
Gussen, J., 213, 229
Gustin, B., 124

Hall, C., 103, 124
Hall, J.C., 7, 19, 41, 42, 43, 73
Hall, R., 122
Hamburg, D.A., 214, 216, 228
Hamelink, M., 106, 107, 125
Hannah, J.T., 16, 20, 155, 172
Hanson, P.G., 10, 19
Hardy, M., 108, 124
Harrand, G., 94, 95, 101
Harris, D., 107, 108, 124
Harris, J., 103, 123
Hart, D.W., 234, 236
Hart, M., 109, 124
Hartog, J., 221, 229
Haven, G.A., 8, 19
Heap, F.R., 10, 13, 19
Heath, D., 151
Heller, K., 213, 228
Hersen, M., 95, 101, 151
Hersen, P., 136, 151
Hershenson, D.B., 192
Hetherington, H., 222, 229
Hinko, E.N., 7, 19
Hinterkopf, E., 95, 101
Hipple, J.J., 212
Hoffman, J.J., 9, 19
Holder, T., 111, 123
Holland, J.L., 18, 72
Holzberg, J.D., 222, 229
Hord, E.J., 10, 19
Hornstra, R.K., 11, 19
Horvath, S., 106, 107, 126
Hoskins, R., 106, 107, 125
Huddelson, J., 106, 107, 125
Hume, K., 225
Hurst, J., 109, 127

Ismail, A., 107, 108, 110, 123
Iven, D., 40, 41, 74
Ivey, A.E., 36, 95, 101

Jacobson, L., 113, 126
Jarmon, B., 110, 123
Johnson, D.L., 9, 19
Johnson, R.G., 10, 19
Johnson, T., 108, 109, 124
Jones, M., 113, 114, 153, 172

Kaden, S.E., 42, 49, 73
Kapland, M.D., 13, 18
Kassebaum, G.G., 189, 192
Kastenbaum, R., 82, 100

258

Subject Index

comparison of clients' reports of gains, Table 10-7, 200
comparison of medication vs skills treatment, Table 10-2, 197
examples of new activities initiated, Table 10-8, 201
examples of skills learned, Table 10-4, 198
test analysis of client reports, Table 10-3, 198
Reinforcement, 80-82
  client as, 82
  learning theory and, 81
  natural reinforcers, 89
  practitioners as, 82; 86; 87
  reprogramming environment to deliver, 88-89
Resume writing, 146. See also Career placement.

Self-actualizing, 103
Self-concept, 108; 137; 202
Skills
  activities of daily living (ADL), 33; 155
  as goals, 31
  assessment skills, special techniques, 62-64
  categorized for comprehensiveness, 31
    examples, 32-33
    Table 3-2, 35
  decision-making skills, 158-61
  definition, 31
  "empathy" in programming, 82
  generalization, 85-86
    vs extendability, 87
  importance in career placement, 145
  information-gathering, 56; 62-63
    "in vivo" observation, 63
    role playing, 62
    simulation, case illustration, 62
  individualizing skill goals, case illustration, 33
  initiative skills, 59-61
  institutionalized juveniles and, 10
  marketing in community rehabilitation, 161-65
  operationalizing skills, 50-55; 56
  quantifying skills, 56; 63
  responsive skills, 57-59. See also Empathy.
  training programs

examples, outcomes, 94-97
in work adjustment, 136
See also Rehabilitation outcome studies.
training vs insight in marital dysfunction, 206-7
State vocational rehabilitation, 138
Stigma reduction, 66; 83; 84; 87; 156
  Appendix B, 243-251
  promise of rehabilitation, 234
  Table 4-4, 67
Supervision. See Training.

Tests
  AAHPER-Youth Fitness, 110
  California Personality Inventory (CPI), 107-8
  Cattell's 16PF, 108
  Edwards' Personality Preference Inventory, 49
  Interpersonal Relationship Rating Scale, 206
  Minnesota Multiphasic Personality Inventory (MMPI), 49; 107; 108
  psychological scores as outcome predictors, 48-49
  Rorschach, 49
  Stanford Binet Intelligence Test, 110-11
  Trainability Index, 224
  Wechsler Intelligence Scale-Children (WISC), 110
  Wide Range Achievement Test (WRAT), 110
Therapies
  modalities, behavior-milieu, 9-10
    chemotherapy (drug), 1; 3; 8; 10-11; 27-28; 133; 193; 232
      in rehabilitation programming, 90-91
    corrective therapy, 103
    counseling, 92; 133; 214
    group therapy, 1; 3; 8; 214
    milieu therapy, 9-10
    token economy, 9-10
    work therapy, 9
  practitioner status and, 2
  rehabilitation interpretations and, 60-61
  theories of psychotherapy
    dynamic (Freud, Jung)/insight, 8; 27; 103; 207; 214; 232